Mental Health and Mental Illness in Paramedic Practice

Mental Health and Mental Illness in Paramedic Practice

Louise Roberts

David Hains

ELSEVIER

ELSEVIER

Elsevier Australia. ACN 001 002 357
(a division of Reed International Books Australia Pty Ltd)
Tower 1, 475 Victoria Avenue, Chatswood, NSW 2067

ISBN: 978-0-7295-4318-7

Notice

National Library of Australia Cataloguing-in-Publication Data

---

 A catalogue record for this book is available from the National Library of Australia

---

Senior Content Strategist: Rachel Simone
Content Project Manager: Kritika Kaushik
Copy edited by Jo Crichton
Proofread by Kate Stone
Cover by Georgette Hall
Index by SPi Global
Typeset by New Best-set Typesetters Ltd
Printed in Singapore by KHL Printing Co Pte Ltd

Last digit is the print number: 9   8   7   6   5   4   3   2   1

Contents

About the Editors

Dr Louise Roberts's main interest and principal research expertise is in the out-of-hospital management of mental health presentations. Her PhD explored how paramedics identify, assess and manage psychiatric presentations in the community. Dr Louise Roberts has led and contributed to narrative literature reviews into the management of low-acuity presentations in the pre-hospital setting for the Victorian Ambulance Service. She has collaborated on national research into men's lived experience with mental health and paramedics' understanding of mental health and AOD presentations (Beyond Blue and Turning Point Drug and Alcohol Centre). She has also conducted research into state and territory Mental Health Acts and how paramedics are represented in those Acts, and how this has informed the development of clinical practice guidelines. Recently, she has contributed to research into PTSD and its effects on partners of veterans and emergency first-responders, and current research addresses the physical, psychological, psychobiological and psychosocial health of operational ambulance staff. She has been lecturing in mental health since 2007, and paramedic science since 2012. She has also published and presented in this area.

David Hains is a registered nurse with almost 20 years' experience working as a mental health nurse consultant in emergency departments in Adelaide. David is also an adjunct lecturer at Flinders University, and has several years' experience teaching nursing and paramedic students in mental health subjects, as well as working as an academic at Toi Ohomai Institute of Technology in New Zealand. His interests include single session therapy, not just as a 'therapist' but also as a clinician, i.e. how to make every interaction a therapeutic one; for example, turning an assessment into therapy/treatment. David is the current President of the Australasian Solution Focused Association, the Chairperson of the International Management Group for the *Journal of Solution Focused Practices* (JSFP), and has an *ex-officio* place on the JSFP Editorial Board. Since 2016 he has run a small business Left Turn Solutions, which conducts training in solution-focused brief therapy.

Preface

'The way you've been brought up to think about mental illness has a huge impact on how you deal with somebody, with a patient with mental illness. Some people don't understand how somebody can have a mental illness, you know you get people that have a "just get over yourself" kind of attitude because they have never been exposed to it in their personal life so they physically don't understand it, whereas some people they may have seen it in someone close to them or experienced it themselves and so they have a better understanding of it, but I don't think that is something you have to have had to be empathetic and to understand.'

Dr Louise Roberts 'Ethnography in the pre-hospital field: An exploration of the culture of how paramedics identify, assess and manage psychiatric presentations in the community' (doctoral thesis, 2013)

When discussing the approach in attending to people with challenges to their mental health, paramedics have told us that 'we tend to deal with what is going to kill you now and not what's going to kill you later'. These stories from paramedics, and listening to those with lived experience of mental ill-health are why we wanted to collaborate with experts in the field to provide a text that is specific to paramedic practice. Hopefully, this book will assist students to develop a strong foundation that will help them understand that being human and communicating in a genuine, empathetic and authentic way will connect you with another human in distress and provide the beginnings of a strong therapeutic relationship. Paramedicine is one of the few health professions that see and care for people in their home environment, usually when they are at their most vulnerable. How you act and respond will influence both patient outcomes and further help seeking by the individual. Just like when you are dealing with a cardiac patient or a trauma, the assessment, treatment and actions of a frontline health professional can make a huge difference to the individual's experience and can be the difference between positive or negative patient outcomes in both the short and the long term. You can definitely be saving a life even though it might not seem so at the time!

The objective of any healthcare provision is to be person-centred, and to endeavour to provide compassionate and timely care. This can be especially difficult in the pre-hospital environment where paramedics are confronted with physical environments that are varied and potentially difficult to navigate, scenes that can be confronting and overwhelming, potential high-level risks to all involved, and behaviour and emotions that can be hard to understand, all of which can generate a wide range of personal emotions and responses. This text hopefully provides knowledge combined with realistic and relevant case studies and strategies to assist paramedics and those working in the pre-hospital environment to be able to recognise, assess and provide high-quality initial care and support.

The hope we all have is to decrease the stigma and discrimination experienced by those with lived experience of mental ill-health, to provide access to care, and be an advocate and facilitator for recovery. Paramedics are, and will continue to be, an essential part of care provision within the mental health system, and deserve to be recognised and supported in this role.

HOW TO USE THIS BOOK

One of the fascinating things about studying mental health is that 'mental health' means different things to different people. As with clinical practice, no two people or situations or scenarios will be the same. Therefore, the way to use this book will require a different approach for different people. The terms 'mental health' and 'mental illness' have a social, cultural and individual context; in other words, the way we exist in the world can influence how we see ourselves as thinking, feeling and interacting human beings.

Within this book you will find things that amaze you, things that fascinate you, things that challenge you, things that disturb you and things that reassure you. There will also be things that you might agree with, and things that you disagree with. For us, that is part of the reason why we enjoy working in this field. It is amazingly challenging and can be amazingly rewarding. You could be in the emergency department, in the back of an ambulance, on the side of the road, or in a house; people will let us into their world, share with us their deepest secrets, and trust us with some of the most intimate things. But by listening, using our whole person and presence, just being there, we are in the right place at the right time. We are only ever one sentence away from starting the healing process.

WHERE DO YOU START?

In business, there are two key things you need to know in order to be successful; the first thing is to know who your customer is, and the second thing is to know what your customer wants. As a clinician, mental healthcare is no different. You can loosely define this as 'person-centred care' – finding out who the person is, and knowing what they want.

The key to this book, and to good clinical practice, lies in Chapters 2 and 3. The rest of the book is predominantly a reference guide. In Chapter 2 we start by learning about the person, not the illness. Chapter 2 is the lens through which we can look at the rest of our book and at our clinical practice. We can learn a lot through the study of history, society and culture, and it is easy to see how this can influence us in our clinical work, but ultimately it is our relationship with our customer; our human presence, our care and our conversation that will provide us with the story.

So, if Chapter 2 is the lens we look through (with our eyes), then Chapter 3 is what we do with our ears, mouth and body – the conversation and language. We develop our relationship through our words, actions and body language. Central to this, however, is our ability to listen, which could be described as 'listening therapy'. We listen not only with our ears, but with our attention, our body, our focus. We attune our senses to what is happening around us, and we focus our attention on finding out what is important for our customer. The focus on 'active listening', 'being present' and the individual's narrative (the story-making and meaning for those we care for) is reinforced by the use of case studies which have questions that encourage reflection on both clinical management and personal, cognitive and emotional responses to the case circumstances. The aim is to encourage both personal and professional reflection and a critical view of how we see those we care for, and how we act and respond, and why.

Chapter 5, Assessment, is where we start to put it all together. 'Assessment' is multifactorial; it is where we start to pull together the person's narrative along with that of others involved (family, carers, other professionals, etc.), as well as our clinical knowledge and understanding. However, one of the key issues or challenges for the clinician is to not lose sight of the person once we start looking through a medical lens. Most emergency-type assessments (e.g. medical, trauma) focus on the presenting or primary problem, and a mental health assessment from a traditional medical model would be the same, with a focus on the problem/deficit/symptom. However, a comprehensive mental health assessment incorporates things that are not actually a problem, such as an examination of a person's strengths, supports, resources and hopes.

Other factors involved in assessment and clinical practice include scene awareness, trauma-informed care, risks, vicarious trauma and challenging behaviours. Information relating to these are found in Chapters 4, 11, 12 and 15. Then of course there are the legal and ethical risks, challenges, restraints and liberties which are covered in Chapter 6, noting of course the complexities of living in a country with multiple jurisdictions.

The remainder of the book is primarily a reference of the various disorders and treatments. However, while we acknowledge that the medical system we work in requires most call-outs and emergency department presentations being summarised by a diagnosis, a diagnosis is predominantly a classification or administrative function. Subsequently, we run the risk of putting a person into a category, often a one-size-fits-all category when we revert to the medical model approach of problem/deficit/symptom focus seen through a medical lens rather than a person-centred one.

We should never lose sight of the individual.

We hope you enjoy this book, the first book written specifically for Australasian paramedics covering the topic of mental health and mental illness. We hope you see why we enjoy working in the area of mental health. While this can be the most challenging work, it can also be the most rewarding. As clinicians we may see good people at their worst, but we should always remember that we are potentially just a few words away from starting the healing process.

Foreword

Mental Health and Mental Illness in Paramedic Practice makes an essential contribution to paramedic education and will help equip future paramedics with the skills and knowledge to provide effective person-centred mental healthcare in the critical role they play. I believe that *Mental Health and Mental Illness in Paramedic Practice* will be a valuable asset that builds on the tool kit paramedics use every day in practice.

Mental illness and mental health mean different things to different people. For some, mental illness is perceived with much stigma, fear and discrimination. For a person experiencing symptoms for the first time, this can be a time of great anxiety with many unanswered questions about their experience. One in two people will either experience mental health issues or care for someone with mental health issues in a lifetime. One in five people each year is diagnosed with a mental health condition. People are also more likely to have their first experience in the key developmental years of the late teens and early adulthood, often leading to questions about their identity and what this will mean for their life. Many people who experience mental health issues are unlikely to need acute inpatient-based care. Many will never experience hospital treatment; however, hospital-based care may be needed for a smaller proportion and may be lifesaving.

Paramedics provide the vital role of first-responders in the health system, and each day their work saves many lives and ensures people get the urgent medical care they need. Almost every paramedic call-out will have a component of mental health support; this may be supporting a patient or family member who is rightly scared in a life-or-death situation, someone experiencing anxiety about their health condition, supporting a person with a chronic illness who is depressed due to multiple frequent hospital admissions, or supporting a person with a mental health condition. Knowledge of signs and symptoms and effective early intervention for people experiencing mental health issues is critical and can significantly improve their experience and outcome. Empathic person-centred care is crucial at this vital time in a person's life, with this first experience potentially shaping their engagement in treatment and future help seeking. A mental health call-out can be very different to other health call-outs. This can be a terrifying time for the person, with feelings of fear and uncertainty about seeking help, and they may not wish to go to a hospital. The call-out may involve other parties, such as bystanders, distressed family members and, potentially, the police. This can make the experience even more anxiety-provoking, as the person may feel they are being threatened or punished and not actually being helped. As a new paramedic, you may also notice systemic stigma towards mental health call-outs. For all of these reasons, knowledge of mental health, mental illness and how paramedics can support people is vital to paramedic care.

I still vividly remember the support provided to me by paramedics when I was last hospitalised for mental illness. This was 17 years ago, and the care I experienced,

I believe, was a critical factor in my mental health recovery. Like many others with mental health conditions this was not my first admission, and, as is common, I have had my share of poor experiences in the mental health system. I still remember how scared I was when the ambulance and police arrived. At the time I was struggling with severe depression and anxiety, and had experienced multiple suicide attempts. If I had not got the help I needed, I would not be here writing this foreword today. What changed that time started with paramedic care. I still remember the calming voice, the compassion shown, and the words used that made all the difference.

> *'I know you are sacred, and life is really tough right now, but we want to help, and we really think you need some help. Can you at least trust us and let us help you?'*

For me, these simple words and the empathic person-centred care I received were truly lifesaving. This paramedic support, along with others, made a difference in my life that many will never know and cannot be expressed in words. It led me to the support I needed, challenged my negative views of the mental health system, helped break the self-stigma I was experiencing and led me to a career in mental health. My lived experience of being shown care and compassion inspired me to want to learn how I could help other people and strive each day to make a difference in a person's life in the way that those paramedics did for me that day.

I hope in reading this, each person sees how vital mental healthcare is in the role of paramedics, and that you treat each person as an individual by providing compassionate, empathic person-centred care. Building a therapeutic relationship starts with your first words. Although your time with the person may only be a single brief support interaction, the respect, dignity and compassion you show will always be remembered.

> *'People will forget what you said, people will forget what you did, but people will never forget how you made them feel.'*
>
> Maya Angelou

Matthew Halpin
Lived Experience Leader
Adjunct Industry Fellow and Lecturer
Mental Health and Suicide Prevention Research Group
University of South Australia

Contributors

Michael Baigent MBBS, FRANZCP, FACHAM
Professor of Psychiatry, Department of Psychiatry, College of Medicine and Public Health, Flinders University, Adelaide, SA, Australia

Sharon Brown BN, GradDipMHN, MHN, MMHSc
Lecturer, Discipline of Behavioural Health, College of Medicine and Public Health, Flinders University, Adelaide, SA, Australia

Scott Brunero RN, DipApSc, BHSc, MA (nurs prac), PhD
Clinical Nurse Consultant, Mental Health Liaison, Prince of Wales Hospital, Sydney, NSW; Sessional Academic, Western Sydney University/University of Technology, Sydney, NSW, Australia

Paul Cammell MA, MBBS(Hons), FRANZCP, PhD
Clinical Associate Professor, Department of Psychiatry, University of Melbourne, Melbourne, Vic, Australia

Georgia Clarkson BA, DipEd, DAPS, GCTE, MEd, PhD
Senior Lecturer – Academic Development, Learning and Teaching Centre, Australian Catholic University, Melbourne, Vic, Australia

Tim J. Crowley RN, NP, BN, GradDipMHN, MNG(NP)
Nursing Director, Manager – Acute and Statewide Services, Nurse Practitioner – Complex Care and Trauma Mental Health, Child and Adolescent Mental Health Services (CAMHS), Women's and Children's Hospital Network, SA Health, Adelaide, SA, Australia

Fiona Glover, BSW, MMHSc, MAASW, DipMgmnt
Lecturer, Discipline of Behavioural Health, College of Medicine and Public Health, Flinders University, Adelaide, SA, Australia

Elizabeth A. Goble RN, BSc(Hons), MMedSc, PhD
College of Nursing and Health Sciences, Sturt Campus, Flinders University, Adelaide, SA, Australia

David Hains BN
Director, Left Turn Solutions; Adjunct Lecturer, Paramedic Unit, College of Medicine and Public Health Flinders University, Adelaide, SA, Australia

Lyza Rachel Helps BN, MMHN
Faculty of Nursing and Medicine, University of Adelaide, Adelaide, SA, Australia

Julie Henderson BA(Hons), GDipIS, PhD
Senior Research Fellow (Academic Status), College of Nursing and Health Sciences, Flinders University, Adelaide, SA, Australia

Madeleine Herd BPsych(Hons)
Project Officer, College of Medicine and Public Health, Flinders University, Adelaide, SA, Australia

Lian Hill BHSc(Hons)
Lecturer, Discipline of Behavioural Health, College of Medicine and Public Health, Flinders University, Adelaide, SA, Australia

Blair Hobbs BPsychNurs, MANP
Team Leader and Nurse Practitioner, Consultation Liaison and Emergency Psychiatry, Alfred Mental and Addiction Health, Melbourne, Vic, Australia

Cate Houen MBBS(Hons II, Sydney), FRANZCP
Deputy Director of Training, South Australian Branch Training Committee, Royal Australian and New Zealand College of Psychiatrists, Adelaide, SA, Australia

Breanna K. Jennings BHSc (Paramedic), GradCertClinEd
Lecturer in Paramedicine, School of Nursing, Midwifery and Paramedicine, Faculty of Health Sciences, Australian Catholic University, Melbourne, Vic, Australia

Michael Keem BBiomed, MD, MPsych
Neuropsychiatry Registrar, Neuropsychiatry, NorthWestern Mental Health, The Royal Melbourne Hospital, Melbourne, Vic, Australia

Scott Lamont RMN, RN, MN(Hons), PhD
Clinical Nurse Consultant, Mental Health Liaison, Prince of Wales Hospital, Sydney, NSW, Australia; Casual Academic, Southern Cross University, Lismore, NSW, Australia

David Lawrence PhD
Principal Research Fellow, Graduate School of Education, The University of Western Australia, Perth, WA, Australia

Bonita C. Lloyd MBBS, FRANZCP, Cert. Psychotherapy Psych.
Consultant Psychiatrist, Flinders Medical Centre; Lecturer, Flinders University, Adelaide, SA, Australia

Prue McEvoy MBBS, Diploma Psychotherapy, FRANZCP, Certificate of Accreditation in Child and Adolescent Psychiatry
Lead Psychiatric Director, Department of Child Protection, and Lead Psychiatrist CAMHS APY Team, Adelaide, SA, Australia

Denise E. McGarry RN, BA, MPM, GCHE, CMHN
Lecturer and Teaching Intensive Scholar, School of Nursing, College of Health and Medicine, Rozelle Campus, University of Tasmania, Sydney, NSW, Australia

Francesca Valmorbida McSteen MBBS, MPM, MPP, FRANZCP
Consultant Psychiatrist, Royal Melbourne Hospital, Melbourne, Vic, Australia

Conrad Newman MBBS, FRANZCP, MPS
Consultant Psychiatrist, Associate Clinical Director, Headspace Early Psychosis Program, Adelaide, SA, Australia

Heidi Newton BMedSc, BMBS, FRANZCP, Cert. Adult Psych., AFRACMA
Consultant Psychiatrist, Noarlunga Hospital, Adelaide, SA, Australia; Lecturer, Flinders University, Bedford Park, Adelaide, SA, Australia

Paula Redpath MMHSc, GCMHSc, BSW(AMHSW), BA(Hons)
Discipline Lead and Course Coordinator Behavioural Health, College of Medicine and Public Health, Flinders University, Adelaide, SA, Australia

Louise Roberts BN, BHSc(Hons) (Paramedic), PhD
Lecturer Bachelor of Paramedic Science, College of Medicine and Public Health, Flinders University, Adelaide, SA, Australia

Jade Sheen SFHEA, MAPS
Clinical/Health Psychologist and Family Therapist; Director of Simulation-based Education, School of Psychology, and Associate Professor in Clinical Psychology, Deakin University, Melbourne, Vic, Australia

Janine Stevenson MBBS(Hons I), MM, PhD, FRANZCP
Clinical Associate Professor, Department of Psychological Medicine, Sydney University, Sydney, NSW, Australia

Richard Summers BPharm, AACPA, GradDipHospPharm
Lecturer and Subject Coordinator, Department of Pharmacy and Biomedical Sciences, College of Science, Health and Engineering, Bendigo Campus, La Trobe University, Melbourne, Vic, Australia

Ellie Taylor BParaMedSc
Advanced Care Paramedic II, Queensland Ambulance Service, Brisbane, Qld, Australia

Ruth Townsend BN, LLB, LLM, GradCertVET, GradDipLegalPrac, PhD
Senior Lecturer – Law, Ethics, Professionalism, Faculty of Science, School of Biomedical Sciences, Charles Sturt University, Bathurst, NSW, Australia

Anthony Venning BSocSc, BHSc(Hons), MPsych(Clin), PhD
Senior Lecturer, Discipline of Behavioural Health, College of Medicine and Public Health, Flinders University, Adelaide, SA, Australia

Reviewers

Sherphard Chidarikire (Shep) RN, MN (Nurse Practitioner), PhD
Lecturer (Mental Health), School of Nursing, College of Health and Medicine, Newnham Campus, University of Tasmania, Hobart, Tas, Australia

Lisa Holmes PhD
Lecturer, Unit Coordinator and Researcher, Paramedicine Team, Allied Health, School of Medical and Health Sciences, Edith Cowan University, Perth, WA, Australia

Fiona Lamont BN, MBehavSc
Lecturer, Rozelle Campus, University of Tasmania, Hobart, Tas, Australia

David Reid BSc (Paramedic), MHM(Hons), GradCertHSM, DipHlthSci (Paramedic), GAICD, MACPara
Senior Lecturer, School of Medical and Health Sciences, Edith Cowan University, Joondalup, WA, Australia

Scott Stewart BSc, MBus, DipEd, DipHealthSci, Registered Paramedic MACPara, PhD(c)
Senior Lecturer, School of Nursing, Midwifery and Paramedicine, Australian Catholic University, Brisbane, Qld, Australia

Introduction to mental healthcare in paramedic practice: The provision and context of mental healthcare in Australia

1

Louise Roberts

LEARNING OUTCOMES

This chapter will:

- outline the context of mental healthcare in paramedic practice
- define and discuss the concepts of mental illness and mental health and wellbeing
- discuss the prevalence of mental illness in the community and emergency settings
- discuss the effects of stigma and discrimination on those with the lived experience of mental illness
- describe the major policy directions internationally and in Australia for mental health service delivery and how they apply to paramedic practice and service delivery.

INTRODUCTION

Paramedics in their role as emergency medical care providers are in a unique position to provide mental health assessment, care and transport for those with mental ill-health. Paramedics, as one of only a few professions which provide immediate emergency medical care and cross boundaries into both primary and tertiary care, attend individuals in their home and in the community. Paramedicine is undergoing a change in service provision as public health needs and demands change (Eaton et al., 2019). The shift for paramedic practice in Australia, New Zealand and internationally is towards models of primary and community care as well as maintaining the traditional emergency service provision as the prevalence of chronic medical conditions (e.g. coronary heart disease, respiratory conditions such as asthma and chronic obstructive pulmonary disease and mental ill-health) increases in the community in which they serve (Elliott & Brown, 2013; Evash-kevich & Fitzgerald, 2014). This unique position and role provides the opportunity to not only offer immediate support but also gather essential information for emergency department staff and mental health professionals that no one else may have witnessed or have been present for in a time of crisis. Paramedics' unique position gives them the opportunity to work collaboratively across multidisciplinary health provision, advocate for the individual to access further care, and be integral in the development of alternative care pathways for those who need mental health support. The advent of online support and resources through organisations such as Beyond Blue, Black Dog Institute, Headspace, Lifeline, ReachOut and government services such as Mental Health Triage and community mental health teams means paramedics have a role in psychoeducation and, in collaboration with mental health services, help the person re-engage with treatment and support services.

The movement of those with mental illness from institutions to community-based care occurred as medical management became more possible with the advent of antipsychotics and antidepressants in the 1950s and 1960s. Changes in medication occurred alongside a greater shift towards human rights for those with mental illness. The change in societal understanding of mental health and mental ill-health and society's recognition of human and civil rights continued to support the movement from institutional and custodial care to community care for those with mental ill-health. The 'deinstitutionalisation' of those with mental ill-health and the integration of mental healthcare into the general health system with a greater emphasis on community care (care provision in the least restrictive means) have increased the number of mental-health-related cases to emergency departments and attendance by paramedics (Broadbent et al., 2020). This increase in demand for mental healthcare affects how ambulance services allocate resources, their operational structures, such as response times and training, and how paramedic clinical practice is delivered.

This chapter outlines how mental health and ill-health are defined, the prevalence of mental ill-health, how the mental health system is structured, and how paramedicine and paramedic practice fit within this system. Understanding how the mental health system is structured and the gaps in service provision gives context to the role of paramedics when caring for those with mental ill-health, and why they are an important part of the initial care and assessment and how crucial their clinical decisions are to the further care of the person.

DEFINING MENTAL HEALTH AND ILLNESS

Defining mental health and ill-health is key to understanding how we identify, assess, manage and care for those who present with mental ill-health in paramedic practice. The World Health Organization provides a broad social and contextual definition of mental health and ill-health. The definition encompasses the concept that mental health is not separate from physical health or wellbeing. This is useful when taking a holistic approach to a person's overall care, and one which requires a whole-of-government response.

> *'Health is a state of complete physical, mental and social well-being and not merely the absence of disease or infirmity.'*
> (Constitution of the World Health Organization)

> *'Good mental health enables people to realize their potential, cope with the normal stresses of life, work productively, and contribute to their communities.'*
> (World Health Organization, 2013, p. 7)

A 'whole-of-government response' means that policy, service delivery and treatment needs to be comprehensive and coordinated. The response needs to include strategies for the promotion of mental wellbeing, the prevention of mental ill-health, equitable access to treatment options and the inclusion of those with mental ill-health in the design and implementation of services (World Health Organization, 2013, p. 7). The Australian Department of Health states 'a person's mental health affects how they feel, think, behave and relate to others' (https://www.health.gov.au/health-topics/mental-health). How a person feels, thinks, behaves and relates to others and their environment affects how we as health practitioners approach the care of those with mental ill-health and define mental wellbeing. The National Mental Health Commission defines mental ill-health as:

> *'a wide spectrum of diagnosable health conditions that significantly affect how a person feels, thinks, behaves, and interacts with other people. Mental illness can vary in both severity and duration'*
> (National Mental Health Commission, 2019)

One of the challenges to the implementation of mental health initiatives, policy and integration into primary healthcare is the lack of a consensus definition on mental health and wellbeing and mental ill-health. Mental health can be viewed within the medical model, where it is the absence of mental disease and is based in the pathophysiology of changes in the brain (Manwell et al., 2015). Alternatively, there are definitions of mental health which describe a state of being which not only address the biological aspects of mental health but incorporate the social, psychological, spiritual and environmental factors that are linked to mental and physical wellbeing. Positive self-perception, self-worth and emotional development extend some of the generally accepted definitions and are important when considering the causes and influences on mental health and wellbeing. The global mental health movement advocates for a policy- and resource-driven focus to addressing mental healthcare needs and service delivery, one which acknowledges that for various social and cultural contexts the strategies to address mental healthcare needs are going to be different, and require different resources and policies to meet the needs of a given population (Bemme & Kirmayer, 2020). Patel and others (2018) suggest that it is important to recognise that service delivery needs to be diverse and flexible to address the complexity and varied nature of mental healthcare needs for individuals and populations.

> '*Mental health problems exist along a continuum from mild, time-limited distress to chronic, progressive and severely disabling conditions. The binary approach to diagnosing mental disorders, although useful for clinical practice, does not accurately reflect the diversity and complexity of mental health needs of individuals or populations.*'
>
> (Patel et al., 2018, p. 1)

To provide flexible and evidence-based mental healthcare therefore requires an understanding of culture, and of the social and policy direction that clinicians and individuals exist within. Culture, how a group and individuals view and position themselves in their society, influences how mental health and mental ill-health are viewed and defined. Culture is constructed through social norms, practices and beliefs which shape the way mental health and ill-health are viewed by the group and the individual, and what is actually seen as being ill. Culture, discussed further in Chapter 2 of this book, also encompasses how families and social networks are used as supports, and what is considered recovery and treatment and how that is delivered. As an example, Australian Indigenous mental health is seen as part of a broader concept of health and wellbeing and includes the concept of intergenerational trauma, and understandings of kinship, family and connection to country and a greater role in leadership and service design (Dudgeon et al., 2016).

> '[For]...*Aborigines, mental health must be considered in the wider Aboriginal concept of health and well-being. This requires that their health issues be approached in the social emotional context, and that both social and emotional health and psychiatric disorders encompass oppression, racialism, environmental circumstances, economical factors, stress, trauma, grief, cultural genocide, psychological processes and ill-health.*'
>
> (Swan & Raphael, 1995, p. 15)

These definitions inform the structure of mental health assessment and history taking, and support the need for a comprehensive and holistic view of the person seeking care and the importance of different key areas. Mental health assessment focuses on the individual's emotional and cognitive state, how they are interacting and behaving within their environment and with others, how they view their circumstances, their thought patterns, flow and content at that time, and how they view their mental state and their ability to make decisions regarding their actions and care needs. Mental state assessment is further detailed in Chapter 5.

Legal definitions of mental illness in the various Mental Health Acts around Australia and New Zealand inform and guide how ambulance services, paramedics and other health services develop, translate and implement policy and practice in conjunction with local jurisdiction agreements between relevant services (e.g. health departments, mental health services, office of chief psychiatrist or equivalent, the police, and Royal Flying Doctor Service). The definitions of mental illness from the states and territories Mental Health Acts, outlined in Table 1.1, cover the key features of what is considered mental illness. Most *Acts* include reference to a *condition* or *medical condition* which *severely affects, impairs or disturbs a person's thoughts, mood, perception, behaviour, cognition, memory and ability to function*. The majority of the *Acts* also feature a reference to whether the change is either *temporary or permanent* in those who are experiencing mental ill-health and provides a list of exclusion criteria which are considered not to be mental illness. These definitions and powers under legislation for paramedic practice are discussed in more detail in Chapter 6 of this book which deals with the legal and ethical issues around mental healthcare.

Table 1.1 Australian and New Zealand Mental Health Acts and the Definitions of Mental Illness

Mental Health Act	Definition of Mental Illness
Australian Capital Territory (2015)	'a condition that seriously impairs (either temporarily or permanently) the mental functioning of a person in 1 or more areas of thought, mood, volition, perception, orientation or memory, and is characterised by— (a) the presence of at least 1 of the following symptoms: (i) delusions; (ii) hallucinations; (iii) serious disorders of streams of thought; (iv) serious disorders of thought form; (v) serious disturbance of mood; or (b) sustained or repeated irrational behaviour that may be taken to indicate the presence of at least 1 of the symptoms mentioned in paragraph (a).'
New South Wales (2007)	'a condition that seriously impairs, either temporarily or permanently, the mental functioning of a person and is characterised by the presence in the person of any one or more of the following symptoms: (a) delusions, (b) hallucinations, (c) serious disorder of thought form, (d) a severe disturbance of mood, (e) sustained or repeated irrational behaviour indicating the presence of any one or more of the symptoms referred to in paragraphs (a)–(d).'
Northern Territory (Mental Health and Related Services Act 1998; as in force at 1 December 2018)	'a condition that seriously impairs, either temporarily or permanently, the mental functioning of a person in one or more of the areas of thought, mood, volition, perception, orientation or memory and is characterised: (a) by the presence of at least one of the following symptoms: (i) delusions; (ii) hallucinations; (iii) serious disorders of the stream of thought; (iv) serious disorders of thought form; (v) serious disturbances of mood; or (b) by sustained or repeated irrational behaviour that may be taken to indicate the presence of at least one of the symptoms referred to in paragraph (a).'
Queensland (2016)	'a condition characterised by a clinically significant disturbance of thought, mood, perception or memory.'
South Australia (2009)	'mental illness means any illness or disorder of the mind.'

Continued

Table 1.1 Australian and New Zealand Mental Health Acts and the Definitions of Mental Illness *continued*

Mental Health Act	Definition of Mental Illness
Tasmania (2013)	'(1) For the purposes of this Act—(a) a person is taken to have a mental illness if he or she experiences, temporarily, repeatedly or continually—(i) a serious impairment of thought (which may include delusions); or (ii) a serious impairment of mood, volition, perception or cognition; and (b) nothing prevents the serious or permanent physiological, biochemical or psychological effects of alcohol use or drug-taking from being regarded as an indication that a person has a mental illness.'
Victoria (2014)	'a medical condition that is characterised by a significant disturbance of thought, mood, perception or memory.'
Western Australia (2014)	'(1) A person has a mental illness if the person has a condition that—(a) is characterised by a disturbance of thought, mood, volition, perception, orientation or memory; and (b) significantly impairs (temporarily or permanently) the person's judgment or behaviour.'
New Zealand (Mental Health (Compulsory Assessment and Treatment Act 1992; reprinted 2017)	'mental disorder, in relation to any person, means an abnormal state of mind (whether of a continuous or an intermittent nature), characterised by delusions, or by disorders of mood or perception or volition or cognition, of such a degree that it—(a) poses a serious danger to the health or safety of that person or of others; or (b) seriously diminishes the capacity of that person to take care of himself or herself;—and mentally disordered, in relation to any such person, has a corresponding meaning.'

Mental health conditions worldwide pose a significant burden on social, economic and health infrastructure (Doran & Kinchin, 2019; Rehm & Shield, 2019; Schofield et al 2019). In Australia the 2015 Australian Burden of Disease Study examined the effect of different diseases on fatal and non-fatal (years of life lived with a disability) people for the Australian population. The study found mental and substance use disorders were responsible for an estimated 12% of the total disease burden in Australia, making it the fourth highest group of diseases behind cancer (18%), cardiovascular diseases (14%) and musculoskeletal conditions (13%) (AIHW, 2019a) (Fig. 1.1).

The World Health Organization measures the economic effect of mental illness through lost labour force participation and lost productivity summarised as lost personal earnings. Estimates made by Levinson and others (2010) using data from the WHO's World Mental Health Surveys found that those experiencing serious mental illness earned a third less, on average, than the median earnings of the whole population in the 10 high-income and 9 low- and medium-income countries included in the study (Levinson et al., 2010). These losses, equating to approximately 0.3%–0.8% of national earnings, may lead to further financial hardship and out-of-pocket expenditure for individuals and loss of revenue through taxes and increased social and health payments for governments (Schofield et al., 2019). In

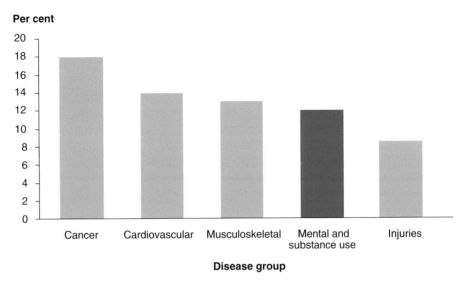

Per cent

FIGURE 1.1

Australia's top five burden of disease groups, 2015: mental and substance use disorders (24%) were the second largest contributor to non-fatal burden, behind musculoskeletal conditions (25%)

AIHW (2019a)

Australia, government spending on mental health services has increased from $5.3 billion in 2004–05 to $8.5 billion in 2014–15. The Australian Productivity Commission Report (2019) into mental health estimates that the cost to the Australian economy of mental ill-health and suicide is $43–51 billion per year with an additional $130 billion associated with diminished health and reduced life expectancy.

HOW PREVALENT ARE MENTAL HEALTH CONDITIONS IN THE COMMUNITY AND WHY IS THIS RELEVANT TO PARAMEDIC PRACTICE?

Mental health conditions, depending on their severity, early intervention and access to treatment, can affect a person's life expectancy, and their ability to engage with their community and significant others, and to partake in work or manage their own physical health and wellbeing (Ilyas et al., 2017). Measuring the prevalence and effect of mental health conditions on individuals, groups and populations is challenging and is widely recognised as being under-reported (Bharadwaj et al., 2017).

In 1997 and 2007 the Australian Bureau of Statistics (ABS) conducted the National Survey of Mental Health and Wellbeing (NSMHWB), which provided governments and service providers with comprehensive estimates for lifetime and previous 12-month prevalence data on mental disorders for Australian adults aged

16 to 85 years. The survey, although now dated, estimated 45% of Australians had experienced a mental disorder in their lifetime, with 20% experiencing a mental disorder in the previous year. These estimates, when based on 2017 population numbers, equate to approximately 8.7 million people who will experience a common mental disorder in their lifetime (AIHW, 2019b). According to the most recent ABS National Health Survey, mental and behavioural conditions were estimated to affect around 4.8 million Australians (20.1% of the population) in 2017–18. These current estimates indicate an increase from 2014–15 of 2.6%, which is believed to be from increased reporting of anxiety-related conditions, depression or feelings related to depression (Department of Parliamentary Services, 2019). The challenge with the most recent data is it only reports on those individuals who currently self-identify as having a mental or behavioural condition, and does not take into account lifetime prevalence or 12-month incidence of mental illness.

In mid-2013 to 2014 the Australian Child and Adolescent Survey of Mental Health and Wellbeing, which was conducted by the Department of Health, estimated that approximately 14% or 560,000 of young people aged between 4 and 17 years had experienced a mental disorder in the previous 12 months (AIHW, 2019b). The following two figures from the Productivity Commission's 2019 report show prevalence with age of common mental health conditions and less common conditions (Figs 1.2 and 1.3).

Figure 1.4, from the Australian Institute of Health and Welfare: Mental Health Services in Brief 2019, shows the difference in gender experience of mental illness, especially for anxiety, affective (mood) and substance use disorders. The figure

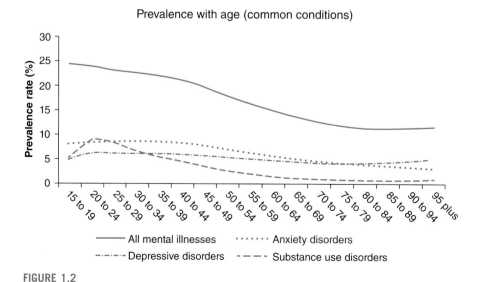

FIGURE 1.2

Prevalence of common mental illnesses with age

Productivity Commission (2019)

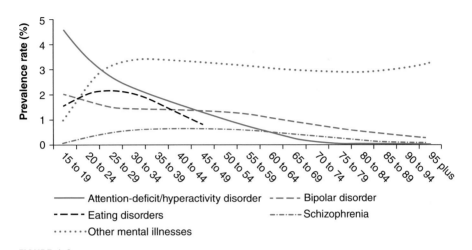

Prevalence with age (less common conditions)

FIGURE 1.3

Prevalence of less common mental illnesses with age

Productivity Commission (2019)

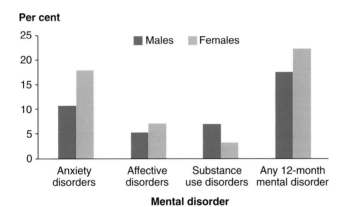

Women experienced a higher prevalence of mental disorders in the preceding 12 months than men (22.3% compared with 17.6%)

FIGURE 1.4

Common mental illnesses by gender

AIHW (2019b)

shows that women experienced a higher prevalence of mental disorders in the previous 12 months compared with males (Fig. 1.4).

To understand the nature of mental health conditions that paramedics are attending in the community, it is also worth considering the use of community mental healthcare services and presentations to emergency departments. As the care of those with mental illness shifted from institutions to community-based and primary care, mental illness and suicidal behaviour – including self-injury, overdose, suicidal ideation and actual attempts at suicide – became a major public health issue (Hickie & McGorry 2007). The increase in need in the community space has led to the coordination of services such the mental health triage service and the instigation of mental health liaison teams within emergency departments. As part of the shift, emergency services such as paramedics, the police and frontline services have taken an increasing role in the provision of services to those with mental illness (Bismah et al., 2017; Parsons et al., 2011; Roberts & Henderson, 2009; Shaban, 2005). The increasing demand for adequate specialist, community and primary mental healthcare services has seen emergency departments (ED) become the entry point for mental healthcare alongside GPs (Bismah et al., 2017).

COMMUNITY MENTAL HEALTHCARE (CMHC)

Recent estimates for community mental healthcare (CMHC), which includes both community and hospital outpatient-based services, showed about 9.5 million contacts were provided in 2017–18 nationally to over 430,000 people. In 2018–19, community mental health services (CMHS) nationally provided approximately 9.7 million community mental healthcare service contacts to around 453,000 patients. Of total patient contacts, 1,768,500 were with people diagnosed with schizophrenia (AIHW, 2020a). The importance of these numbers for pre-hospital care is on average people were accessing care 22 times a year with a national average of 17.6 patients per 1000 population receiving community mental healthcare (AIHW, 2019a). The implication is that those needing mental healthcare often need medium- to long-term help, have regular contact with mental healthcare services, and the ambulance service and paramedics provide the immediate and stop-gap care to those experiencing mental illness in the community.

MENTAL HEALTH SERVICES PROVIDED IN PUBLIC HOSPITAL EMERGENCY DEPARTMENTS

The important role of public hospital EDs as an initial point of care for those with acute mental healthcare needs, those experiencing mental health concerns for the first time, and for those seeking after-hours mental healthcare is well established. According to the Australian Institute of Health and Welfare (2019b), the number of recorded mental-health-related ED occasions of service has increased as a proportion of total ED presentations from 3.3% in 2013–14 to 3.6% in 2017–18.

The national number of ED mental-health-related presentations per 10,000 population increased by 10.3% between 2013–14 and 2017–18, with Western Australia having the largest increase over this period. In 2017–18 there were an estimated 286,985 mental-health-related ED presentations (3.6% of all ED occasions of service). On initial assessment, almost 4 in 5 (78.6%) mental-health-related ED presentations were classified as being either urgent (requiring care within 30 minutes) or semi-urgent (requiring care within 60 minutes). Approximately a

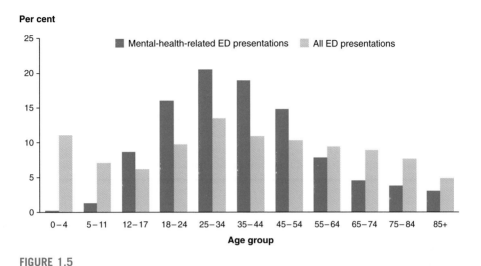

FIGURE 1.5

Presentations to public hospital emergency departments, by age group (years), 2017–18

AIHW (2019b)

further 14.4% of presentations were classified as emergency (requiring care within 10 minutes) and 1.0% as resuscitation (requiring immediate care). These statistics indicate that those needing mental healthcare through the ED are in significant need, require urgent care and support, and paramedics are crucial in the initial assessment and care provided (Fig. 1.5).

These estimates are recognised as being under-reported due to the lack of uniformity across jurisdictions in data reporting and the classification of mental-health-related occasions of service. Even though it is difficult to estimate the provision of emergency care in the pre-hospital and emergency setting, paramedics – as the primary pre-hospital emergency medical care providers – have been forced to consider role changes with their increasing responsibility in the care of those with mental illness.

Another relevant part of the picture for paramedics is the average length of stay in the ED. The AIHW (2019b) reported that the average length of stay for mental-health-related presentations in the ED was approximately 3.5 hours (213 minutes). The most recorded discharge or end status for mental-health-related presentations in the ED was departed without being admitted or referred to another hospital (58.1%). Approximately 4 in 10 (39.1%) presentations resulted in admission to a hospital, either to the hospital where the emergency service was provided (34.9%) or referred to another hospital for admission (4.2%) (AIHW, 2019b). This suggests that paramedics are often managing the presentation at the scene and taking the person to hospital where the person is most commonly not admitted, after being in the ED for an average of 3.5 hours. Paramedics may re-attend these individuals within the same shift or within a short period of time depending on follow-up mental health services and access to community care (colloquially known as the revolving-door syndrome).

Paramedics and ambulance services are in a position where they provide not only acute crisis care for those with mental health conditions, but find they are also the link between those with primary mental healthcare needs and community services. Paramedics are increasingly required to be able to assess and make clinical decisions around the need for hospital and intensive mental healthcare or the appropriateness of alternative referral to community mental health services. One example of these changes in responsibility is the extended powers provided to paramedics and other accredited health practitioners under the various state and territory Mental Health Acts. Under the Mental Health Acts, for example those of South Australia (2009, s56), Victoria (2014, s350) and New South Wales (2007, ss19, 20 and 23), paramedics and accredited health professionals are authorised to restrain and transport those experiencing suspected mental illness to either a designated mental health facility or a healthcare facility where appropriate assessment and further care can be arranged (e.g. an ED). The Mental Health Acts provide for the use of 'reasonable force', physical and mechanical restraint and sedation, by those trained to provide it, for the individual under their care. As these roles and responsibilities expanded, the aim was to reduce the role of the police as de-facto community mental health providers and allow their role to return to managing behaviour more in line with the justice system, providing support as requested. The increased responsibility required ambulance services to allocate training time and resources (allocative efficiency) and create flexibility while roles and responsibilities were redistributed or negotiated through memorandums of understanding between frontline services and health departments (dynamic efficiencies). The initiation of mental health co-responder service delivery in several jurisdictions has also demonstrated an organisational shift to accommodate these changes in demand and expectations in service delivery. (Ambulance services have joined with mental health services and professionals to provide specific multidisciplinary teams to manage mental health presentations within the home and offer referral to community or acute services as needed.)

The next section in this chapter describes the historical and policy context for mental healthcare in Australia. The section begins with a case study and questions for reflection as a foundation for discussion on the effects of the move to community care, the access to mental healthcare, and the role of stigma and help-seeking for those experiencing mental illness.

CASE STUDY

Jared

You have been called late on a Friday night to a 21-year-old male, Jared, who has contacted his friend because of feelings and thoughts of suicide, stating he doesn't know how to cope.

On arrival: Jared is sitting with his friend in the kitchen with the medications temazepam, Endep (Amitriptyline), and paracetamol laid out on the kitchen bench and a bottle of scotch whiskey. Jared's friend informs you that he has known Jared since high school and that over the past three to four years he has been supporting Jared through episodes of depression.

Jared's mother has been contacted and is on her way home from her afternoon shift at the local aged care residential facility. His older sister is his only sibling and is currently living interstate for work.

On assessment: Jared is dressed in an old shirt and jeans. He is approximately 170 cm tall with short brown hair and brown eyes. He is barefoot and sitting on a kitchen stool leaning on the kitchen bench with his head down, hands partially covering his face, and when he looks up you can see tears in his eyes. He is softly spoken, and has little eye contact with paramedics. He tells you in a quiet voice that he has not taken any of the medications on the bench, but has had a couple of beers before he thought about taking an overdose of the medications with the bottle of whiskey.

Jared lets you conduct a series of vital sign observations which all appear to be within normal range.

You notice as you try to build a rapport with Jared that he has old burn marks on his upper arms and scars on his wrists. You ask Jared about the scars on his arms and wrists. Jared immediately gets defensive and withdraws (stops answering questions, becomes very quiet with closed body language) from you. He reluctantly explains the scars were just a joke and prank from a year ago, and that he intends to get them covered with a tattoo when he has enough money.

Background

You find out from Jared's friend that his parents divorced about three years ago, and he has lost contact with his father, who had become more involved with methamphetamine use with periods of paranoia, and was verbally abusive to his mum, his older sister and Jared before he left the family.

After his father left the family, Jared found he struggled to cope and became more despondent and used self-harm as a means of coping. His mother and sister became more concerned and accessed help for Jared via their general practitioner, who was very supportive and referred Jared to a psychologist. After several sessions with the psychologist and his general practitioner, Jared began to feel able to continue his university studies, playing the guitar, which he had played for several years before his father left, and he found he could reconnect with his friends and family.

Two months ago, Jared's psychologist was no longer able to see Jared as they were moving to a new practice and were not able to continue providing mental healthcare. The psychologist recommended and referred Jared to a colleague, but they could not see Jared for a month, and on their first appointment Jared felt very uncomfortable and considered the appointment a waste of money and time. Jared felt that he was being judged for the scars on his wrists, and his thoughts of self-harm, and that he should be stronger, and was told that his father was not worth getting so emotionally involved with since it had been a number of years and he was no longer a part of the family.

Jared and his mother have been trying to access services since then, and Jared has increasingly become disconnected and despondent, with increasing feelings of worthlessness and hopelessness.

CRITICAL REFLECTION

1. Discuss how de-institutionalisation and the movement from institutionalised care to community mental healthcare might have affected how Jared and his family access mental health services, and what role stigma plays in Jared's willingness to seek mental health services.
2. What acute and community services are available for Jared, and how as paramedics might you use this information in your communication with Jared, his friend and family?
3. What social, family and psychological factors would you note, and how would this inform your history taking and your communication with Jared and his family/friend?
4. Consider what factors might be protective of Jared's mental health, and what might be challenging and worsen his mental health.

MENTAL HEALTHCARE IN AUSTRALIA: HISTORICAL CONTEXT

Traditionally, mental healthcare was provided by the state with the penal system initially being tasked with the management of the mentally ill. Mental illness was not historically seen as a medical problem, and asylums were often run by lay rather than medical superintendents. Medical diagnosis and certification of mental illness were not introduced into law until 1839 in New South Wales, followed by other jurisdictions (Cummins, 2003). In the 1880s a series of government inquiries changed the landscape of mental healthcare and increased the involvement of the medical profession to provide what was considered 'scientific' management of the mentally ill. This change led to increased numbers of psychiatric patients, and the increased building of psychiatric hospitals to accommodate those considered mentally ill (Coleborne, 1996; Lewis & Garton, 2017). In the early 1950s the federal government reported that psychiatric hospitals were overcrowded and often housed those such as the elderly and intellectually disabled who could be housed in alternative institutions (Stoller & Arscott, 1955). The recommendation from the federal government at that time was to provide more psychiatric hospitals to manage the increased demand within the system, the use of the general health system and outpatient services, and provision of care in separate services for the elderly and intellectually disabled (Stoller & Arscott, 1955).

DE-INSTITUTIONALISATION

'Community awareness about mental illness has come a long way, but the mental health system has not kept pace with needs and expectations of how the well-being and productive capacity of people should be supported. The treatment of, and support for, people with mental illness has been tacked on to a system that has been largely designed around the characteristics of physical illness. And while service levels have increased in some areas, progress has been patchy. The right services are often not available when needed, leading to wasted health resources and missed opportunities to improve lives.'

(Productivity Commission Report, 2019, p. 4)

De-institutionalisation is a term used to describe the shift from the institutionalised provision of care to community and outpatient service delivery models of care. In Australia this move in service provision in mental healthcare began around 1955, and was driven by the changing belief that mental illness could be prevented by early intervention and the increasing evidence that long-term institutionalisation was having negative effects on mental health outcomes (Lamb & Bachrach, 2001). These changes in beliefs, in conjunction with the shortcomings in institutionalised care, created the 'first wave' of de-institutionalisation and involved the development of community services in the form of state-funded day hospitals, community housing and centres, earlier discharge from psychiatric hospitals and initial models of outpatient care for the newly diagnosed and acutely ill. During this time the separation of older persons and those with intellectual disabilities into alternate separate services was also occurring, which continued to shift care and generated a separation of drug- and alcohol-related issues, mental healthcare and cognitive needs for those with intellectual disability. There was also investment into the development of child psychological services, with the beginning understanding that mental illness could be modified and prevented through early intervention when changes in behaviour were first recognised. During this first wave of de-institutionalisation those with severe or chronic mental illness were not included in these social and service delivery changes.

As de-institutionalisation gained greater prominence in the 1980s, the focus shifted to those who were chronically ill and the development of services for them to live outside the confines of psychiatric hospitals and integrate into the community. The other major change during this time was a move from inpatient treatment being provided in psychiatric hospitals to specific psychiatric wards in general hospitals. The objective was to reduce the separation of mental healthcare from other forms of healthcare and address the disparity and failures in service provision. The shift to the development of community mental healthcare and the integration into general mental health services took time to establish and was not uniform across Australia. To address the varied success of jurisdictions towards the coordination and development of community services and resource allocation to mental health services, the national government called for a coordinated and national mental health policy. The National Mental Health Strategy, as this policy is known, was established and agreed upon by state, territory and federal health ministers in 1992.

NATIONAL MENTAL HEALTH STRATEGY (1992–)

The three documents that originally made up the National Mental Health Strategy were the National Mental Health Strategy and the first National Mental Health Plan, which were released in 1992. The other key document was the Mental Health Statement of Rights and Responsibilities, which was initially released in 1991 and re-released in 2012. Subsequent to the initial National Mental Health Strategy, two five-year National Mental Health Plans were released in 1998 and 2003 (the Second and Third National Mental Health Plans). The aim of these two policy plans was to focus on: the development of service partnerships to broaden the provision of mental health services; the development of pathways to facilitate consumers and carer participation in service design and delivery; research and evaluation; and most significantly funding and creation of prevention and early intervention strategies (Australian Health Ministers 1998, 2003). The shift to include those with lived experience of mental health concerns (consumers) and carers in policy development and service delivery led the Commonwealth to implement monitoring and evaluation of the level of their involvement in both government and non-government services' management boards.

The original National Mental Health Strategy aimed to facilitate the move of service delivery and funding for mental health services from psychiatric hospitals to general hospitals and the community, and to foster better links between government support services and non-government organisations (NGOs). The second main aim was to generate uniform mental health legislation across the country (Australian Health Ministers, 1992). As a result, the number of psychiatric hospitals fell from 59 in 1989 to 20 in 2005. By 2012–13, there were 6768 mental-health hospital beds available in public hospitals in Australia. In 2015–16, 161 public hospitals (7057 public hospital beds) and 66 private hospitals (2754 private mental health beds) provided specialised mental health services for admitted patients. Public psychiatric services provided around 2.2 million patient days to people in hospital and 2385 residential mental health beds, of which almost two-thirds were operated by government services. Almost three-quarters of these (73%, or 4937 beds) were in specialised psychiatric units or wards within public acute hospitals, with the remainder in public psychiatric hospitals (1831 beds) (AIHW, 2014).

Psychiatric beds in private hospitals also grew in number, increasing by 40% between 1992–93 and 2010–11 (Department of Health and Ageing, 2013). In 2011–12, there were 11,113 psychiatric beds available in Australia, of which 2072 were in private hospitals (AIHW, 2014). Closure of psychiatric beds was accompanied by the development of community mental health services. Services ranged from community mental health teams, which assessed, monitored and maintained people in the community, to residential services, such as supported accommodation, and services that provided social and employment activity. Spending on services provided in general hospitals and in the community in Australia increased by 283% by 2011, while spending on stand-alone psychiatric hospitals decreased by 35% (Department of Health and Ageing, 2013).

DISTRIBUTION OF MENTAL HEALTH SERVICES (2017–18)

More recently, the distribution of mental health services in 2017–18 showed 12,616 specialised mental health beds available nationally, with 6920 beds provided by public hospital services, 3146 by private hospitals, and 2550 by residential mental healthcare services (Fig. 1.6). The majority of the 6920 public sector specialised mental health hospital beds were found in specialised psychiatric units or wards within public acute hospitals (76.7%, or 5307 beds), with the remainder in public psychiatric hospitals (1613 beds). The largest proportion of specialised mental health services beds were in general services (4932 beds, or 71.3%), with 976 beds (14.1%) in older person services, 658 (9.5%) in forensic services and 295 (4.3%), provided in child and adolescent services. A small number of beds were located in youth services (59 beds, or 0.9%); a service category that was introduced in 2011–12.

One of the challenges with specialist mental health services is that they specifically target chronic mental illness, which leaves a gap in service provision for people experiencing depression and anxiety disorders and younger people with

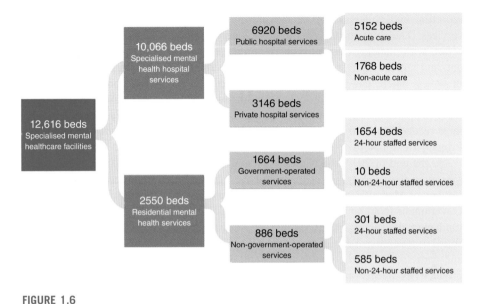

FIGURE 1.6

Distribution of specialised mental health beds in Australia, 2017–18

https://www.aihw.gov.au/reports/mental-health-services/mental-health-services-in-australia/report-contents/

specialised-mental-health-care-facilities/mental-health-beds-and-patient-days

first presentation of mental health symptoms (McGorry, 2007). To address these growing concerns and gaps in services, the government implemented Medicare funding changes encouraging a greater role for primary mental healthcare. General practitioners (GPs) in particular were given a greater role, and have become a first point of call for primary mental healthcare (Department of Health and Ageing, 2009a). Targeted programs such those provided by Headspace, Beyond Blue, Sane, and ReachOut, and established crisis support services such as Lifeline, have become increasingly important as online and alternative services and pathways to face-to-face interaction are needed to manage the demand and the changing ways people engage in healthcare.

The Fourth National Mental Health Plan: An agenda for collaborative government action in mental health 2009–2014 targeted the need for collaborative government action in mental health, and attempted to provide a framework to guide funding and the development of a system of care that was able to intervene early and provide integrated services across health and social domains. The National Mental Health Policy 2008 and the Fourth National Mental Health Plan also moved the focus to recovery-based services and social inclusion through promoting access to housing, education and employment opportunities for people with mental illness. The 2019 National Report on Mental Health and Suicide Prevention outlines that there is still concern regarding consumer engagement and the reporting and collection of data exploring consumer and carer experience with services. The implementation of the recovery approach is often seen as a token effort, with standards not rigorously applied, payment for participation inconsistent, and human rights and a recovery-orientated approach not being reflected well in policy. There has also been a greater focus on integrated community care in this period, with Medicare Locals providing leadership for integration at a regional level (Department of Health and Ageing, 2009b). This model was revised by the most recent Coalition Government, with Medicare Locals being amalgamated into Primary Health Networks (PHNs) and put to tender in late 2014.

At the end of 2014, the National Mental Health Commission (the Commission) submitted their report 'Contributing Lives, Thriving Communities – The National Review of Mental Health Programmes and Services' (the Review) to the Australian Government (National Mental Health Commission, 2018). The Review identified fundamental structural shortcomings in Australia's approach to mental health and suicide prevention. Several factors were contributing to a huge drain on wellbeing and participation in the community – and on jobs, on families, and on Australia's productivity and economic growth. The key findings showed that mental health resources were not distributed equitably across geographic regions, population groups and levels of need. Resources were concentrated in expensive acute-care services, and not enough resources were invested in prevention and early intervention. Patterns of mental ill-health, suicide and suicide attempts differ across regions of Australia and across different population groups, and this was not recognised in the service planning or delivery. At that time the gaps in services for people with serious mental illness were significant, and uncertainty about whether this would be improved or exacerbated by the National Disability Insurance Scheme (NDIS) was a major concern. Aboriginal and Torres Strait Islander people continue to have a higher risk of suicide and mental ill-health than other Australians. Low-intensity services, particularly self-help and e-mental health services, were largely underused, and were still evolving to meet need. Evaluation and research findings were not well translated into practice. There were large information gaps about what was working. There were no agreed or consistent national measures of whether efforts were leading to effective outcomes and better lives for people with mental illness.

The Fifth National Mental Health and Suicide Prevention Plan (the Fifth Plan) and its implementation were endorsed by the Council of Australian Governments Health Council (COAG Health Council) in August 2017. The Fifth Plan foundation has eight targeted priority areas, aligning with the aims and policy directions of the National Mental Health Policy (COAG, 2017). The eight priority areas are:

- Priority Area 1: Achieving integrated regional planning and service delivery.
- Priority Area 2: Effective suicide prevention.
- Priority Area 3: Coordinating treatment and supports for people with severe and complex mental illness.
- Priority Area 4: Improving Aboriginal and Torres Strait Islander mental health and suicide prevention.

- Priority Area 5: Improving the physical health of people living with mental illness and reducing early mortality.
- Priority Area 6: Reducing stigma and discrimination.
- Priority Area 7: Making safety and quality central to mental health service delivery.
- Priority Area 8: Ensuring that the enablers of effective system performance and system improvement are in place.

The Fifth Plan aims to support service reform and policy development until 2022. In an interim report in 2018, PHNs commonly reported that funding and resourcing was a major barrier to implementing the priorities in the Fifth Plan. The key areas lacking in funding and resources included integrated planning and delivery (Priority Area 1), coordinated treatment and supports (Priority Area 3), meaningful engagement with Aboriginal and Torres Strait Islander people (Priority Area 4), and improving the physical health of people living with mental illness (Priority Area 5). Another significant barrier to achieving the aims of the Fifth Plan involved state and territory government health departments not readily receiving guidance from the Australian Government Department of Health on integrated regional planning and service delivery (Priority Area 1) before they could progress with implementation.

PRIVATISATION AND INTEGRATION

Underpinning many of the changes associated with the National Mental Health Strategy has been a movement away from a reliance on government services to more use of private, for-profit services. This marks a shift towards a market model of care that is underpinned by viewing people with mental illness as consumers who can exercise control over their care through deciding between services. Privatisation has resulted in the use of a greater array of service providers and greater complexity in service delivery. To overcome complexity, mental health policy has promoted integration between services. Integrated care is seen as a means of managing the demands on the healthcare budget while improving access to, and the quality of, services, and addressing gaps in service delivery (Petrich et al., 2013). Banfield and colleagues (2012) argue that while service and interprofessional partnerships have been on the policy agenda from the first National Mental Health Plan, they have become a priority area from the Fourth Plan. Examples of schemes created to increase the integration of mental health services include shared care where care is shared between specialist mental health services and general practitioners, and Partners in Recovery which provide case managers to link people with severe and persistent mental illness with health and social services (Smith-Merry & Gillespie, 2016).

In practice, service integration has had mixed results. Petrich and colleagues (2013) argue that services are currently fragmented due to the dispersion of the population, to federalism resulting in two layers of government and blurred lines of accountability between the federal and state governments, and to differences in approach to private services between the major political parties. The dispersion of the population leads to poorer access to services for people living in rural and remote areas. In a joint submission from the national and state mental health commissions to the Accessibility and Quality of Mental Health Services in Rural and Remote Australia senate inquiry in May 2018, the commissions associated ongoing issues with access to mental health services for rural and remote populations with disproportionate spending on metropolitan services, limited access to social support services, and difficulties in attracting and retaining staff. These issues are compounded by the social determinants of health, as rural populations are older, have fewer educational opportunities and greater economic uncertainty (Australian Mental Health Commission, 2018).

Federalism results in the state governments providing specialist mental health services and the federal government funding NGOs and primary care, leading to difficulties in coordinating services as political differences have led to changes in service funding (Petrich et al., 2013). Carey and others (2012) identify two approaches to governance of social services within Australia: an approach favouring social inclusion and one favouring market approaches. Social inclusion involves addressing social inequities through creating the conditions for people with mental illness to participate in economic, political and social life. A market approach favours the neoliberal values of privatisation, deregulation, reliance on the market and mutual obligation, i.e. consumer choice of services through the NDIS. The first approach is most commonly associated with the Australian Labor Party, and the second with the Coalition.

Creating partnerships between public and private services has also been identified as difficult. McDonald and colleagues (2011) argue that collaborations are formed to meet mutual or complementary goals, but that goals and ways of working may not be compatible between public and private services. Private service providers, such as GPs, seek results for specific patients, whereas government services have a population approach. Furthermore, GPs and other private service providers may have difficulty in negotiating existing bureaucratic systems (McDonald et al., 2011).

USE OF PRIVATE SERVICES TO DELIVER COMMUNITY MENTAL HEALTHCARE

In the discussion that follows, we outline some of the non-government and private, for-profit services involved in service delivery for people with mental health disorders.

Primary care

The changes outlined above have increased the role of primary care in delivering services to the mentally ill. A move towards primary care has been promoted by strategies to increase collaboration between primary care and specialist mental health services. Better Outcomes in Mental Health Care (BOiMHC) was launched in July 2001 to improve access to primary mental healthcare (Fletcher et al., 2009). The first cycle of reforms allowed GPs to claim through Medicare for psychological interventions and referrals to psychologists and social workers for people with depression and anxiety disorders (Fletcher et al., 2009; Hickie & Groom, 2002). This was extended in November 2006 through the Better Access program, which allowed psychologists, and some social workers and occupational therapists, to claim services under the Medicare Benefits Scheme upon referral by a GP (Fletcher et al., 2009). The 2011 Budget lowered the number of consultations available through the Better Access program and reduced Medicare rebates for GP mental healthcare planning, opting instead to target resources through Medicare Locals and NGOs (Henderson & Fuller, 2011), and from 2015 governance of these services passed to PHNs (Henderson et al., 2019).

PHNs are regional primary healthcare organisations that are responsible for undertaking needs assessment and planning primary care services within a region. The National Mental Health Commission's *National Review of Mental Health Programs and Services*, released in 2014, identified a lack of integration between primary, secondary and tertiary services and a need to redirect funding away from inpatient services towards community and private-for-profit primary care services. Among the recommendations made by the review were an increased role for PHNs in regional planning for primary mental healthcare, and the adoption of a stepped care model (Henderson et al., 2019). Stepped care makes efficient use of existing resources through reserving more intensive treatments for people with the greatest need, and providing cost-effective options for people defined as having fewer needs (Bower & Gilbody, 2005).

The PHNs took responsibility for planning primary mental health and the development of stepped care service delivery from 2015. As part of this they assumed responsibility for managing budgets for existing federally funded mental health programs such as Headspace. General practice is at the centre of primary mental healthcare stepped care. GPs have become a major source of care because they are viewed as the first point of contact for someone with a mental health disorder. According to the BEACH data, 12.4% of all GP encounters were mental-health-related, equating to just under 18 million contacts, with depression being the most common at approximately one-third, or 32.1%, during 2015–16 (AIHW, 2020b). The capacity of general practice to manage mental health is enhanced by the Mental Health Nurse Incentive Program (MHNIP), which provides a payment to general practices and other primary care services to employ a mental health nurse to 'assist in the provision of coordinated clinical care for people with severe mental illness' (RHealth, 2016). Earlier data suggests, however, that uptake of this funding is uneven, undermining capacity to deliver healthcare to people with chronic mental illness. Data from 2015 demonstrates that Victoria and Queensland record significantly higher proportions of patients receiving services under the MHNIP than other states (Henderson et al., 2019).

Non-government organisations

A second source of care has been the use of non-government services to provide support services for people with mental illness. The original National Mental Health Strategy (Australian Health Ministers, 1992) argued for the use of a combination of government and NGO service providers to meet the needs of the mentally ill. For Carson and Kerr (2014), the use of NGOs is associated with the 'hollowing-out' of government departments in an effort to achieve value-for-money with public funds. This process has consequences for NGOs, which experience difficulties in retaining staff, due to insecure funding, and with excessive reporting mechanisms (Carson & Kerr, 2014).

Social support services for people with mental illness are currently primarily managed through the NDIS, supplemented by state and Commonwealth funding for people who are ineligible for NDIS services. Critics have also noted that mental illness does not fit comfortably within a disability model as it is often episodic, leading to concerns with continued eligibility for social services (MIND, 2014). It is evident that many people with severe mental illness may not be eligible to access these services. On 30 June 2019, only 25,192 people who had a disability associated with a mental health issue had an approved management plan under the NDIS (AIHW, 2020c) while Smith-Merry and colleagues (2018) noted that based on government figures in 2018 nearly 20% of people with psychosocial disability who requested access into NDIS were not accepted.

Informal carers

Families and friends of the mentally ill also provide a major source of care. The original National Mental Health Strategy document stated that 'many people with mental disorders are cared for in the community by "unpaid" carers' (Australian Health Ministers, 1992, p. 26), where a carer was defined as 'a person whose life is affected by virtue of his or her having a close relationship with a consumer, or who has a chosen and contracted caring role with a consumer' (Australian Health Ministers, 1991, p. 23). There is currently little data on the number of people caring for people with mental health disorders, although estimates suggest that 2.6 million Australians are caring for someone with a disability of some sort (AIHW, 2009). Of these people, one-third are primary carers. Responsibility for providing day-to-day care falls disproportionately on women, with two-thirds of primary carers being women. This is sometimes referred to as the feminisation of care. Adoption of a carer role has been associated with poorer mental and physical health. Pirkis and others (2010) found that the carers of people with mental illness were more likely to be women, to be aged between 55 and 64 years old, and to experience significant levels of depression and distress. Despite this, government policy presumes that carers are not only willing but able to provide care to families and friends with mental illness, and that people with mental illness want to be cared for by their families. Currently, the National Mental Health Commission is working with state and territory bodies to establish a Lived Experience Steering Group to engage and co-design policy, practice and research priorities with service providers and policy groups.

CONCLUSION

The aim of this chapter has been to introduce and define mental health and mental illness, the associated challenges with those definitions, and how they affect policy, service design and delivery, and their relevance to paramedic practice. The prevalence of mental illness, and the types of mental illness that are most common in the community and their burden, gives context to mental health policy, service design and delivery, and where and how paramedic practice fits into a complex mental health system. The development of community mental healthcare and the increasing availability of online mental health services and NGO involvement have changed the way people engage with mental health services. These structural and delivery changes have influenced how paramedics and ambulance services engage with the community, and their care provision for those experiencing mental illness.

The chapters in this book outline the clinical skills required to assess and identify those experiencing mental ill-health. Clinical skills include communication skills, mental state assessment and examination, legal and ethical considerations, and managing challenging behaviour and risk. The characteristics of the various mental disorders are covered in separate chapters, with case studies and discussion points to provide the foundations for understanding and building paramedic clinical practice.

LINKS AND RESOURCES

Beyond Blue: https://www.beyondblue.org.au/
Black Dog Institute: https://www.blackdoginstitute.org.au/
Headspace: https://headspace.org.au/
SANE: https://www.sane.org/
Lifeline: https://www.lifeline.org.au/
ReachOut: https://au.reachout.com/
Head to Health: https://headtohealth.gov.au/
Australian Institute of Health & Welfare Mental Health Services: https://www.aihw.gov.au/
 reports-data/health-welfare-services/mental-health-services/overview

REFERENCES

Australian Health Ministers, 1991. Mental health statement of rights and responsibilities. AGPS, Canberra.
Australian Health Ministers, 1992. National mental health strategy. AGPS, Canberra.
Australian Health Ministers, 1998. Second national mental health plan. Commonwealth Department of Health and Family Services, Canberra.
Australian Health Ministers, 2003. Third national mental health plan. Commonwealth Department of Health and Family Services, Canberra.
Australian Institute of Health and Welfare (AIHW), 2009. Carers national data repository scoping study: final report. AIHW, Canberra.

Australian Institute of Health and Welfare (AIHW), 2014. Mental health services—in brief 2014. Cat. no. HSE 154. AIHW, Canberra.

Australian Institute of Health and Welfare (AIHW), 2019a. Australian Burden of Disease Study: Impact and causes of illness and death in Australia 2015. Australian Burden of Disease Study series no. 19. Cat. no. BOD 22. AIHW, Canberra.

Australian Institute of Health and Welfare (AIHW), 2019b. Mental health services – in brief 2019. Cat. no. HSE 228. AIHW, Canberra.

Australian Institute of Health and Welfare (AIHW), 2020a. Community mental health care services. Online. Available: https://www.aihw.gov.au/reports/mental-health-services/mental-health-services-in-australia/report-contents/state-and-territory-community-mental-health-care-services.

Australian Institute of Health and Welfare (AIHW), 2020b. General practice. Online. Available: https://www.aihw.gov.au/reports/mental-health-services/mental-health-services-in-australia/report-contents/general-practice.

Australian Institute of Health and Welfare (AIHW), 2020c. Psychiatric disability support services. Online. Available: https://www.aihw.gov.au/reports/mental-health-services/mental-health-services-in-australia/report-contents/psychiatric-disability-support-service.

Australian Mental Health Commission, 2018. Submission to the Senate Inquiry into Accessibility and Quality of Mental Health Services in Rural and Remote Australia. Online. Available: https://www.mentalhealthcommission.gov.au/monitoring-and-reporting/submissions/accessibility-and-quality-of-mental-health-service.

Banfield, M., Gardner, K., Yen, L., et al., 2012. Co-ordination of care in Australian mental health policy. Aust. Health Rev. 36 (2), 153–157.

Bemme, D., Kirmayer, L.J., 2020. Global mental health: interdisciplinary challenges for a field in motion. Transcult. Psychiatry 57 (1), 3–18.

Bharadwaj, P., Pai, M.M., Suziedelyte, A., 2017. Mental health stigma. Econ. Lett. 159 (C), 57–60.

Bismah, V., Prpic, J., Michaud, S., et al., 2017. P018: prehospital diversion of mental health patients to a mental health center vs the emergency department: safety and compliance of an EMS direct transport protocol. CJEM 19 (S1), S83–S84.

Bower, P., Gilbody, S., 2005. Stepped care in psychological therapies: access, effectiveness and efficiency: narrative literature review. Br. J. Psychiatry 186 (1), 11–17.

Broadbent, M., Moxham, L., Dwyer, T., 2020. Understanding nurses perspectives of acuity in the process of emergency mental health triage: a qualitative study. Contemp. Nurse 56 (3), 1–25.

Carey, G., Riley, T., Cramming, B., 2012. The Australian government's 'social inclusion agenda': the intersection between public health and social policy. Crit. Public Health 22 (1), 47–59.

Carson, E., Kerr, L., 2014. Australian Social Policy and the Human Services. Cambridge University Press, Port Melbourne.

Coleborne, C., 1996. The 'scientific management' of the insane and the problem of 'difference' in the asylums in Victoria, 1870s–1880s. Aust. J. Vict. Stud. 2 (1), 126–137.

Council of Australian Governments (COAG), 2017. The fifth national mental health and suicide prevention plan. Commonwealth of Australia, Canberra.

Cummins, C.J., 2003. A history of medical administration in NSW 1788–1973. NSW Department of Health, North Sydney. Online. Available: https://www.health.nsw.gov.au/about/history/Publications/history-medical-admin.pdf.

Department of Health and Ageing, 2009a. Fourth national mental health plan – an agenda for collaborative government action in mental health 2009–2014. Commonwealth of Australia, Canberra.

Department of Health and Ageing, 2009b. National mental health policy 2008. Commonwealth of Australia, Canberra.

Department of Health and Ageing, 2013. National mental health report 2013: tracking progress of mental health reform in Australia 1993–2011. Commonwealth of Australia, Canberra.

Department of Parliamentary Services, 2019. Mental health in Australia: a quick guide. Parliament of Australia, Canberra.

Doran, C.M., Kinchin, I., 2019. A review of the economic impact of mental illness. Aust. Health Rev. 43 (1), 43–48. doi:org/10.1071/AH16115.

Dudgeon, P., Calma, T., Brideson, T., et al., 2016. The Gayaa Dhuwi (Proud Spirit) Declaration – a call to action for Aboriginal and Torres Strait Islander leadership in the Australian mental health system. Adv. Ment. Health 14 (2), 126–139.

Eaton, G., Williams, V., Wong, G., et al., 2019. Protocol for the impact of paramedics in NHS primary care: application of realist approaches to improve understanding and support intelligent policy and future workforce planning. Br. Paramed. J. 4 (3), 35–42.

Elliott, R., Brown, P., 2013. Exploring the developmental need for a paramedic pathway to mental health. J. Paramed. Pract. 5, 264–270.

Evashkevich, M., Fitzgerald, M., 2014. A Framework for Implementing Community Paramedic Programs in British Columbia. Ambulance Paramedics of British Columbia, Richmond, BC.

Fletcher, J., Pirkis, J., Kohn, F., et al., 2009. Australian primary mental health care: improving access and outcomes. Aust. J. Prim. Health 15 (3), 244–253.

Henderson, J., Fuller, J., 2011. 'Problematising' Australian policy representations in responses to the physical health of people with mental health disorders. Aust. J. Soc. Issues 46 (2), 183–203.

Henderson, J., Javanparst, S., Baum, F., et al., 2019. The governance of primary mental health planning by Primary Health Networks. Aust. J. Soc. Issues 54 (3), 267–284.

Hickie, I., Groom, G., 2002. Primary care-led mental health service reform: an outline of the Better Outcomes in Mental Health Care initiative. Australas. Psychiatry 10 (4), 376–382.

Hickie, I., McGorry, P., 2007. Increased access to evidence-based primary mental health care: will the implementation match the rhetoric? Med. J. Aust. 187 (2), 100–103.

Ilyas, A., Chesney, E., Patel, R., 2017. Improving life expectancy in people with serious mental illness: should we place more emphasis on primary prevention? Br. J. Psychiatry 211 (4), 194–197.

Lamb, H.R., Bachrach, L.L., 2001. Some perspectives on deinstitutionalization. Psychiatr. Serv. 52 (8), 1039–1045.

Levinson, D., Lakoma, M., Petukhova, M., et al., 2010. Associations of serious mental illness with earnings: results from the WHO World Mental Health surveys. Br. J. Psychiatry 197 (2), 114–121.

Lewis, M., Garton, S., 2017. Mental Health in Australia, 1788–2015: a history of responses to cultural and social challenges. In: Minas, H., Lewis, M. (Eds.), Mental Health in Asia and the Pacific. Springer, Boston, MA, pp. 289–313.

McDonald, J., Davies, G., Jayasuriya, R., et al., 2011. Collaboration across private and public sector primary health care services: benefits, costs and policy implications. J. Interprof. Care 25 (4), 258–264.

McGorry, P., 2007. The specialist youth mental health model: strengthening the weakest link in the public mental health system. Med. J. Aust. 187 (7), S53–S56.

Manwell, L.A., Barbic, S.P., Roberts, K., et al., 2015. What is mental health? Evidence towards a new definition from a mixed methods multidisciplinary international survey. BMJ Open 5 (6), e007079.

MIND, 2014. Mental health and the NDIS: a literature review. Online. Available: https://www.ndis.gov.au/html/sites/default/files/files/Mental-health-and-the-NDIS-Literature-Review.pdf. 16 May 2017.

National Mental Health Commission, 2018. Monitoring mental health and suicide prevention reform: Fifth national mental health and suicide prevention plan, 2018. National Mental Health Commission, Sydney.

National Mental Health Commission, 2019. Monitoring mental health and suicide prevention reform: national report 2019. NMHC, Sydney. Online. Available: www.mentalhealthcommission.gov.au. 17 February 2020.

Parsons, V., O'Brian, L., O'Meara, P., 2011. Mental health legislation: an era of change in paramedic clinical practice and responsibility. Int. Paramed. Pract. 1 (2), 9–16.

Patel, V., Saxena, S., Lund, C., et al., 2018. The Lancet Commission on global mental health and sustainable development. Lancet 392 (10157), 1553–1598.

Petrich, M., Ramamurthy, V.L., Hendrie, D., et al., 2013. Challenges and opportunities for integration in health systems: an Australian perspective. J. Integr. Care 1, 347–359.

Pirkis, J., Burgess, P., Hardy, J., et al., 2010. Who cares? A profile of people who care for relatives with mental disorder. Aust. N. Z. J. Psychiatry 44 (10), 929–937.

Productivity Commission, 2019. Mental health, draft report. Productivity Commission, Canberra. Online. Available: https://www.pc.gov.au/inquiries/current/mental-health#report. 17 February 2020.

Rehm, J., Shield, K.D., 2019. Global burden of disease and the impact of mental and addictive disorders. Curr. Psychiatry Rep. 21 (2), 10. doi:org/10.1007/s11920-019-0997-0.

RHealth, 2016. Mental Health Nurse Incentive. Online. Available: http://www.rhealth.com.au/page/Programs__Services/Services_for_Health/Mental_Health_Nurse_Incentive/. 15 November 2017.

Roberts, L., Henderson, J., 2009. Paramedic perceptions of their role, education, training and working relationships when attending cases of mental illness. J. Emerg. Prim. Heal. Care 7 (3).

Schofield, D., Cunich, M., Shrestha, R., et al., 2019. Indirect costs of depression and other mental and behavioural disorders for Australia from 2015 to 2030. BJPsych Open 5 (3), e40.

Shaban, R., 2005. Accounting for assessments of mental illness in paramedic practice: a new theoretical framework. J. Emerg. Prim. Heal. Care 3 (3).

Smith-Merry, J., Gillespie, J., 2016. Embodying policy-making in mental health: the implementation of partners in recovery. Health Sociol. Rev. 25 (2), 187–201.

Smith-Merry, J., Hancock, N., Gilroy, J., et al., 2018. Mind the Gap: The National Disability Insurance Scheme and psychosocial disability. The University of Sydney, Sydney.

Stoller, A., Arscott, K., 1955. Mental Health Facilities and Needs of Australia. Government Printing Office, Canberra.

Swan, P., Raphael, B., 1995. National Consultancy Report on Aboriginal and Torres Strait Islander mental health, part 1: 'ways forward'. National Mental Health Strategy. Australian Government Publishing Service, Canberra.

World Health Organization, 2013. Mental Health Action Plan 2013–2020. Online. Available: https://www.who.int/mental_health/publications/action_plan/en/. 17 February 2020.

Caring and person-centred mental healthcare: Stigma, discrimination and the role of culture

2

Breanna K. Jennings, Denise E. McGarry and Georgia Clarkson

LEARNING OUTCOMES

After reading this chapter and completing the associated activities, you should be able to:

- outline the concepts of person-centred care, stigma, discrimination, culture and recovery-oriented care
- explain how the concepts defined influence the provision of care by paramedics and others for those experiencing mental health problems
- apply, as a student or beginning paramedic, these understandings to the care of people experiencing mental health problems.

INTRODUCTION

The work of paramedics includes a significant amount of responses to people experiencing mental health concerns or crises. It also involves supporting people during distress that arises from the other health circumstances that have necessitated paramedic response. Additionally, paramedics are recognised as working in an environment that significantly jeopardises their own mental health (Courtney et al., 2013; New South Wales Ambulance, 2016; Parsons & O'Brien, 2011). Mental health presentations are often very different from other areas of paramedic practice as they can be highly ambiguous. Clear clinical decisions may not initially be readily apparent following assessment. This is a common feature for those working with people experiencing mental health problems. However, sound authentic communication that is person-centred represents the basis of all mental health interventions that produce positive outcomes.

For the person who is experiencing mental health problems that are so distressing as to trigger seeking help from paramedics, their experience can be very different from those reported by other people seeking the support of paramedics for non-mental health issues. It can be characterised by misunderstanding, ambivalence and suspicion on the side of all parties. Many health workers, including paramedics, have a series of stereotypes about mental illness that may at times be misplaced.

Historically, Western society has tended to be stigmatising about those who have lived experience of mental illness. These ideas are indiscriminate in their application to individuals, and emphasise differences in a way that rejects the person with mental health problems as being irreconcilably different. These differences are explained commonly as being unpredictable, dangerous, unsuccessful, isolated, unintelligent, incomprehensible and untreatable. This is reflected in the manner in which language referring to mental health problems often becomes pejorative. Examples of this usage include 'mad', 'insane' or 'schizo', which are used to insult. Other cultures also have beliefs about mental health problems that can be negative. In multicultural countries such as Australia and New Zealand, not only those experiencing mental health problems but also those supporting them may be impacted by a range of different preconceptions of the nature of mental health problems.

That fear is commonly a response to mental health distress is self-evident. This fear can often undermine the centrality of a person-centred approach to help. Other areas of paramedic practice and healthcare are characterised by procedural approaches that lend themselves to standardisation. However, when communication with those experiencing mental health distress may be negatively affected by fear, stigma and complexity, often resulting in time-consuming interventions, it is unsurprising that mental health call-outs may be unpopular with paramedics. Yet the response from paramedics can represent the first step of the journey towards recovery for the person in mental distress. Recovery (rarely meaning cure) in mental health contexts means a reworking of one's self-understanding to live a meaningful life with or without continuing mental health problems. The paramedic response is pivotal to this. This response relies on the capacity to communicate and support the person and their carers to maintain dignity and hope in the face of significant challenges to their autonomy. Legislative frameworks and common medical interventions emphasising the role of pharmaceuticals can be experienced as traumatising. Those who experience mental health problems and who seek help from mental health services include large numbers of people who have histories of complex trauma (Varese et al., 2012). It is critical that paramedic practice does not further traumatise people seeking help. These issues are explored in depth later in this text, but here their importance in the context of person-centred care, stigma, discrimination and the role of culture is acknowledged.

This chapter will explore these concepts in great detail. By developing the skill of self-reflection, professional critical reflection plus curiosity about mental health, your paramedic practice will positively influence recovery outcomes for those experiencing mental health problems. Self-reflection will also become a key skill that will be central to maintaining your own mental health in such a critical and challenging professional practice.

REFLECTION

- Consider the reasons you were attracted into paramedicine.
- Now reflect on the statistics provided in Chapter 1 on the mental-health-related workload. Did you realise just how much mental-health-related work there would be? How does this change the way you think about your future career?

- Consider your own personal understanding and beliefs on mental health, mental illness, culture, religion and sexuality. How will your personal beliefs influence the way you do your work? Are there any potential conflicts with your belief system that you might be faced with?
- Why is self-awareness of our own beliefs and responses as a paramedic important when interacting with the people we attend?

CASE STUDY

The following is an account of a lived experience of mental health crisis as told in the words of the carer. Carers (those who provide support and assistance to people with mental health problems) may or may not be a family member. In this account, Mary tells the story of an incident with her daughter. The account in her own words is termed the Lived Experience. This means it is free from a third party imposing a formation of the way in which the experience is relayed. However, it is true that the understandings of Mary's lived experience and that of her daughter are formed by the dominant social paradigms. Additionally, the lived experience of a carer is distinct from that of the person experiencing mental health problems.

Mary

What made this period of my life so confusing at the time is that there is no rule book or map for carers to follow. After our daughter's initial diagnosis we read the literature, watched the films, encountered other carers, but no two incidents will be the same. No matter how prepared I thought I was, in the middle of a crisis things become confusing and the mind numbs: it can often be so difficult to respond quickly, sensibly and appropriately. At the particular time I'm recalling, our daughter, then in her twenties, had already experienced quite a traumatic time in a mental hospital, so she would try any means to avoid another episode there. She wanted me to promise I would never send her there again, and yet the time arrived when her father and I could see that it was unavoidable as she was becoming unwell once more. Although she was compliant with medicine, it was not really effective and, mainly at night, she was tormented by hearing voices. She was complaining that even while in bed she could hear the neighbours, in their house across the road, talking about her (it made no difference me pointing out that our neighbours were Korean with no English at all); or it was police who were flashing lights into her bedroom; another time she claimed her brother was in danger from 'the man with the gun'.

Despite the above signs, there were times throughout the days when our daughter somehow pulled herself together, appearing rational for a while, seemingly defying us to say that anything was wrong. This made it the hardest time, trying to judge whether she was really in need of medical intervention or it was just a blip on her recovery path. Through all this, while we were watching her, she was watching us. She monitored us consistently to ensure we did not ring 000. My first attempt at alerting the police (as they had been involved when she was scheduled once before) had to be aborted. She guessed I was going to the police station, and burst into the interview room behind me, declaring that there was no problem.

In our home, conditions were escalating as we were woken at night with the sound of our daughter weeping in her shower. She would tear at her skin, saying she was ugly. I rang 000, and by the time an ambulance arrived she had dried and dressed herself, ordering me to send the ambulance away. The paramedics were confronted with the two of us at the front door, she insisting that I (her mother) had a heart problem and that she (the daughter) had no problem at all, just concern for her mother. Very conscious that it was about midnight, the whole street was in silence but the neighbours' houses were all around us, I could only think to repeat 'but, there's nothing wrong with me'. The older of the two paramedics kept requesting me to come and sit in the ambulance with him so he could 'check my blood pressure'. For a while I was confused – he had the wrong person! Then somehow I dimly realised the ploy to separate me from my daughter so they could really gauge the whole situation. While the other paramedic had my daughter engaged, I was able to spell out my concerns within the ambulance. When we emerged from the ambulance reporting that my blood pressure had been checked and, accepting my assurance that I was coming to the hospital, we were able to finally induce our daughter to come along too for a doctor to see us.

If it had not been for the paramedics' ability to sum up the situation at a glance and respond accordingly, our daughter would not have received the help she needed that night.

CRITICAL REFLECTION

Mary's account of this incident of support and understanding by paramedics relies on the expertise in the paramedics' ability to assess and identify relationship dynamics and observe interaction between people, and then communicate effectively. Consider the following aspects:

1. What observations and communication skills were employed by the paramedics that contributed to the successful outcome of transporting Mary's daughter for further assessment and care?
2. What stereotypes and prejudgements (by paramedics and societal norms) might have influenced the outcome for Mary and her daughter? Consider the story and where these stereotypes and preconceptions might have changed the outcome.
3. Mary had the perception that the paramedic 'summed up her situation at a glance'. What may have been the paramedic's process in reaching the conclusions that they did?

ETHICAL DILEMMA

In the above case study, Mary is the main carer and is obviously concerned for her daughter's wellbeing. While talking to Mary's daughter, she tells you a number of things about herself that sound delusional; furthermore, she advises you that she has not been taking her medication for several months, but she insists that you do not tell her mum or the doctor/hospital. Later, Mary asks you for detailed content of your discussion.

- Under what circumstances can you tell Mary details of the confidential conversation?
- Under what circumstances can you withhold information from Mary?
- Is there a difference between you disclosing information without the person's consent to a doctor, or to a carer? Discuss.

THE CONTEXT OF CARING AND DEFINING PERSON-CENTRED CARE

Consistent with all healthcare practice, current understandings of pre-hospital mental healthcare provision acknowledge that practice should be centred on the needs, preferences and circumstances of each individual. People accessing mental healthcare are entitled to a caring, safe, respectful and empowering experience, the same as those accessing healthcare for other reasons. This concept, commonly known as person-centred care (PCC – sometimes referred to as *patient*-centred care) is prioritised in healthcare policy and planning and legislation in Australia. Literature on how it can be implemented and its benefits are widely documented (Sommaruga et al., 2017).

> *'Provision of patient centred care is integral to quality care and used as a quality indicator by private and public healthcare organisations all over the world'*
>
> (Sommaruga et al., 2017, p. 974)

Although referring to the person on whom the episode of care is centred as 'the patient' is common in paramedic and broader healthcare practice, the term 'patient' has connotations that can disempower an individual, particularly in mental health contexts. As such, the term 'person-centred care' is adopted within the current discussion.

Historically in mental healthcare, people experiencing mental health issues were often viewed as being 'unfit' or legally 'incompetent' to be involved in the decision-making processes around their care (Szmukler et al., 2014). More-recent Australian mental healthcare legislation and policy prioritise the involvement and autonomy of the individual within mental health practice, regardless of their 'capacity' to make safe decisions regarding the care they receive or refuse. This necessitates the incorporation of person-centred mental healthcare within the pre-hospital setting, as even those who are found to be unfit or 'without the capacity' to refuse transport or treatment should still be given appropriate opportunity to be autonomous and be involved in decisions.

The provision of person-centred care in the pre-hospital setting can be challenging, as paramedics are faced with difficult circumstances, minimal resources and often only basic mental healthcare training. In order to provide care that is centred on the individual, paramedics must take the time to listen and understand from the perspective of the person, and allow this to guide the clinical decisions that need to be made.

An example of how person-centred care can be incorporated into the pre-hospital mental healthcare environment is in the case of a person who is considered to require compulsory transport to hospital from a legal perspective. This indicates that the person has been identified as high risk or unsafe to be left at a scene without appropriate support, however they are not consenting to transport (see Chapter 11 'Michael'). In this case, paramedics and perhaps police can collaboratively provide person-centred care, even though the person is required to accept transport against their will. The development of therapeutic rapport and the skilled use of communication skills is critically important in such a scenario. Listening to the concerns and preferences of the person being transported is critical within such a situation. Addressing such concerns while protecting the person's right to privacy, particularly from neighbours and bystanders, can improve the person's perception of the event. Effective use of these skills is critical to individualising the care experience and ensuring the situation is managed in an ethical, legal and positive manner.

Ways in which paramedics may individualise the person's experience may include encouraging the person to bring belongings that are familiar and provide comfort for them, explaining the processes and legislation honestly and carefully, or assisting the person to complete a task at home that may distract them if left incomplete. Such tasks could include feeding or securing a pet, locking the house or turning off the heater. Although these examples may seem simple, it is important to remember that person-centred care is based around the concerns and priorities of the person at the time, and achieving this can be simple. In the longer term, this approach reduces distress and can empower the individual, and should be prioritised over paramedic or operational priorities.

Understanding and empathising with a person who requires mental healthcare empowers the paramedic to act in a way that is centred on that person, and this has the potential to create an experience based on respect and dignity. Conversely, when a person feels they are unheard or not in control of their own healthcare, negative experiences for both the paramedic and the person can occur. Negative experiences impact on the likelihood that a person will call for help in the future, and potentially reduces their cooperation with care providers. These experiences can negatively affect their recovery. It is therefore imperative that as the first line of healthcare, paramedics provide a safe, person-centred experience.

There are many benefits to person-centred care in all healthcare presentations; however, it is particularly pertinent in a pre-hospital mental health crisis. According to Rathert and colleagues (2012) there is a positive correlation between person-centred care and individual outcomes for those seeking support. This study found that specific benefits of person-centred care include:

- improved personal satisfaction for individuals being cared for
- improved diagnostic accuracy
- enhanced cooperation and fewer incidences of hostility
- more-effective communication
- improved empowerment and trust for individuals
- decreased physical symptoms of anxiety, such as increased respiration and heart rate, allowing for a more accurate assessment
- willingness to access multiple healthcare providers, and improved chances of addressing health concerns.

In mental healthcare, particularly in the first line of care within the pre-hospital setting, it is imperative that the person is provided a safe, positive experience that is tailored to their needs. Person-centred care is a well-known concept in the hospital and medical setting, although it is new to the pre-hospital mental healthcare environment, where time and resources can be restricted. Person-centred care can be an enabler of better person–paramedic interactions, and certainly better personal outcomes. This approach can be adopted with simple changes to attitude and communication that give preference to the needs of individuals experiencing mental illness.

THE ROLE OF CULTURE: SOCIETAL AND PERSONAL FACTORS THAT INFLUENCE MENTAL HEALTH

Many factors affect a person's mental health and wellbeing across the life span. The biopsychosocial model has been the dominant modern paradigm in healthcare, and it reflects an understanding that health is a product of complex and highly individualised biological, psychological and social factors (Wade & Halligan, 2017). The societal factors that can affect a person's mental health include societal status and inequities, religion and community identity (Hussain, 2017). The range of factors that impact on an individual's health are complex and varied. Social determinants of health (WHO, 2017) have been discussed and researched among healthcare providers for many years; however, the practice of accommodating these factors is relatively new, particularly in mental healthcare. Social determinants such as a person's socio-economic status and cultural-linguistic status have a large impact on their understanding of mental health issues and their willingness or knowledge of how to access mental health services. Social inequities can also have an impact on understanding and access. These include gender, sexuality, education and geographical location.

The following are examples of how social inequities can impact on a person's ability and willingness to access mental health services.

ETHICAL DILEMMA

You are attending a person who is unemployed and lives in a low socio-economic area. You are concerned for their mental health and wellbeing, and you insist that they need to come to hospital. However, the person is refusing on the basis that they do not have ambulance insurance and will not be able to afford the ambulance bill. Your colleague thinks you should 'load and go' and let someone else worry about the details and cost later.

- How will you resolve this situation so that the person can still obtain the care they need?
- Does the person's socio-economic status influence how you approach the care provision for this patient? If so, how?

ETHICAL DILEMMA

You are attending a case where the original dispatch was due to chest pain, but after your initial assessment you think it is more likely non-cardiac and related to anxiety. The person you are assessing is transgender. In the past, their family has said that their gender belief and sexual orientation is a result of a mental illness. Subsequently, the person has been reluctant to attend hospital or see a psychiatrist. You would like to take the person to hospital for further cardiac medical tests, and hope that they can also see the mental health team.

- How will you resolve this situation so that the person can still obtain the care they need for both their physical and mental health?
- Does a person's gender/sexual identification affect how you engage and communicate with a patient? Would your communication and engagement differ in this case. If so, why?
- How would you explain the situation and your plan to the person's family?

In both of these situations it is essential that paramedics consider the individual and societal context of the person's situation. In doing this, a paramedic can provide care that is empathetic, person centred and effective, thereby contributing to a more positive experience.

Cultural factors are important in protecting a person from developing mental illness and assisting in their recovery. It is important that paramedics recognise, respect and respond to the individual cultural needs of people experiencing mental health problems in the community, and accommodate for cultural needs during all pre-hospital assessment and care processes. In doing so, it is imperative that a person is treated as an individual and that assumptions are not made about them on the basis of general understandings about a group they may belong to. For example, it may be assumed that someone from a specific ethnic background holds a specific set of religious beliefs. Where this is based on assumption and with little engagement or communication with them as an individual, a number of issues can arise.

When considering culture and mental health, it is important to consider both the individual and the societal factors in a person's life at the time care is required. Factors that contribute to a person's mental health include a knowledge of mental health and health literacy in general, including understanding of the services available to them and the skills they have to cope with challenges. These may have been acquired throughout life via previous experience, through observation of presentations of mental health problems and recovery in others, their attitude towards mental health, the attitude of the people who have an influence on them, and their beliefs surrounding mental health and health services. Other factors also include a person's personality, the way they naturally cope with feelings and emotions, and also their resilience, which is reliant on their previous experiences and support networks. Personal factors play a large role in a person's protection from, and also risk of developing, mental health issues. Importantly, personal factors also play a large role in a person's recovery, which is why each individual should be treated in a way that is tailored to them, with person-centred care. As a paramedic it is not possible to be aware of or understand all of the cultural beliefs and practices of the people you attend. Being sensitive to personal preferences and beliefs is a good starting point, however. This sensitivity, combined with good communications, can help foster a good therapeutic relationship.

Assessment of the personal, protective and risk factors that affect a person's mental health is a skill that all paramedics need to develop using observational and interpersonal communication skills. Although this can be very easy with people who are willing to share personal information and answer questions with care providers, it can be very difficult when dealing with people who do not wish to interact with others, including paramedics. Careful selection of questions and active listening on the part of the paramedic can assist in developing a strong understanding of a person's situation in a short amount of time. This must be put into the context of limitations related to commonly short interactions for gaining insight into the complexity of many people's situations.

CULTURAL SAFETY AND PROVIDING CULTURALLY AWARE MENTAL HEALTH CARE

Although the provision of culturally competent and safe mental healthcare in the pre-hospital setting can be challenging, it is central to the experience of the individual and process of recovery. Cultural safety may be defined as the act of providing a place or situation where a person's cultural needs are respected and acknowledged

(Australian Human Rights Commission, 2010). In the pre-hospital setting, the paramedic should quickly ascertain the cultural beliefs and requirements of a person, and adapt to their needs where possible. This is best done through communication and the involvement of the person using a collaborative approach. Putting the person at the centre of their care experience is critical. As such, while understandings of different cultural beliefs and practices can assist a paramedic here, this is only as a starting point. Developing a thorough understanding of them as an individual relies on communication.

Culture has impacts on illness, behaviour and experience (Ang, 2017); therefore, in the case of challenges to mental health, it can have an impact that is positive and protective or negative. Cultural variations affect the way in which people express their problems, such as the way in which they express frustration or cope with grief, and the likelihood of them complaining, reporting or seeking assistance for these problems. The recognition and response to mental health issues in different cultures will vary. This means it may be difficult in some cases for paramedics to ascertain the problem or experience of individuals. This is because they may be responding in ways paramedics are not familiar with due to their cultural beliefs. Using a collaborative approach between paramedics and carers or significant others can promote the development of a clearer understanding of the presenting issue. It can also assist to identify the desired outcome for an episode of care and make this consistent for both parties. For example, a person of one culture who is experiencing symptoms of depression and suicidal thoughts may not be able to verbalise this to paramedics in the presence of family members due to a cultural belief that suicide is wrong. In contrast, another person may be unable to discuss their symptoms at all with paramedics unless a senior family member is present. In both instances, a paramedic must recognise and respond to the cultural needs of the individual.

How might paramedics provide culturally safe care?

- LISTEN to what is important to the individual and their carers/significant others, and include them in a collaborative approach.
- OBSERVE cultural cues and practices.
- ADAPT to the situation and provide person-centred care, and negotiate guidelines and follow legislative requirements as required.
- COMMUNICATE when cultural needs cannot be met, and how you can accommodate them in other ways.
- DOCUMENT AND HAND OVER cultural preferences and requirements clearly and accurately when arriving at hospital to ensure continuity of care.
- DON'T assume a person's culture or cultural needs or dismiss the cultural needs of people, as this can lead to negative experiences and outcomes.

STEREOTYPES, STIGMA AND DISCRIMINATION

In the past a range of views of people with mental health issues impacted on people's interaction with them. Whether the interaction took place in general social contexts or in active assessment, intervention and support episodes, a number of underlying beliefs influenced these experiences. Such beliefs included understandings that presentations were produced by supernatural forces, views that people were unable to recover, beliefs that people were inherently dangerous, and fears that experiences were contagious, self-induced or inauthentic. For example, in Middle Ages England it was not uncommon for women presenting with mental health issues to be labelled as 'witches'. Such people were often segregated and cruelly punished, tortured or executed. Cultural beliefs that mental health problems are related to witchcraft exist in some cultures even today (Ofori-Atta et al., 2010).

These underlying beliefs have influenced the policy and practice framework around management of mental health problems. For example, prior to the widespread acceptance of recovery frameworks, people presenting with mental health issues tended to be isolated from others. Such isolation was facilitated by means of separate mental health 'systems' and also segregation from other people. Historically, there was a greater propensity to use more aggressive or invasive procedures such as restraint, insulin therapy and even lobotomy. Not only were such practices limited in their effectiveness, they reinforced existing beliefs and misunderstandings. Isolation also compounded some of the issues of social disconnection that commonly contributes to mental health problems (Green et al., 2018).

Historically, these myths and misconceptions have been informed by negative stereotypes of people with mental health issues. Stereotypes can be defined as widely held but fixed and oversimplified images or ideas of a particular type of person or thing. Whether stereotypes are positive or negative in nature, they tend to overgeneralise. As such, they can work against an individualised 'person-centred' approach to providing care and support. This can present challenges for paramedics who are often limited in the information they have about a person to whom they are attending. In these situations, it is not uncommon to 'default' to stereotypes as a way of trying to make sense of a situation. While this can provide some direction as a starting point, it is critical to ensure that a person-centred approach is taken to respond to the unique needs of the individual. Communication skills are critical to ascertaining these needs.

In addition to tending to oversimplify care, where a stereotype takes on a negative connotation it almost invariably has a negative consequence. This is known as stigmatisation. While some may define a stigma as essentially a negative stereotype, there is more complexity to the process of stigmatisation. It involves a societal construct of what is different and not fitting in the social norm and how that is applied to the 'other'. This can potentially be as a mark of disgrace associated with a particular circumstance, quality or person. Negative stereotypes can have an impact on intellectual function, stress levels and tension between people (Steele, 2010). Stigmatisation devalues people who have attributes seen as inferior or unacceptable, the impacts of which include reduced social status and discrimination (Willis & Elmer, 2011). This impact is often amplified by the fact that such stigmatised people often anticipate stigma and can experience feelings of anxiety as a result (Quinn & Earnshaw, 2013).

There are different types of stigma associated with mental illness (Beyond Blue 2015:2) including:

- Personal stigma – a person's stigmatising attitudes and beliefs about other people ('People with depression should snap out of it')
- Perceived stigma – a person's beliefs about the negative and stigmatising views that other people hold ('Most people believe that a person with depression should snap out of it')
- Self-stigma – the stigmatising views that individuals hold about themselves ('I should be able to snap out of my depression')
- Structural stigma – the policies of private and governmental institutions and cultural norms that restrict the opportunities of people with depression and anxiety ('Mental health services and research don't deserve as much funding as other health problems').

Choice plays a part in an individual's decision to disclose an 'invisible' attribute which may be stigmatised (Quinn & Earnshaw, 2013). As people who are stigmatised often encounter discrimination, it follows that people with mental health issues can be reluctant to disclose their experiences to others. This can be particularly challenging for people with mental health problems as they may perceive that the potential benefits of seeking support may be outweighed by the anticipated costs in the form of discrimination. For paramedics, who are often the first source of assistance for these individuals, this means initial interactions are acutely important. Any interaction seen as discriminatory by the individual seeking support has the potential to impact negatively on their disclosure and consequently their interaction with those in a position to support them. It is important to recognise that an individual will also commonly 'self-stigmatise' and already hold negative views of mental health issues (Corrigan, 2004; Davidson et al., 2011). This self-stigmatisation may mean that they are reluctant to seek support as they anticipate stigma (Quinn & Earnshaw, 2013). This means that the interaction with paramedics is critical as negative experiences at an early point of disclosure can influence the degree to which an individual is prepared to continue to engage with sources of support.

When considering the concept of discrimination, it is important to be aware of the forms this may take. In recent times, understandings of discrimination have evolved. In this time it has become increasingly understood that discrimination is not limited to more overt and direct forms. More commonly, in societies with legislative and social mechanisms in place to counter discriminatory practices, they tend to be subtle and less tangible. Some have referred to these discriminatory acts as 'microaggressions' (Sue, 2010). The fact that these microaggressions are less tangible makes them difficult to identify or 'call out'. In fact, a person may even be unaware of the way in which their behaviour is being interpreted and perceived by another as subtly negative or discriminatory. This is because inequalities are often invisible, especially to those who are advantaged by them (Acker, 2011). Further to this, indirect discrimination may be a product of a number of socio-legal structures (Corrigan, 2004) that restrict opportunities for those with mental illness. A good example of this is refusing to sell an insurance policy to someone with a mental illness.

The significance of this for paramedics is that they must maintain an acute awareness of how their attitudes and beliefs may play out in interactions with people experiencing mental health issues. Increased awareness of mental health issues has been a product of contemporary public education programs. While there is increased awareness, it is still debatable as to whether the underlying issues of inequity for those experiencing mental illness have been addressed and whether support has improved. Although debate exists, some would assert that contemporary understandings of mental health issues means that there tends to be less negativity than in the past. Regardless of this, individual paramedics may hold negative attitudes and beliefs. In these situations it is critical that these are not projected onto the episode of care. Although this applies to all people a paramedic may attend to, it is of particular significance in the context of a person with mental health issues. As with all people, construction of identity is a continuous process involving ongoing renegotiation (Willis & Elmer, 2011). Negative interactions with paramedics at an acute stage may mean that people integrate negative understandings of mental health issues into their identity. This can compound issues and inhibit recovery as such internalised stigma has been positively associated with symptom severity, and negatively associated with treatment adherence (Livingston & Boyd, 2010). When a person feels valued, has their differences respected and needs met, they are more likely to live with dignity (Keleher & MacDougall, 2011) and have a better chance of recovery.

These understandings have informed a range of public health measures to increase awareness and combat stereotypes. The trend towards de-institutionalisation has also correlated with trends towards least restrictive practices, which are minimally invasive and protect the human rights of people with mental health issues. Furthermore, public awareness campaigns have become more common in Australian society. Overall, both these education programs and inclusivity leading to contact with people with mental health issues have had positive effects on reducing stigma (Corrigan et al., 2012).

These shifts in understandings of mental health issues, their causes and management, combined with knowledge of some of the subtleties of stigma and discrimination, have underpinned changes in the culture and practice associated with supporting people experiencing mental health issues. This is evident in the discourse within the field of practice and legislative and policy instruments governing the area. Recent drives to refer to people in this category as 'consumers' have been met with mixed reactions. Although these terms are better aligned to recovery approaches of mental health, the terminology is still contentious and a matter of continued discussion in the field. Currently there has been a move to the term 'those with lived experience' to engender a sense that those who live with mental health problems are best positioned to explain and collaborate in their own care. The tendency for paramedics to refer to all of those they attend to as 'patients' can compound this issue in the context of the discipline. Although the term 'consumer' remains contentious, the label 'patient' can infer disempowerment, which, within the mental health context, does not put the individual at the centre of their care. This can therefore add to a discourse that does not promote recovery (Russo et al., 2018).

THE RECOVERY MODEL AND HOW IT APPLIES TO PRE-HOSPITAL CARE

Previous understandings of mental health issues tended to be premised on the belief that people would be unable to recover from mental illness and therefore unlikely to fully participate in society. The Recovery Model, however, directly challenges this premise.

What we now know as the Recovery Model developed from a range of different sources that were critical of mental health services as they existed. These critiques did not arise in a vacuum; rather, they were influenced by a range of contemporary forces. The groundwork for these changes could be argued to have arisen in part from the development of a range of psychotropic medications through the 1940s and 1950s and their introduction into widespread use. This saw a marked reduction in the average length of stay experienced by those admitted as inpatients to hospital, and increased capacity for people to stay in their own homes while receiving treatment (Caton & Gralnick, 1987; Johnstone & Zolese, 2000; Stein & Test, 1980).

Coinciding with these developments was an increased interest in mental health matters and treatment, in part due to the large numbers of US military servicemen who returned from both World War I, and especially World War II, with emotional and psychological damage. This created a greater visibility of mental health issues and a pressure that pre-existing mental health services adapt to be able to meet these needs.

The antecedents for the development of the human rights movement of the 1960s and 1970s were numerous. A range of previously marginalised groups in Western societies sought redress and greater opportunities to participate in society on terms inclusive of their values. Leading groups in these movements, often operating under the banner of liberation, included African American groups in the USA and women's liberation movements. Groups of people with physical disabilities, perhaps because of the visibility of returned military servicemen, had significant recognition of their rights. Provisions of physical accommodation for their needs were legislated, along with a range of anti-discrimination legislation around the Western world. Examples include Australia's Racial Discrimination Act 1975, the UK Disability Discrimination Act 1995 and New Zealand's Human Rights Act 1993.

The United Nations (UN) took a role in developing a range of human rights statements that were ratified by member nations through adoption by government into policy and law. Of significance in the history of the Recovery Model was the Convention on the Rights of Persons with Disabilities (CRPD) negotiated from

2002 to 2006. This enshrined a range of principles with relevance to mental health with synergy to the Recovery Model. This includes the protection of human rights and dignity, and the guarantee of full equality under law. All people are to be regarded as full and equal members of society (United Nations, 2007).

The developments known as the 'Anti-psychiatry Movement' particularly focused on the abuses of psychiatric treatments. Although displaying fresh impetus in the 1960s, it had existed in varying forms at least for two centuries prior. Indeed, the Quakers in the eighteenth and nineteenth centuries are credited with developing models for supporting people with mental health problems that preferenced total holistic frameworks emphasising dignity and purpose. This approach, known as 'Moral Treatment' had association with Phillipe Pinel in France, and William Tuke at the York Retreat (Charland, 2007). This was in contrast to some contemporaneous approaches that employed punitive models of workhouses. These 'asylums', employing models of 'moral treatment', were widely adopted. This was especially so in the USA, where Quaker influence through migration was strong.

Over time, the asylums had become oppressive and lost this philosophy of supporting dignity and purpose in life. The interest of the medical community in the problems of people experiencing mental illness arose in the mid-nineteenth and early twentieth centuries, building on the success the medical model had demonstrated in relieving the suffering of people with various physical health problems. The promise of this approach in the field of mental health, however, fell short of many of the expectations. The medical model of treatment for mental illness was also recognised as having the potential to mistreat those experiencing mental health problems.

The Anti-psychiatry Movement arising in the 1960s argued that the root of the abuse of those experiencing mental health problems turned on inequities in power. Socio-political analyses such as those of Foucault emphasised the way in which these inequities achieved social order and protected the interests of those who currently held power (Foucault, 2006). Other theorists questioned the veracity of regarding mental health experiences as invalid or pathological expressions of human experience (Szasz, 1960). Some argued that such phenomenon was intelligible when put in the context of social power distribution (Cooper, 2013). In this context, the range of options for the powerless and oppressed is narrow, and in times of abuse may make certain behavioural manifestations comprehensible or indeed adaptive. The symptoms of dissociation witnessed among people exposed to traumatising events are an example of this.

Other theorists of significance in the Psychiatric Survivor's movement included those who explored the impact of stigma arising from false stereotypes that served to marginalise those experiencing mental health problems. Goffman conceptualised this in terms of the other being regarded as 'spoilt' (Goffman, 1963). The persistence and transmission of such misconceptions was examined by other theorists and suggested the powerful impact of cultural understandings perpetuated within cultural artefacts such as media and indeed language itself (Link et al., 2017; Rodwell et al., 2017; Sampogna et al., 2017). Scheff (1971) applied the tenets of labelling theory to mental health and argued that as society tends to label people who exhibit some incomprehensible experiences and behaviours as 'mentally ill', those referred to in this way will, over time, tend to adopt these behaviours and characteristics.

Recovery principles emerged from this multitude of influences. It has been consolidated into a set of principles or a movement in the writing of various people with a lived experience of mental health problems, and adopted by governments as policy (Anthony, 1993; Australian College of Mental Health Nurses Inc, 2013; Australian Government Department of Health, 2010, 2013; Australian Health Ministers' Advisory Council and National Mental Health Strategy, 2013; Davidson et al., 2011; Deegan, 1988, 1996, 2014; Jacob et al., 2017; Macpherson et al., 2016; Mental Health Coordinating Council, 2013).

The central tenet of recovery is the observation that for many people the experience of mental health problems differs in many aspects from that of physical ill-health. Essentially, clear understanding of causation that indicates a sure course of treatment resulting in a cure is uncommon. The aetiology of mental health problems is elusive. Biomarkers that confirm the presence of a pathological process have not been identified. Diagnoses are based on symptoms and are contentious. Experiences are common across different diagnoses.

Recovery principles recognise this and articulate the significant difference between clinical recovery and personal recovery (Corrigan, 2004). Clinical recovery is conceptualised as conforming to recovery as understood in some acute physical health paradigms. Recovery in this context is the resolution of symptoms – effectively a cure. This is an uncommon experience for those experiencing mental health problems. Rather, mental health problems are more often experienced as having periods of remission. Reoccurrence of mental health problems with their associated manifestations or symptoms, such as unusual beliefs (delusions) or perceptions (hallucinations), may happen at different periods in a person's life, often at periods of stress. Hence what is often referred to as a 'journey' is recognised as highly individual and defying the surety of a standardised notion of the 'progression of the disease'.

The notion of 'Personal Recovery' encompasses this (Corrigan et al., 2011). The unique accommodation to the individual's experience of mental health problems is central. However Personal Recovery is more than this. It recognises that people comprise many more elements than the mental health experience alone. It is person centred and holistic, and seeks an appreciation of the strengths of each person instead of focusing on the deficits or difficulties an individual experiences. Even with ongoing mental health problems, recovery principles assert that all people desire and find value in a 'contributing life', and that this can exist with or without continuing mental health symptoms or problems. A person remains a friend, a parent, an artist even when experiencing mental health problems (Australian Government Mental Health Commission, 2012).

The Australian Government formulated these understandings into a formal policy document: 'A national framework for recovery-oriented mental health services: guide for practitioners and providers' (Australian Health Ministers' Advisory

Council and National Mental Health Strategy, 2013). This policy obligates all those who work with people experiencing mental health problems to adopt this set of guidelines to their practice.

All people employed in health services, regardless of their role, profession, discipline, seniority or degree of contact with consumers, will use the framework to guide their recovery-orientated practice and service delivery. This includes practitioners, leaders, volunteers and people in administrative, policy development, research, program and service planning and decision-making positions (Australian Health Ministers' Advisory Council and National Mental Health Strategy, 2013, p. 1).

This policy embeds a critical tenet of the recovery approach – collaboration. It was the result of genuine collaboration between state, territory and national government, professions and those who have 'lived experience of mental health' problems, their families, loved ones and carers.

The Guidelines (Australian Health Ministers' Advisory Council and National Mental Health Strategy, 2013) offer a number of features (domains) that characterise practice that is recovery orientated. The principle domain, and the one that provides the underlying framework for the entire document, is Domain 1: Promoting a Culture and Language of Hope and Optimism (Australian Health Ministers' Advisory Council and National Mental Health Strategy, 2013, p. 12). This encompasses the other four domains:

1. Person first and holistic
2. Supporting personal recovery
3. Organisational commitment and workforce development
4. Action on social inclusion and the social determinants of health, mental health and wellbeing.

Clearly, however, there are many challenges to implementing such practice guidelines in the field, especially in pre-hospital environments when people may be experiencing extreme distress and disorganisation. The requirement that healthcare workers like paramedics balance a range of other service and practice imperatives is recognised. These might include minimising risk, the maintenance of safety, and the efficient delivery of services. The Guidelines (p. 11) nominate the following as representing particular challenges:

1. the offering of choice
2. support of risk taking
3. the dignity of risk
4. medico-legal requirements
5. duty of care
6. promoting safety.

As Slade (2009, pp. 176–179) has argued clearly, the capacity to balance risk in a complex and changing environment that may regard risk as unacceptable to services is difficult to reconcile.

CONCLUSION

This chapter has explored the concept of person-centred care and its interaction with culture, stereotypes, stigma and discrimination. Exploration of the Recovery Model of mental health has highlighted the relationship between the care experience and promotion of recovery. All healthcare workers, including paramedics, have a critical role to play in promoting recovery. As a paramedic may enter into interactions with an individual at a critical point in time, a respectful and individualised approach is essential.

LINKS AND RESOURCES

Trauma-informed care and practice – Blue Knot

- Blue Knot Foundation's Practice Guidelines for Treatment of Complex Trauma and Trauma Informed Care and Service Delivery provide a summary of the understanding of trauma from research of the past two decades. These guidelines address the needs of the large numbers of people with unresolved 'complex trauma' – child abuse in all its forms, neglect, family and community violence and other adverse childhood events. The guidelines argue that optimism for recovery from complex trauma is justified, and that childhood trauma can be resolved. Paramedic practice can play a significant role by being informed by the insights available from these.
https://www.blueknot.org.au/ABOUT-US/Our-Documents/Publications/Practice-Guidelines

Standards for practice – Australian National Practice Standards for the Mental Health Workforce 2013

- These standards outline the capabilities that are expected to be achieved by all mental health professionals in their work. These complement discipline-specific practice. http://www.health.gov.au/internet/main/publishing.nsf/content/mental-pubs-n-wkstd13

Recovery-oriented language guide

- The NSW Mental Health Coordinating Council (MHCC) has published a Recovery Oriented Language Guide. This Guide helps to challenge common ways of speech, and suggests alternatives in order to support recovery orientation and hope. http://www.mhcc.org.au/resource/recovery-oriented-language-guide-2nd-ed/

Pat Deegan

- Dr Patricia E Deegan is a seminal figure in the recovery movement worldwide. She has published extensively and remains an activist in the field, drawing from her own lived experience. In this recording, Dr Deegan recounts some of her critical insights into the importance of the recovery movement, drawing on her lived experience of a diagnosis of schizophrenia. She is an Adjunct Professor at Dartmouth College School of Medicine and Boston University, Sargent College of Health and Rehabilitation Services. https://www.youtube.com/watch?v=yawlKbOvHHo

Eleanor Longden

- In her TED talk, Eleanor Longden recounts eloquently her lived experience of hearing voices, which started when she was a university student. She describes the challenges she encountered and the strategies that she found supportive to her recovery. https://www.youtube.com/watch?v=syjEN3peCJw

Fay Jackson

- Fay Jackson was a deputy commissioner with the NSW Mental Health Commission when this item was recorded in 2017. She held this position as a person with a diagnosis of bipolar schizoaffective disorder, and fulfilled the responsibilities of highlighting stigma and the real possibility of recovery. This recording clearly elucidates the multiple challenges experienced by a person experiencing mental health problems.
- Watch: ABC News: *One Plus One: Fay Jackson* http://www.abc.net.au/news/2017-04-06/one-plus-one:-fay-jackson/8422958

Convention on the Rights of Persons with Disabilities (CRPD)

- The Convention follows decades of work by the United Nations to change attitudes and approaches to persons with disabilities. The Convention was negotiated during eight sessions of an Ad Hoc Committee of the General Assembly from 2002 to 2006, making it the fastest negotiated human rights treaty. https://www.un.org/development/desa/disabilities/convention-on-the-rights-of-persons-with-disabilities.html

A contributing life: the 2012 national report card on mental health and suicide prevention

- This first report card casts an independent eye over how Australia as a nation supports the estimated 3.2 million Australians each year who live with a mental health difficulty, their families and support people, and how we provide and coordinate the services they need. http://www.mentalhealthcommission.gov.au/our-reports/our-national-report-cards/2012-report-card.aspx
- The videos from this document, which include stories of lived experience and recovery from consumers and carers, can be found at: https://www.youtube.com/user/ausmentalhealth

---

GLOSSARY

carer A **carer** is someone who voluntarily provides ongoing **care** and assistance to another person who, because of **mental health** issues or **psychiatric** disability, requires support with everyday tasks. (Queensland Government Health https://www.qld.gov.au/health/mental-health/carers)

clinical recovery Synonymous with cure, it refers to the resolution of those mental health problems and experiences regarded diagnostically as symptoms, such as auditory hallucinations (voices), and resumption of the life led prior to these experiences.

consumer This term is used to refer to those receiving mental health services (in the UK known as **service users**). This term was adopted to empower people experiencing mental health problems and support their agency in terms of their treatment by mental health services. Adopted widely in government policy, the term is rejected by many with a lived experience as misrepresenting their lived experience of disempowerment.

lived experience The term **lived experience** is used to describe the first-hand accounts and impressions of living as a member of a minority or oppressed group. In the field of mental health, this refers to people's accounts of their own mental health problems and knowledge of treatments, interventions and consequences of this. Increasingly, the experience of living with mental health problems is regarded as a source of particular expertise. The phrase **Lived Experience Expert** incorporates this recognition of unique insights unavailable to those without this experience.

personal recovery This refers to an individual's journey to a self-reconciliation with the challenges and features of mental health problems and incorporation into an individual's new self-image. This does not require the resolution of the mental health problems, but rather reaching an accommodation with these problems such that the person's life is not defined by these problems alone. Frequently this also will mean that the person achieves means by which to have a life that incorporates contribution – **a contributing life.**

recovery Rarely meaning cure – in mental health contexts means a reworking of one's self-understanding to live a meaningful life with or without continuing mental health problems.

REFERENCES

Acker, J., 2011. Theorizing gender, race and class in organizations. In: Jeanes, E.L., Knights, D., Martin, P.Y. (Eds.), Handbook of Gender, Work, and Organization. Wiley, West Sussex, pp. 65–80.

Ang, W., 2017. Bridging culture and psychopathology in mental health care. Eur. Child Adolesc. Psychiatry 26 (2), 263–266.

Anthony, W., 1993. Recovery from mental illness: the guiding vision of the mental health service system in the 1990s. Psychosoc. Rehabil. J. 16 (4).

Australian College of Mental Health Nurses Inc, 2013. Scope of practice of mental health nurses in Australia, standards. Online. Available: http://www.acmhn.org/career-resources/workforce-standards. 28 June 2018.

Australian Government Department of Health, 2010. National standards for mental health services. Online. Available: http://www.health.gov.au/internet/publications/publishing.nsf/Content/mental-pubs-n-servst10-toc. 8 June 2018.

Australian Government Department of Health, 2013. National practice standards for the mental health workforce. Online. Available: http://www.health.gov.au/internet/publications/publishing.nsf/Content/mental-pubs-n-wkstd13-toc. 28 June 2018.

Australian Government Mental Health Commission, 2012. A Contributing Life: The 2012 national report card on mental health and suicide prevention. Online. Available: http://www.mentalhealthcommission.gov.au/our-reports/our-national-report-cards/2012-report-card.aspx. 28 June 2018.

Australian Health Ministers' Advisory Council and National Mental Health Strategy, 2013. National framework for recovery-oriented mental health services: guide for practitioners and providers. Online. Available: http://www.health.gov.au/internet/publications/publishing.nsf/Content/mental-pubs-n-recovgde-toc. 28 June 18.

Australian Human Rights Commission, 2010. Social Justice Report 2010. Online. Available: https://www.humanrights.gov.au/our-work/aboriginal-and-torres-strait-islander-social-justice/publications/social-justice-report-1. 13 July 2018.

Beyond Blue, 2015. *beyondblue* Information Paper: Stigma and discrimination associated with depression and anxiety. Online. Available: https://www.beyondblue.org.au/docs/default-source/policy-submissions/stigma-and-discrimination-associated-with-depression-and-anxiety.pdf. 11 November 2019.

Caton, C., Gralnick, A., 1987. A review of issues surrounding length of psychiatric hospitalization. Psychiatr. Serv. 38, 858–863.

Charland, L., 2007. Benevolent theory: moral treatment at the York Retreat. Hist. Psychiat. 18, 61–80.

Cooper, D., 2013. Psychiatry and Anti-Psychiatry. Routledge, London.

Corrigan, P., 2004. How stigma interferes with mental health care. Am. Psychol. 59, 614.

Corrigan, P., Roe, D., Tsang, H., 2011. Challenging the Stigma of Mental Illness: Lessons for Therapists and Advocates. Wiley-Blackwell, Sussex.

Corrigan, P., Morris, S., Michaels, P., et al., 2012. Challenging the public stigma of mental illness: a meta-analysis of outcome studies. Psychiatr. Serv. 63 (10), 963–973.

Courtney, J., Francis, A., Paxton, S., 2013. Caring for the country: fatigue, sleep and mental health in Australian rural paramedic shiftworkers. Community Health (Bristol) 3 (1), 178–186.

Davidson, L., Rakfeldt, J., Strauss, J., 2011. The Roots of the Recovery Movement in Psychiatry: Lessons learned. Wiley-Blackwell, Hobeken.

Deegan, P., 1988. Recovery: the lived experience of rehabilitation. Psychosoc. Rehabil. J. 11, 11–18.

Deegan, P., 1996. Recovery and the conspiracy of hope. The Sixth Annual Mental Health Services Conference of Australia and New Zealand. Brisbane.

Deegan, P., 2014. Commentary: shared decision making must be adopted, not adapted. Psychiatr. Serv. 65 (12), 1487.

Foucault, M., 2006. History of Madness. Routledge, Abingdon.

Goffman, E., 1963. Stigma: Notes on the management of spoiled identity. Prentice-Hall, New Jersey.

Green, M., Horan, W., Lee, J., et al., 2018. Social disconnection in schizophrenia and the general community. Schizophr. Bull. 44 (2), 242–249.

Hussain, M., 2017. Protective and risk socio-economic – environmental factors affecting mental health. Eur. Psychiatry 41, S572.

Jacob, S., Munro, I., Taylor, B., et al., 2017. Mental health recovery: a review of the peer-reviewed published literature. Collegian 24 (1), 53–61.

Johnstone, P., Zolese, G., 2000. Length of hospitalisation for people with severe mental illness. Cochrane Database Syst. Rev. (2), CD000384.

Keleher, H., MacDougall, C., 2011. Understanding Health, third ed. Oxford University Press, South Melbourne.

Link, B., Phelan, J., Sullivan, G., 2017. Mental and physical health consequences of the stigma associated with mental illnesses. In: Major, B., Dovidio, J., Link, B. (Eds.), The Oxford Handbook of Stigma, Discrimination, and Health. Oxford University Press, Oxford.

Livingston, J., Boyd, J., 2010. Correlates and consequences of internalized stigma for people living with mental illness: a systematic review and meta-analysis. Soc. Sci. Med. 71 (12), 2150–2161.

Macpherson, R., Pesola, F., Leamy, M., et al., 2016. The relationship between clinical and recovery dimensions of outcome in mental health. Schizophr. Res. 175, 142–147.

Mental Health Coordinating Council (MHCC), 2013. Trauma Informed Care and Practice: Towards a cultural shift in policy reform across mental health and human services in Australia, a national strategic direction, position paper and recommendations of the National Trauma – Informed Care and Practice Advisory Working Group. Mental Health Coordinating Council, Sydney.

New South Wales Ambulance, 2016. NSW Ambulance Year in Review 2015/16. Online. Available: http://www.ambulance.nsw.gov.au/Media/docs/Year%20in%20Review%20 2015-2016-a3ac8fbd-c795-4576-a363-6bd41448d811-0.pdf. 13 July 2018.

Ofori-Atta, A., Cooper, S., Akpalu, B., et al. The MHaPP Research Programme Consortium, 2010. Common understandings of women's mental illness in Ghana: results from a qualitative study. Int. Rev. Psychiatry 22 (6), 589–598.

Parsons, V., O'Brien, L., 2011. Paramedic clinical decision-making in mental health care: a new theoretical approach. J. Paramed. Pract. 3 (10), 572–579.

Quinn, D., Earnshaw, V., 2013. Concealable stigmatized identities and psychological well-being. Soc. Personal. Psychol. Compass 7 (1), 40–51.

Rathert, C., Wyrwich, D., Boren, S., 2012. Patient-centered care and outcomes: a systematic review of the literature. Med. Care Res. Rev. 70 (4), 351–379.

Rodwell, J., Cole, J., Grogan, S., 2017. Language and labelling used by university students when discussing mental health. Br. J. Sch. Nurs. 12 (8), 380–385.

Russo, J., Beresford, P., O'Hagan, M., 2018. Commentary on: Happell, B., Scholz, B., Doing what we can, but knowing our place: being an ally to promote consumer leadership in mental health. Int. J. Ment. Health Nurs. doi:10.1111/inm.12520.

Sampogna, G., Bakolis, I., Evans-Lacko, S., et al., 2017. The impact of social marketing campaigns on reducing mental health stigma: results from the 2009–2014 Time to Change programme. Eur. Psychiatry 40, 116–122.

Scheff, T., 1971. Being Mentally Ill: A sociological theory. Transaction Publishers, Chicago.

Slade, M., 2009. Personal Recovery and Mental Illness: A guide for mental health professionals. Cambridge University Press, Cambridge.

Sommaruga, M., Casu, G., Giaquinto, F., et al., 2017. Self-perceived provision of patient centered care by healthcare professionals: the role of emotional intelligence and general self-efficacy. Patient Educ. Couns. 100 (5), 974–980.

Steele, C., 2010. Whistling Vivaldi And Other Clues to How Stereotypes Affect Us. WW Norton, New York.

Stein, L., Test, M., 1980. Alternative to mental hospital treatment. Arch. Gen. Psychiatry 37 (4), 392–397.

Sue, D., 2010. Microaggressions in Everyday Life. Wiley, Hoboken.

Szasz, T., 1960. The myth of mental illness. Am. Psychol. 15 (2), 113–118.

Szmukler, G., Daw, R., Callard, F., 2014. Mental health law and the UN Convention on the Rights of Persons with Disabilities. Int. J. Law Psychiatry 37, 245–252.

United Nations, 2007. UN General Assembly, Convention on the Rights of Persons with Disabilities: resolution / adopted by the General Assembly, 24 January 2007, A/RES/ 61/106. Online. Available: http://www.refworld.org/docid/45f973632.html. 3 October 2018.

Varese, F., Smeets, F., Drukker, M., et al., 2012. Childhood adversities increase the risk of psychosis: a meta-analysis of patient-control, prospective-and cross-sectional cohort studies. Schizophr. Bull. 38 (4), 661–671.

Wade, D., Halligan, D., 2017. The biopsychosocial model of illness: a model whose time has come. Clin. Rehabil. 31 (8), 995–1004.

Willis, K., Elmer, S., 2011. Society, Culture and Health, second ed. Oxford University Press, South Melbourne.

World Health Organization (WHO), 2017. Social Determinants of Health. Online. Available: http://apps.who.int/iris/bitstream/handle/10665/206363/B3357.pdf?sequence=1&isAllowed=y. 13 July 2018.

Communication and the therapeutic relationship

3

Jade Sheen

'The single biggest problem in communication is the illusion that it has taken place.'
George Bernard Shaw

LEARNING OUTCOMES

This chapter will assist the paramedic to:

- understand the key principles of the therapeutic relationship and of effective patient communication
- understand the early indicators of aggression and escalation
- detail the principles of verbal de-escalation
- discuss the role of reflection in paramedic practice.

INTRODUCTION

The Australian Safety and Quality Framework for Health Care (ASQFHC, 2010) identifies person-centred care as the first of three dimensions required for a safe and high-quality health system in Australia. Person-centred care in this context relies on three pillars: care that is easy for patients to get when they need it; making sure that healthcare staff respect and respond to patient choices, needs and values; and forming partnerships between patients, their family, carers and healthcare providers. It is argued that all three pillars of person-centred care rely on respectful and effective communication between a healthcare provider and their patient.

Person-centred care describes a standard of care delivery that ensures that the patient and their family are at the centre of care delivery (Kornhaber et al., 2016). Person-centred care also represents a shift from patient to person, from disease to illness (Finset, 2010). Practically, this means that clinical decisions are made with the unique needs of the individual person and their support system in mind. It also suggests that we allow time to communicate openly with the person and to listen to their concerns, needs and hopes for treatment. In this context, communication is defined as the sending of information from one person or place to another.

As a healthcare professional, your communication with your patients will typically rely on a combination of verbal, non-verbal and paraverbal cues (Ranjan et al., 2015) and, in some instances, written information. Verbal cues focus on the content of the message, including word selection (Ranjan et al., 2015). Non-verbal cues include body language, such as your posture, facial expression and spatial distance (Ranjan et al., 2015). Paraverbal cues include matters such as the tone, pitch and volume of your voice (Ranjan et al., 2015). Effective delivery across each delivery mode is vital to ensure that the intended messages are conveyed.

It could be argued that effective communication is the cornerstone of clinical practice. Establishing open and respectful communication from the start of patient care increases the probability that important information will be disclosed during your assessment, resulting in improved patient outcomes. Positive outcomes of effective communication can include an improved clinician–patient relationship (Hardee & Platt, 2010), increased clinician and patient satisfaction (Brody et al., 1989; Suchman et al., 1993), improved engagement with treatment regimens (Kim et al., 2004; Stewart, 1984), improved health outcomes (Stewart, 1995), improved diagnostic accuracy (Hardee & Platt, 2010) and decreased medico-legal risk (Beckman et al., 1994).

COMMUNICATION AS A CLINICAL INTERVENTION

As noted above, communication is the foundation of every successful clinical encounter. While medical interventions learnt through training are often a focus, open communication with your patient ensures that you have the necessary information to inform your treatment plan, and may also alter the course of your treatment by providing an accurate feedback loop. Communication is essential, for example, when taking a patient history. If communication is established well, your patient should feel able to disclose necessary medical information even if it is considered embarrassing or stigmatising. Communication is thereby an intervention in itself.

Good communication can also improve patient engagement with treatment (Thompson & McCabe, 2012). Engagement with treatment is a crucial outcome for many medical and mental health disorders, with deviations from prescribed regimens potentially resulting in relapse, rehospitalisation and poor prognosis (Thompson & McCabe, 2012). A link between communication and engagement in treatment has been observed in general practice. A meta-analysis by Haskard-Zolnierek and DiMatteo (2009) synthesised the results from correlational and experimental studies and found that the odds of a patient adhering to their treatment plan are 2.16 times greater if their doctor is a good communicator. Good communication between a clinician and their patient can therefore improve history taking through improved trust and transparency and also patient engagement.

Conversely, when communication between a clinician and their patient is poor, the results can be catastrophic. The Institute of Medicine (IOM) highlighted the critical importance of communication in healthcare in their 2001 monograph 'Crossing the quality chasm: a new health system for the 21st century' (Institute of Medicine [IOM], 2001). Of significant concern, the IOM estimated that between 44,000 and

98,000 lives are lost in hospitals every year due to preventable errors. Further, it was suggested that 80% of these errors could be traced back to breakdowns in communication (Frankel & Sherman, 2015).

CASE STUDY

Paramedics have been dispatched to a home address in the early evening to a 25-year-old female who has cut herself on the upper thighs. The call comes from the patient's sister. Laney has gone to live with her older sister while she finds a new place to rent. Laney is in-between jobs. The sister reports that Laney has a history of depression and anxiety from early in her teens after their parents separated and later divorced.

Laney

I am home lying in bed with the lights off and under the blankets. I hear the front door open and my sister and her husband talking to the paramedics in low voices. I am scared, I don't know what is going to happen next so I move to the far corner of my bed and pull my sheets up around me. The paramedics knock but don't wait for a response, they just stride in. They turn on the lights and start to ask me a lot of questions, really quickly. I blink my eyes as I try to adjust. The paramedics don't seem to see how intimidated I feel, lying here in my bed. It's like all control has been taken away from me. It won't be long and they will be telling me what I've been doing wrong.

The paramedics are both men. It seems odd to have two grown men, strangers, in my room asking me personal questions. They are moving all over the place getting gear out of their bags. They want to know if I have taken anything and what is happening and I don't know how to answer them. There doesn't appear to be any time or space to answer or tell them what I am really thinking or, for that matter, feeling. One of them tries to make a joke after he stumbles on the clothes on my floor. I feel embarrassed and ashamed and look away from him. I can't bear to make eye contact now.

I don't know the answers to a lot of their questions. They ask me why they have been called out (I don't know, my sister did it), what is my concern (I don't know what to name it exactly, I just feel as if the walls are closing in on me) and what might have caused the problem (if I knew that I probably wouldn't need you). When I finally come up with some description for them, overwhelmed and scared, they don't respond, just keep taking out more equipment.

I am feeling ill, stomach cramps are curling me up into a ball and I cannot stop the groaning or the tears that I am embarrassed for them to see. The paramedics want me to take off my pants and tell me it is 'all right' and that it is 'something they see all the time'. Perhaps, but this is not something I experience often. I try to stop shaking and tell them what's in my mind, but my voice is soft and so tightly controlled they find it difficult to hear me.

I am tired of telling people that I don't want to be forced into taking the antidepressants that my GP prescribed. I just want some time to try and work things out. My GP suggested, in not a subtle way, that it was my reluctance to get better which was preventing me from being sensible, taking medication and getting on with my life. I guess everyone thinks the same.

REFLECTION

1. What assumptions do you make as a paramedic when you first walk onto a scene?
2. What impressions do you think patients have when you walk onto a scene?
3. What might change your patient's impression of you, and how would that affect the development of communication and a therapeutic rapport?
4. In the case of Laney, what barriers exist to developing therapeutic rapport and communication?
5. What observations and initial impressions of Laney would influence your approach and communication with her?

THE THERAPEUTIC RELATIONSHIP

Open communication allows both parties to engage and express their needs, thereby improving the clinician–patient or therapeutic relationship. The importance of the therapeutic relationship is highlighted across a range of therapy movements, from the early days of psychoanalytic therapy to humanistic therapy and more recently solution-focused therapies (Shattell et al., 2007). While views regarding the action of the therapeutic relationship differ, each school of thought highlights the importance of this construct.

There have been several previous reviews focusing on the effect of the therapeutic relationship in healthcare (Bultman & Svarstad, 2000; Hamann et al., 2003; Horvarth & Greenberg, 1989; Joosten et al., 2008; Priebe & McCabe, 2008). Overall, the literature suggests that a strong therapeutic relationship between the healthcare professional and their patient is associated with improvements in patient satisfaction, engagement with treatment, quality of life, reduced levels of anxiety and depression, and decreased healthcare costs (Kelley et al., 2014; Kornhaber et al., 2016; Shay et al., 2012; Step et al., 2009). Conversely, increased psychological distress and feelings of dehumanisation are associated with negative clinician–patient relationships (Step et al., 2009).

One study investigating patient perceptions of the therapeutic relationship through qualitative interviews with 20 adults with a mental illness (Shattell et al., 2007) identified three central themes. They were: relate to me, know me as a person and get to the solution. The first theme, *relate to me*, centred on the notion that in an effective therapeutic relationship the patient feels heard and understood. Clinician traits such as warmth, empathy and respect were raised, as was the importance of touch, such as a hand on the shoulder or a gentle pat on the back. In addition to personal attributes, communication strategies such as summarising and clarifying the patient's perspective were deemed to be useful. The second theme, *know me as a person*, centred on the notion that the individual is a person not a diagnosis. In this theme, personal knowledge was deemed important, knowledge that paramedics in the pre-hospital sector may not hold. This can be addressed through other comments in the theme, however, which suggested that showing an interest in the person and asking them occasional non-clinical questions (such as their school or their favourite football team) implied an interest beyond the task at hand. The final theme, *get to the solution*, centred on the notion that helpful healthcare providers provide some form of problem solving or solution in addition to comfort and engagement. Central themes included the importance of communicating a treatment plan and being honest about the options. These findings are echoed throughout the therapeutic relationship literature (Bedi, 2006; Bedi et al., 2005; Littauer et al., 2005; Shattell et al., 2007).

Use the case study of 'Laney' to reflect on the following issues:
- Shattell and colleagues (2007) identified three themes common in the positive therapeutic relationship (see above). Use these themes to make suggestions that will enhance the therapeutic encounter described and repair potential rifts.

DEVELOPING THE THERAPEUTIC RELATIONSHIP

The therapeutic relationship is widely acknowledged as being central to the development of a constructive clinician–patient experience (Ross, 2013). Achieving an optimal therapeutic relationship in the unpredictable pre-hospital environment can seem a daunting task. Studies in the acute care sector for example suggest that the high-pressure, task-oriented nature of the environment can act as a barrier to the establishment of this relationship (Kornhaber et al., 2016). The same may seem true for the pre-hospital sector. In an emergency context, even the most person-centred clinician can overlook engagement in favour of urgent medical intervention.

The patient–clinician relationship has both emotional and informational components – what Di Blasi and colleagues have termed emotional care and cognitive care (Di Blasi et al., 2001). Emotional care includes mutual trust, empathy, respect, genuineness, acceptance and warmth (Ong et al., 1995). Cognitive care includes information gathering, sharing medical information, and patient education and expectation management (Kelley et al., 2014). Additional elements of the therapeutic relationship highlighted in the literature include listening, responding to patient emotions and unmet needs, and person centeredness (Kornhaber et al., 2016).

INTERPERSONAL AND COMMUNICATION SKILLS

The main way for a clinician to influence the relationship and communication with a patient in a given clinical setting is through the way they behave towards the patient. As noted previously, communication occurs in verbal, non-verbal and para-verbal domains. Verbally, we can engage patients through the following techniques.

SET A COLLABORATIVE AGENDA

Agenda setting at the commencement of the clinical encounter is a core clinical skill that can have a significant impact on the course, direction and outcome of the care episode (Frankel & Sherman, 2015). The critical aspect of agenda setting in this instance is collaboration – there should be an opportunity for each person to state and prioritise their concerns. This collaborative agenda setting is consistent with the principles of patient-centred care, discussed earlier in the chapter (Frankel & Sherman, 2015). A range of studies highlight the benefits of collaborative agenda setting; for example, Williams and colleagues (1998) reported increased patient and clinician satisfaction; Beckman and Frankel (1984) described a reduction in premature hypothesis testing on the part of the clinician and also fewer 'hidden' concerns at the end of the visit. Early collaborative agenda setting has also been associated with improved clinical outcomes, such as the resolution of chronic headaches at the 12-month follow-up (Headache Study Group of The University of Western Ontario, 1986).

In the case of Laney, the attending paramedics could approach her in the following way: *'I understand that your sister has contacted us today. She has told us about her concerns, but I am interested in your ideas and opinions. What, if anything, do you think we could help you with today?'*

USE ACTIVE AND REFLECTIVE LISTENING

This involves paraphrasing and summarising the patient's report, both to demonstrate that you have heard them and also to ensure that your understanding is accurate. An illustration of this concept might include the following: '*Mrs Jones, so far you have told me that you injured your ankle when you fell in the bathroom* (summarising statement). *I can see that there is a lot of tenderness and swelling in the ankle, and we are going to manage that as soon as we can* (observation and empathy). *You also told me that before the fall you felt dizzy and lightheaded. Does that sound correct to you?* (checking for accuracy)'.

The importance of checking in with patients was highlighted in a study by Zandbelt and colleagues (2007). These researchers established that patient satisfaction was positively associated with doctors' facilitating patients' expression of their perspective. Facilitative behaviours included attentive silence, verbal and non-verbal encouragements, summarising patients' words, and reflections of facts, emotions and processes.

MIRROR THE PATIENT'S LANGUAGE

Mirroring the patient's language (or a close approximation, wherever possible) and particularly the adjectives used to describe their experience, demonstrates to the patient that you have listened carefully and that you respect their unique expertise with respect to their experience. This technique also removes the temptation to use overtly clinical language with a patient, just because we can! This technique can be seen in the following scenario: You attend a 16-year-old female with chest pain and laboured breathing in a shopping centre. During your interview the patient describes '*pins and needles*' in her fingers and toes. You suspect that this symptom is parathesis, which commonly occurs during a panic attack. While you could label the experience for the patient using this clinical term, it would be far more engaging to use her term, '*pins and needles*'.

Paraverbally we can engage patients through the following techniques:

MODERATE YOUR VOICE

Vocal modulation is an important aspect of communication. The tone of your voice can convey specific emotions like empathy or urgency. The same is true of the pace, pitch and volume of your voice. The importance of non-verbal cues in patient management was highlighted by Milmoe and colleagues in 1967. These authors suggested that the tone of voice used by a clinician early in the visit could predict satisfaction and follow-up with treatment recommendations (Milmoe et al., 1967).

In an urgent situation, paramedics are encouraged to use a low, calm tone of voice to reassure patients and help them to calm themselves. Your pace should not be so fast that they lose the message, but should also convey the importance of timely action. Verbal techniques such as short, simple statements also help to communicate your message in an emergency.

Non-verbally we can engage patients through the following techniques:

IDENTIFY AND MANAGE YOUR BODY LANGUAGE

Another fundamental aspect of non-verbal communication is your body language. In this area the terms 'closed' and 'open' body language are often used. Closed body language is generally thought to convey disinterest, defensiveness or disengagement. Signs of closed body language include crossing arms or legs, hunched posture, turning away from the person, and so on. By contrast, open body language is thought to express interest, openness, engagement and transparency. Open body posture includes hands by sides or behind the back, open stance if standing, uncrossed or loosely crossed legs if sitting. Clearly, if you are trying to engage a patient or their family in the treatment plan, the latter is preferable.

It is important to note that most people are not consciously aware of their body language. In some instances, this may be due to a lack of education regarding the factors that influence body language and/or the importance of body language in our communication. At times, body language may also be reflexive. For example, if you feel threatened or defensive you will likely change your body language to mirror this emotion.

As a clinician it is important to bring these unconscious actions into conscious awareness by reflecting on your internal state and then reflecting on your stance, position and other aspects of body language. When you start your training, one way to do this would be to include it as a part of your patient assessment, asking yourself internally at designated intervals: how am I feeling right now, where is my body in relation to the room and the patient, and what non-verbal cues am I giving. Making this a part of your routine will allow you over time to bring unconscious actions into conscious awareness and thus your control, and make it easier to manage your responses at difficult times. Requesting feedback from your peers, educators and simulated patients is also highly recommended, as each of these parties brings a unique perspective to the scenario.

MANAGE DISTANCE

The notion of proximity and touch in healthcare can be contentious. It is obviously important to ensure that you act in a professional and appropriate manner when working. In an effort to maintain boundaries and professionalism, however, we can lose sight of the power of human contact to reassure and connect with others. This element of communication is particularly important in the pre-hospital context; consider instances where you may be consoling a grief-stricken relative, reassuring a trapped patient following a motor vehicle accident or engaging an elderly man when he is in pain. In these examples, closer proximity and occasional touch may be useful engagement tools. Examples of appropriate contact may include a light touch on the back of the hand, a hand on the shoulder, or moving closer to a family member as they grieve. For a mental health patient in distress, gentle tactile stimulation may be enough to distract a person from their distressing thoughts, or reassure them that you are there to offer your support.

In some instances, however, distance should be maintained to ensure the safety of all parties. For example, if a patient is exhibiting paranoia, fear or delirium, or has a history of abuse, they should be warned before contact is made for any purpose. Procedures should be explained wherever possible and permission sought. This notion is explored further below in the section on de-escalation.

MODERATE FACIAL EXPRESSIONS

Facial expressions are another aspect of non-verbal communication that reflect our emotional state. When you are trying to manage a scene or comfort a patient, care should be taken to moderate your facial expressions so that signs of anger or fear are managed and, wherever possible, you display an open expression conveying interest and curiosity.

EMPATHY AND RESPONDING TO EMOTIONS

Warmington (2011) describes empathy as a process of attuning to or attempting to perceive a patient's inward process and then attempting to match the patient's emotions, demonstrating curiosity and actively checking interpretations. Clinician empathy is a key communication skill that forms a part of person-centred care (Williams et al., 2015).

In the paramedic context, positive empathetic behaviours have been found to be of substantial importance and comfort for grieving parents in cases of sudden infant death syndrome (Nordby & Nøhr, 2008). Williams and colleagues (2012) also note that empathy displayed by paramedics can affirm how the patient will perceive subsequent health professionals through the course of their treatment.

Despite this acknowledgement of the importance of empathy, recent literature suggests that undergraduate health students today display less empathy than did previous generations (Konrath et al., 2011) and fail to acknowledge the importance of empathy (Fields et al., 2011). Further, multidisciplinary studies investigating the empathy levels of paramedic students compared with nursing, midwifery, occupational therapy, physiotherapy and health sciences students, have suggested that paramedic students exhibit lower empathy scores on validated rating scales compared with those of fellow healthcare students, though it is important to note that all of the disciplines surveyed experienced struggles with empathy (Boyle et al., 2009). These findings highlight the need to address empathy in the training and education of paramedics.

While the benefits of empathy are clear, clinicians maintain reservations regarding the application of empathy in time-poor, highly intense clinical environments such as the pre-hospital sector. According to Hardee and Platt (2010), concerns are typically centred on four themes: not enough time, Pandora's Box, burnout, and what to say. Each of these perceived barriers is addressed below.

1 NOT ENOUGH TIME

Within the emergency services, time is at a premium. Paramedics must balance the demands of medical management in a dynamic and unpredictable environment, and provide an effective and efficient intervention for the issue of concern, all the while being cognisant of the needs of other service users. As with accident and emergency departments, these demands often leave clinicians with the concern that they are time poor and thus must focus on efficiency at all costs.

Efficiency at the expense of communication and empathy would be a significant concern. As noted before, empathy has many benefits both in terms of patient outcomes and, arguably, the efficiency of the clinical exchange. If your patient does not feel heard or they have a sense that you do not understand their emotional space, they may limit their own engagement, which can limit your ability to gain important treatment information. It could also be argued that leaving the patient feeling heard and respected is as important an outcome of the clinical encounter as treating a fracture or stabilising a wound. With this in mind, empathy seems essential, particularly when attending cases relating to mental health and emotional issues.

Further, research suggests that empathetic communication actually increases efficiency and saves time (Hardee & Platt, 2010).

2 PANDORA'S BOX

The fear of a flood of difficult emotions can often lead clinicians to avoid some lines of questioning and communication (Hardee & Platt, 2010). This is often seen in novice clinicians when they suddenly defer to closed questions and appear less curious. While you cannot manage everything in the pre-hospital sector, questions such as *'Can you tell me a little about your day so far?'* or *'How do you normally manage your anxiety?'* show that you are interested in the patient, and can potentially elicit clinical information such as triggers or events prior to your attendance, while also demonstrating empathy. Should you find yourself in a situation where you cannot address all of the patient's concerns, statements like *'It sounds like things have been very difficult for you. While I would like to help you as best as I can, I am not sure we can manage all of that right now, so let's see if we can focus in on … (reason for referral)'* let the person know you are interested in and value them, that you have empathy, but also that there are limits to your role.

3 BURNOUT

The notion of empathy burnout or compassion fatigue has often been raised (Figley, 2002). Some argue that empathy, if given freely throughout all shifts, may leave clinicians with little left for their private life (Sabo, 2006). Others argue that empathy can be both depleting and re-energising (Hunsaker et al., 2015). Caring for others clearly requires that you engage in enough self-care activities to balance the scales. On the other hand, connecting with another person and caring for them in a difficult moment can be highly rewarding, so burnout must not be assumed in all instances.

4 WHAT TO SAY

Clinicians often cite uncertainty and a fear of saying the 'wrong thing' as barriers to open empathetic questioning. Hardee and Platt (2010) assert that empathy can be conveyed through the following devices:

- Listen to the patient, attend to non-verbal cues, and try to come to an understanding of what is important to the patient (values).
- Try to understand the patient's conceptualisation of the problem (what do they think re: diagnosis and intervention).
- Attend to feelings (in the pre-hospital context, often a mix of sadness, anger and/or fear).
- Summarise for the patient what you think you have heard, and seek clarification to make sure you have understood correctly.

It is now accepted that empathy is a teachable skill and a cornerstone of the clinical encounter. Improvements in empathy have been demonstrated in programs that teach empathetic skills lasting only one hour (Guastello & Frampton, 2014; Stepien & Baernstein, 2006). How this skill set is maintained and then applied clinically, however, remains unclear. What is clear is the need for empathetic communication, and for genuine interest in and curiosity around patients' experiences and needs.

INTRODUCTION TO DE-ESCALATION

De-escalation refers to the active adoption of a range of psychosocial techniques, with an aim to reduce disruptive or aggressive behaviour (NICE, 2005). This approach is sometimes referred to as 'talking someone down' (NICE, 2005). The significant role that de-escalation can and should play in the management of disruptive behaviour was highlighted following several high-profile deaths involving restraint (Blofeld et al., 2003). De-escalation also aligns well with the philosophy of person-centred care using the least restrictive means available.

Despite the importance of de-escalation across the health field, there is a lack of consensus regarding the undertaking or parameters of de-escalation (Price & Baker, 2012). This concern was highlighted in a systematic review of training programs undertaken by Richter and Whittington (2006), who noted that there was significant heterogeneity in the content and duration of the available training programs. A related review conducted by Graj and colleagues (2019) noted that students in the healthcare field are exposed to adverse events like agitation and aggression while undertaking work placement, but there is a dearth of de-escalation training programs that focus on the experience level, roles and responsibilities of students. This gap has since been addressed by programs such as *Risk Aware* (Graj et al., 2018), but further work is required to ensure that students learn de-escalation skills early in their training.

De-escalation is recognised as an important part of Clinical Practice Guidelines (CPGs) for paramedics; however, the CPGs reviewed in Australia reflected a distinct lack of detail for trainees. For example, the South Australian Clinical Practice Guideline for Challenging Behaviours suggests in step 2 that the paramedics de-escalate the challenging patient where possible. Unfortunately, further steps to undertake this action are not provided. NSW Ambulance protocols (2016) also indicate that communication and de-escalation are first-line management for behavioural concerns, but again additional data is limited.

The Victorian CPGs suggest the following considerations for verbal de-escalation (Ambulance Victoria, 2018):

- Listen to the patient.
- Use the patient's name to personalise the interaction.
- Use open-ended questions.
- Use a calm, consistent, even tone of voice, even if the patient's communication style becomes hostile or aggressive.
- Avoid 'no' language which may prompt an aggressive response; for example, 'I'm sorry, our policy doesn't allow me to do that but I can offer you other assistance'.
- Allow the patient as much personal space as possible while maintaining control of the scene.
- Avoid too much eye contact as this can increase fear in some paranoid patients.

The section below details additional considerations when de-escalating patients, and attempts to provide a practical framework for trainees should they be required to engage this skill (see Fig. 3.1). You will note that many of the examples outlined as de-escalation strategies have also been highlighted above. This is because active listening, empathic engagement and open communication are essential to all patients, but particularly so when patients feel threatened or fearful.

PRINCIPLES OF DE-ESCALATION
STAFF CHARACTERISTICS

Effective de-escalators are viewed as transparent, supportive, self-aware, non-judgmental and confident without appearing arrogant (Carlsson et al., 2000, Delaney

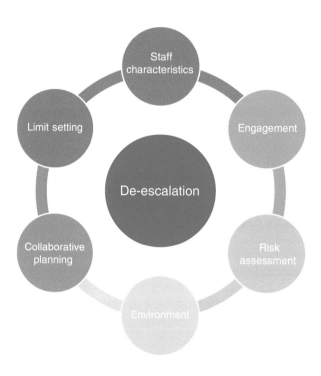

FIGURE 3.1

Six principles of de-escalation in the pre-hospital environment

& Johnson, 2006; Duperouzel, 2008; Gertz, 1980; Johnson & Hauser, 2001; Lane, 1986; Lowe, 1992). They express genuine concern for their patient and have a non-threatening, non-authoritarian manner (Price & Baker, 2012). These character-istics allow the patient to feel supported and for rapport to develop.

Effective de-escalators are also able to remain calm in the face of escalation (Duperouzel, 2008; Lowe, 1992). This means that even if the staff member is experiencing anxiety internally, they maintain a calm exterior. In principle, it is thought that this calm presence allows others to match the staff member's affect, and provides a sense of safety and security for the agitated individual (Price & Baker, 2012).

The staff characteristics outlined can be conveyed through both your verbal and non-verbal communication. Verbally it is important to maintain a calm tone of voice and low volume, rather than raising your voice to match the agitated individual's. Humour can also be used in some instances to diffuse tension and establish rapport. Non-verbally, it is important to manage your facial expressions to convey calm, to match levels with your patient (i.e. if they are sitting, do not stand over them but squat down to their level), and to allow the person adequate space to ensure your safety and theirs while also being close enough to establish rapport (Carlsson et al., 2000).

ENGAGEMENT

Carlsson and colleagues (2000) suggest that aggression is often a response to a loss of dignity, highlighting the importance of respectful engagement and empathy. As part of this communication, paramedics should endeavour to support the autonomy of the patient by minimising restriction wherever possible (Delaney & Johnson, 2006; Duperouzel, 2008; Lowe, 1992).

Active listening is also an essential engagement tool. Active listening involves the use of summaries and paraphrasing to check in with your patient and make sure that you have heard their concerns correctly. This process allows for clarification in the event of a miscommunication and, potentially, problem solving of the concerns identified. Importantly, this approach focuses on working together to find a mutual path forward.

RISK ASSESSMENT

Effective de-escalation involves an element of ongoing risk assessment to ensure that you are aware of the risks within your environment and any fluctuations in the state of the agitated person. Importantly, your responses must be calibrated to this risk assessment. For example, if the agitated person moves from verbal agitation to pacing and large hand gestures, the person's agitation has clearly escalated. This shift indicates the need for your own recalibration, perhaps by creating a safe space between yourself and the individual or discreetly moving closer to the exit. Conversely, a lowering in the person's agitation may allow you to move closer. This change could be prefaced with a comment such as *'Do you mind if I move closer now to examine you?'*

ENVIRONMENT

Managing the environment is an important component of de-escalation, and pre-hospital care more broadly. In the case of agitation, a person's environment can be a trigger for agitation or can present a range of risks to the healthcare professional. Common environmental triggers for aggression include other people (such as partners or family members), noise, extreme temperatures, etc. Consider the person's response to these environmental cues and, where possible, either remove them or, if necessary, move yourself and your patient.

COLLABORATIVE PLANNING

An important component of de-escalation is coming to some form of resolution to the problems/concerns experienced. Resolution can often be achieved by asking the patient:

- What is the problem of concern?
- What does the patient think can be done about the problem?
- Is the patient open to other ideas or solutions?
- What normally helps the patient to feel calmer?

If the agitated patient is able to engage in this discussion, you should be able to identify a management plan together.

LIMIT SETTING WHERE NECESSARY

On some occasions, individuals are reluctant to engage in problem solving and, despite your best efforts, remain agitated. In these instances, you might suggest an alternate coping skill yourself. For example, '*I can see that you are very frustrated right now and I would like to understand more about it. Can I ask that you take a moment to take a few deep breaths with me? This will help us both to calm ourselves and make a plan.*'

If this does not work or the individual is using aggression as a form of control, setting limits like the following may be useful: '*I understand that you are frustrated, but we can't work together effectively when you are yelling at me. Can I ask you to lower your voice so that I can understand what you want to happen right now?*' Remember that every step that we take towards authoritarian approaches typically increases the chances of agitation escalating to aggression, so use these options as a last resort. These options can also be combined with the use of positive reinforcement; for example, praising non-violent behaviour (Gertz, 1980).

REFLECTIVE PRACTICE

Reflective practice is commonly viewed as the process of learning through and from experience, of gaining new insights into yourself and your practice (Boud et al., 1985; Finlay, 2008). This often involves examining our assumptions of everyday practice, being self-aware and critically evaluating our own responses to practice situations (Finlay, 2008).

It could be argued that strong reflective process is fundamental to the undertaking of many of the skills detailed in this chapter. The varied communication approaches described here typically highlight the importance of open, honest and active communication, calibrated to the needs of the patient. The skills detailed are ones that develop throughout our professional careers, requiring the ability to assess our skills and responses and make modifications. From my own perspective I note that as I learn more, I realise that I know very little!

Sobral (2000) asserts that reflection is associated with a more positive learning experience, while Glaze (2001) found that reflective practice has the capacity to improve understanding of learning content, transform perspective and engagement with healthcare and improve clinical practice (although this paper was based on the views of experienced clinicians, not a randomised control trial evaluating skill sets). Mann and colleagues (2009) argue that there are two primary dimensions to the varied models of reflective practice that exist:

1. An **iterative dimension** within which the process of reflection is triggered by experience, which then produces a new understanding, and the intention to think

or act differently in future related experiences (e.g. *I saw a patient experiencing mania the other day. She was quite delusional and refused to get in the ambulance. She thought she was going to the Academy Awards ceremony. I got so frustrated that I kept arguing with her, trying to make her see sense. It did not work. Then her mum came out and didn't really argue with her so much as talk about it while getting her in the ambulance and calming her down. It worked so much better that I think next time I will try it her way*).

2. A **vertical dimension**, which suggests that there are different levels of reflection on experience. Generally, the surface levels are more descriptive (i.e. *I noted that I felt anxious when I performed CPR in front of the family*) and less analytical, and then deeper levels of reflection that require analysis and critical synthesis (i.e. *I noted that I felt anxious when I performed CPR in front of the family because I felt their sadness and anxiety and wanted a good outcome for them. It also reminded me of my grandfather's recent ambulance visit, which made me sad. These feelings resulted in me focusing on CPR for far too long and promising the family a good outcome instead of preparing them for the patient's likely death. In the future I will be more aware in these situations, focus on my clinical guidelines for optimal CPR, and make sure that myself or my partner engages with the family in an honest and transparent manner.*)

Work within the Open University's Health and Social Care faculty has put forward a model whereby reflective practice is seen as a synthesis of *reflection, self-awareness* and *critical thinking* (Eby, 2000). Within this model, reflective practice is seen as the intersection between self-awareness, reflection and critical thinking (Finlay, 2008).

Barriers to reflective practice include years of practice (i.e. there is a decrease in reflective practice with greater years of experience) (Mamede & Schmidt, 2005), time pressure in a busy clinical environment (Dornan et al., 2002; Mamede & Schmidt, 2005), and working in an environment where reflective thinking is not reinforced (Mamede & Schmidt, 2005) and mentoring and support is not reinforced (Platzer et al., 2000).

If reflective practice is considered to be integral to healthcare practice, the question remains: how do we develop reflective practice in novice clinicians? In their review of the literature, Mann and colleagues (2009) identified four studies addressing the development of reflective practice. Collectively these studies suggest that reflective practice can be developed over time. Having an avenue for development, like a logbook or portfolio or supervision, appears to enhance the development of this skill (Mann et al., 2009). Moreover, having a workplace context that encourages reflection also allows for the development of this skill (Mann et al., 2009). Using models of reflective practice like those above is also useful.

While reflective practice is ingrained in the professional development of many healthcare disciplines, paramedicine still has some work to do in this space to ensure that novice paramedics are encouraged to discuss their practice and to reflect not only the clinical nature of the encounter but all aspects of patient care.

CONCLUSION

Communication is fundamental to the delivery of safe and effective healthcare. Communication allows us to work in a person-centred fashion as we seek the opinions and goals of the patient and their family. Effective communication can also facilitate the development of a strong and trusting therapeutic relationship. Insufficient or closed communication, however, has been linked with lower satisfaction and increased errors. Reflection can facilitate the development of this skill as we strive to make healthcare efficient, effective and *engaging*.

LINKS AND RESOURCES

- Australian Commission on Safety and Quality in Health Care (ACSQHC), 2010. Australian safety and quality framework for health care. Online. Available: https://www.safetyandquality.gov.au/wp-content/uploads/2012/01/32296-Australian-SandQ-Framework1.pdf

REFERENCES

Ambulance Victoria, 2018. Clinical practice guidelines ambulance and MICA paramedics. Online. Available: https://www.ambulance.vic.gov.au/wp-content/uploads/2018/11/Clinical-Practice-Guidelines-2018-Edition-1.5.pdf.

ASQFHC, 2010. Australian Safety and Quality Framework for Health Care. Sydney, Australia. Online. Available: https://www.safetyandquality.gov.au/wp-content/uploads/2012/01/32296-Australian-SandQ-Framework1.pdf. 21 May 2019.

Beckman, H., Frankel, R., 1984. The effect of physician behaiour on the collection of data. Ann. Intern. Med. 101, 692–696.

Beckman, H., Markakis, K., Suchman, A., et al., 1994. The doctor–patient relationship and malpractice: lessons from plaintiff depositions. Arch. Intern. Med. 154 (12), 1365–1370.

Bedi, R., 2006. Concept mapping the client's perspective on counseling alliance formation. J. Couns. Psychol. 53 (1), 26–35.

Bedi, R., Davis, M., Williams, M., 2005. Critical incidents in the formation of the therapeutic alliance from the client's perspective. Psychother. (Chic.) 42 (3), 311–323.

Blofeld, J., Sallah, D., Sashidharan, S., et al., 2003. An Independent Inquiry Set Up Under HSG (94)27 Into the Death of David 'Rocky' Bennett. Norfolk, Suffolk and Cambridgeshire Strategic Health Authority, Cambridge, UK.

Boud, D., Keogh, R., Walker, D., 1985. Promoting reflection in learning: a model. In: Boud, D., Keogh, R., Walker, D. (Eds.), Reflection: Turning experience into learning. Kogan Page, London.

Boyle, M., Williams, B., Brown, T., et al., 2009. Levels of empathy in undergraduate health science students. Internet J. Med. Educ. 1 (1), 1–7.

Brody, D., Miller, S., Lerman, C., et al., 1989. The relationship between patients' satisfaction with their physicians and perceptions about interventions they desired and received. Med. Care 27 (11), 1027–1035.

Bultman, D., Svarstad, B., 2000. Effects of physician communication style on client medication beliefs and adherence with antidepressant treatment. Patient Educ. Couns. 40 (2), 173–185.

Carlsson, G., Dahlberg, K., Drew, N., 2000. Encountering violence and aggression in mental health nursing: a phenomenological study of tacit caring knowledge. Issues Ment. Health Nurs. 21 (5), 533–545.

Delaney, K., Johnson, M., 2006. Keeping the unit safe: mapping psychiatric nursing skills. J. Am. Psychiatr. Nurses Assoc. 12 (4), 198–207.

Di Blasi, Z., Harkness, E., Ernst, E., et al., 2001. Influence of context effects on health outcomes: a systematic review. Lancet 357, 757–762.

Dornan, T., Carrol, C., Parboosingh, J., 2002. An electronic learning portfolio for reflective continuing professional development. Med. Educ. 36 (8), 767–769.

Duperouzel, H., 2008. 'It's OK for people to feel angry': the exemplary management of imminent aggression. J. Intellect. Disabil. 12 (4), 295–307.

Eby, M., 2000. Understanding professional development. In: Brechin, A., Brown, H., Eby, M.A. (Eds.), Critical Practice in Health and Social Care. Sage Publications, London.

Fields, S., Mahn, P., Tillman, P., et al., 2011. Measuring empathy in healthcare profession students using the Jefferson Scale of Physician Empathy: health provider – Student version. J. Interprof. Care 25 (4), 287–293.

Figley, C., 2002. Compassion fatigue: psychotherapists' chronic lack of self care. J. Clin. Psychol. 58 (11), 1433–1441.

Finlay, L., 2008. Reflecting on 'reflective practice.' The Open University (January): 1–27.

Finset, A., 2010. Emotions, narratives and empathy in clinical communication. Int. J. Integr. Care 10 (5), 53–56.

Frankel, R., Sherman, H., 2015. The secret of the care of the patient is in knowing and applying the evidence about effective clinical communication. Oral Dis. 21 (8), 919–926.

Gertz, B., 1980. Training for prevention of assaultive behavior in a psychiatric setting. Hosp. Community Psychiatry 31 (9), 628–630.

Glaze, J., 2001. Reflection as a transforming process: student advanced nurse practitioners' experiences of developing reflective skills as part of an MSc programme. J. Adv. Nurs. 34 (5), 639–647.

Graj, E., Sheen, J., Dudley, A., et al., 2018. Enhancing student competency in risky clinical environments: evaluating an online education program. Aust. Psychol. 54 (1), 68–79.

Graj, E., Sheen, J., Dudley, A., et al., 2019. Adverse health events associated with clinical placement: a systematic review. Nurse Educ. Today 76, 178–190.

Guastello, S., Frampton, S., 2014. Patient-centered care retreats as a method for enhancing and sustaining compassion in action in healthcare settings. J. Compassionate Health Care 1 (1), 2.

Hamann, J., Leucht, S., Kissling, W., 2003. Shared decision making in psychiatry. Acta Psychiatr. Scand. 107 (6), 403–409.

Hardee, J., Platt, F., 2010. Exploring and overcoming barriers to clinical empathic communication. J. Commun. Healthc. 3 (1), 17–23.

Haskard-Zolnierek, K.B., DiMatteo, M.R., 2009. Physician communication and patient adherence to treatment: a meta-analysis. Med. Care 47 (8), 826–834. doi:10.1097/MLR.0b013e31819a5acc.

Headache Study Group of The University of Western Ontario, 1986. Predictors of outcome in headache patients presenting to family physicians – a one year prospective study. Headache 26 (6), 285–294.

Horvath, A., Greenberg, L., 1989. Development and validation of the Working Alliance Inventory. J. Couns. Psychol. 36 (2), 223–233.

Hunsaker, S., Chen, H., Maughan, D., et al., 2015. Factors that influence the development of compassion fatigue, burnout, and compassion satisfaction in emergency department nurses. J. Nurs. Scholarsh. 47 (2), 186–194.

Institute of Medicine (IOM), 2001. Crossing the Quality Chasm: A new health system for the 21st century. National Academies Press, Washington, DC.

Johnson, M., Hauser, P., 2001. The practices of expert psychiatric nurses: accompanying the patient to a calmer personal space. Issues Ment. Health Nurs. 22 (7), 651–668.

Joosten, E., Defuentes-Merillas, L., de Weert, G., et al., 2008. Systematic review of the effects of shared decision-making on patient satisfaction, treatment adherence and health status. Psychother. Psychosom. 77 (4), 219–226.

Kelley, J., Kraft-Todd, G., Schapira, L., et al., 2014. The influence of the patient–clinician relationship on healthcare outcomes: a systematic review and meta-analysis of randomized controlled trials. PLoS ONE 9 (4).

Kim, S., Kaplowitz, S., Johnston, M., 2004. The effects of physician empathy on patient satisfaction and compliance. Eval. Health Prof. 27 (3), 237–251.

Konrath, S., O'Brien, E., Hsing, C., 2011. Changes in dispositional empathy in American college students over time: a meta-analysis. Pers. Soc. Psychol. Rev. 15 (2), 180–198.

Kornhaber, R., Walsh, K., Duff, J., et al., 2016. Enhancing adult therapeutic interpersonal relationships in the acute health care setting: an integrative review. J. Multidiscip. Healthc. 9, 537–546.

Lane, F., 1986. Utilizing physician empathy with violent patients. Am. J. Psychother. 40 (3), 448–456.

Littauer, H., Sexton, H., Wynn, R., 2005. Qualities clients wish for in their therapists. Scand. J. Caring Sci. 19 (1), 28–31.

Lowe, T., 1992. Characteristics of effective nursing interventions in the management of challenging behavior. J. Adv. Nurs. 17 (10), 1226–1232.

Mamede, S., Schmidt, H., 2005. Correlates of reflective practice in medicine. Adv. Health. Sci. Educ. Theory Pract. 10 (4), 327–337.

Mann, K., Gordon, J., MacLeod, A., 2009. Reflection and reflective practice in health professions education: a systematic review. Adv. Health. Sci. Educ. Theory Pract. 14 (4), 595–621.

Milmoe, S., Rosenthal, R., Blane, H., et al., 1967. The doctor's voice: postdictor of successful referral of alcoholic patients. J. Abnorm. Psychol. 72 (1), 78–84.

National Institute for Health and Clinical Excellence (NICE), 2005. Violence: The short-term management of disturbed/violent behaviour in in-patient psychiatric and emergency departments. National Collaborating Centre for Nursing and Supportive Care, London.

Nordby, H., Nøhr, Ø., 2008. Communication and empathy in an emergency setting involving persons in crisis. Scand. J. Trauma Resusc. Emerg. Med. 16 (1), 1–6.

NSW Ambulance, 2016. 2016 Protocol and Pharmacology. NSW Ambulance, New South Wales.

Ong, L., de Haes, J., Hoos, A., et al., 1995. Doctor–patient communication: a review of the literature. Soc. Sci. Med. 40 (7), 903–918.

Platzer, H., Blake, D., Ashford, D., 2000. Barriers to learning from reflection: a study of the use of group work with post-registration nurses. J. Adv. Nurs. 31 (5), 1001–1008.

Price, O., Baker, J., 2012. Key components of de-escalation techniques: a thematic synthesis. Int. J. Ment. Health Nurs. 21 (4), 310–319.

Priebe, S., McCabe, R., 2008. Therapeutic relationships in psychiatry: the basis of therapy or therapy in itself? Int. Rev. Psychiatry 20 (6), 521–526.

Ranjan, P., Kumari, A., Chakrawarty, A., 2015. How can doctors improve their communication skills? J. Clin. Diagn. Res. 9 (3), 1–4.

Richter, D., Whittington, R. (Eds), 2006. Violence in Mental Health Settings: Causes, consequences, management. (Springer-Verlag, New York).

Ross, L., 2013. Facilitating rapport through real patient encounters in health care professional education. Australas. J. Paramed. 10 (4), 1–12.

Sabo, B., 2006. Compassion fatigue and nursing work: can we accurately capture the consequences of caring work? Int. J. Nurs. Pract. 12 (3), 136–142.

Shattell, M., Starr, S., Thomas, S., 2007. 'Take my hand, help me out': mental health service recipients' experience of the therapeutic relationship: feature article. Int. J. Ment. Health Nurs. 16 (4), 274–284.

Shay, L., Dumenci, L., Siminoff, L., et al., 2012. Factors associated with patient reports of positive physician relational communication. Patient Educ. Couns. 89 (1), 96–101.

Sobral, D., 2000. An appraisal of medical students' reflection-in-learning. Med. Educ. 34 (3), 182–187.

Step, M., Rose, J., Albert, J., et al., 2009. Modeling patient-centered communication: oncologist relational communication and patient communication involvement in breast cancer adjuvant therapy decision-making. Patient Educ. Couns. 77 (3), 369–378.

Stepien, K., Baernstein, A., 2006. Educating for empathy: a review. J. Gen. Intern. Med. 21 (5), 524–530.

Stewart, M., 1984. What is a successful doctor–patient interview? A study of interactions and outcomes. Soc. Sci. Med. 19 (2), 167–175.

Stewart, M., 1995. Effective physician–patient communication and health outcomes: a review. Can. Med. Assoc. J. 152 (9), 1423–1433.

Suchman, A., Roter, D., Green, M., et al., 1993. Physician satisfaction with primary care office visits. Med. Care 31 (12), 1083–1092.

Thompson, L., McCabe, R., 2012. The effect of clinician–patient alliance and communication on treatment adherence in mental health care: a systematic review. BMC Psychiatr. 12 (1), 87.

Warmington, S., 2011. Practising engagement: infusing communication with empathy and compassion in medical students' clinical encounters. Health 16 (3), 327–342.

Williams, B., Boyle, M., Brightwell, R., et al., 2012. Paramedic empathy levels: results from seven Australian universities. Int. J. Emerg. Serv. 1 (2), 111–121.

Williams, B., Brown, T., McKenna, L., et al., 2015. Student empathy levels across 12 medical and health professions: an interventional study. J. Compassionate Health Care 2 (1), 4.

Williams, S., Weinman, J., Dale, J., 1998. Doctor–patient communication and patient satisfaction: a review. Fam. Pract. 15 (5), 480–492.

Zandbelt, L., Smets, E., Oort, F., et al., 2007. Medical specialists' patient-centred communication and patient-reported outcomes. Med. Care 45 (4), 330–339.

Stress, arousal and emotions

Julie Henderson and Elizabeth Ann Goble

LEARNING OUTCOMES

By the end of this chapter you should be able to:

- recognise the role of stress in the presentation of mental illness
- identify the connection between the stress response and the hypothalamus, pituitary and adrenal axis
- identify the physiological manifestations of the stress response
- outline the concept of trauma-informed care and how it guides practice in the pre-hospital setting
- identify communication and management strategies to mitigate stress when providing care.

INTRODUCTION

We have all experienced stress at some time in our lives from our studies, work, or relationships with friends, family and partners. Exposure to stress can improve our performance in the short term, but if it goes on for too long it can become chronic and lead to stress overload. When stress becomes chronic it can impair concentration, motivation and sleep, and can lead to behaviours such as social isolation, excessive alcohol use, smoking, over-eating and lack of exercise, all of which impair health. Long-term exposure to stress can, therefore, contribute to physical and mental health problems.

This chapter discusses acute and chronic stress. It commences with a case study of a paramedic who experiences chronic stress followed by an acute stress reaction, and asks you to consider treatment options. It then outlines research about stress, providing information about our current understanding of the physiology of a stress reaction. Following this, we discuss some of the physical and behavioural manifestations of acute and chronic stress, and explore evidence for the impact of stress on the development of other mental and physical health problems. The section after that discusses some of the life events that contribute to stress, and identifies some of the social determinants of stress. The chapter then moves to the management of stress. It highlights recent data about the level of stress-related illness among paramedics and other first-responders, and provides information about techniques for self-management of stress for both paramedics and patients. The chapter concludes with a discussion of trauma-related care and how this can be applied to the management of patients exhibiting symptoms of acute and/or chronic stress or stress overload.

CASE STUDY

Josie

Josie is a paramedic working out of a small station in rural Australia. She has worked as a paramedic for many years and is generally well liked and respected by her colleagues at the station. Recently, there has been turnover of staff and they are short of experienced paramedics. As Josie has worked at the station for a while, she has been asked to take extra shifts. Working extra shifts has compromised the time she has with her partner and children, and her partner Matt has been complaining that he feels like a single parent. In addition, the extra shifts that Josie is working have made it difficult for her to get to the gym, and she is starting to get tired and irritable and to snap at her family and colleagues.

One day she is called out to a car accident in the next town. When she arrives, she realises that the person in the car is the mother of her son's classmate at school. Despite the best efforts of the paramedics, the woman dies while being transported to hospital. After the accident, Josie finds that she is unable to sleep through the night. She has trouble concentrating and is short-tempered with her children. She is becoming socially isolated and is drinking more in the evening. She is also starting to make excuses to call in sick for work. Matt is concerned about her, but doesn't know what to do. There is a formal peer-support program at Josie's workplace, but Josie has had conflict with the person providing peer support and doesn't want to approach them. They do not provide support to family members.

A few weeks later, Josie is on duty when they are called to the town where the accident occurred. As they approach the site of the accident, Josie's heart begins to race and she starts to hyperventilate. You are working with Josie on that shift and you are driving the ambulance.

CRITICAL THINKING

- What can you do to help Josie manage her acute stress reaction?
- What can the organisation/employer do to support Josie?
- What impact is Josie's stress having on her family? What support might her family need?
- What can Josie do to help herself manage stress?

WHAT IS STRESS?

Stress has been studied by both biologists and psychologists in the past 150 years. The research fields developed independently of each other and make different assumptions about the nature of stress and the goal of stress research. Biological studies of stress have traditionally focused on the mechanisms by which the body responds to external or internal challenges (Faraday, 2006). Two researchers who have been instrumental in biological studies of stress are Walter B. Cannon and Hans Selye. Cannon explored the manner in which the sympathetic nervous system acted in response to external stimuli. He was particularly interested in the way the body responded to strong emotions such as rage and fear. He associated the experience of strong emotion with the release of adrenaline and bodily changes such as: release of blood sugar; reduction in peripheral circulation and increased circulation to the heart, lungs, brain and large muscles; reduced digestion; and increased thresholds for muscular exhaustion. He viewed these changes as an adaptive response that allowed the organism to respond to threat, with the sympathetic nervous system maintaining the body within narrow homeostatic boundaries (Faraday, 2006).

In the 1930s, a young physician called Hans Selye used the term 'stress' and applied it to human physiology. Stress was originally used in the field of physics to mean a force applied to a physical material. Selye rejected the idea of homeostasis, and expanded our understanding of stress to include any external stimulus that leads to bodily changes, e.g. physical trauma. He is credited with the development of the concept of the 'general adaptation syndrome'. He argued that the stress response had three phases. During the initial phase, 'alarm', the body responds by the release of corticotropin-releasing factor (CRF) by the hypothalamus. This, in turn, promotes the production of adrenocorticotropic hormone (ACTH) by the pituitary gland, which prompts the release of corticoids by the adrenal glands. The corticoid released is cortisol, which increases blood sugar levels by increasing the production of glucose molecules. It also modifies fat and protein metabolism and, when combining with glucocorticoid receptors, influences cardiovascular function, inflammation, arousal and learning and memory (Stephens &Wand, 2012). The second phase, the 'resistance phase', occurs when the body adapts to the stress response. This phase is associated with a reduction in cortisol levels. If the stress continues, however, a third phase, 'exhaustion', occurs where the body can no longer resist the bodily changes associated with stress, and cortisol levels rise again, precipitating 'diseases of adaption' arising from prolonged exposure to high cortisol levels (Faraday, 2006; Selye, 1956).

In contrast, psychological theories focused on psychological and behavioural mechanisms for managing stress. The methodologies used to study stress (e.g. surveys) enabled comparison and identification of differences in stress response across populations (Faraday, 2006). The work of two researchers is of note. Kurt Lewin's contribution is a separation of the event that causes stress, the stressor, from the way in which the individual experiences stress. He argued that a person's reaction to stress depends on their 'life space', which is the subjective psychological world of the individual. This may include things like belief systems, previous experiences and coping mechanisms. How the individual experiences stress depends upon their life space (Faraday, 2006).

This approach informed the work of Richard S. Lazarus. Lazarus and Folkman (1984, p. 19) define psychological stress as 'a particular relationship between the person and the environment that is appraised by the person as taxing or exceeding his or her resources and endangering his or her well-being'. They found that response to stress was mediated by subjective factors. These include: 'cognitive appraisal' in which the individual considers the potential impact of the event and their capacity to overcome or prevent harm; 'coping strategies', which are the cognitive and behavioural strategies the individual uses to manage demands that exceed the person's resources; and immediate outcome, which is a judgment of the extent to which the issue has been resolved (Folkman et al. 1986).

Our current understanding of stress draws upon the work of these pioneers. Stress can be understood as an essential and characteristic response when we are faced with challenging or threatening situations that can affect the body's wellbeing and homeostasis, whether the threat is perceived or real, and whether it is internally or externally generated. Our initial reaction is triggered by the sympathetic arm of the autonomic nervous system preparing for a fight, flight or freeze response: hormones such as epinephrine (adrenaline) and norepinephrine (noradrenaline) increase heart rate, respiratory rate and blood pressure, redirecting energy and oxygen to muscles to enable us to either escape (flight) to avoid the situation, or to defend ourselves (fight) if we must face the situation which is, or is perceived to be, threatening to our wellbeing. If the situation is too overwhelming, we may be faced with a situation that means we cannot react to either flight or fight and we may freeze. Other physiological mechanisms include mobilisation of energy in the form of glucose to provide the energy to flight or fight, decreases in digestive activity and gut motility (hence the feeling of nausea that often accompanies stress), and alterations in blood composition where platelet levels increase to more rapidly close a potential wound (Martini et al., 2015).

A second reaction occurs through the hypothalamic-pituitary-adrenal (HPA) axis. This builds on work originally undertaken by Selye. According to Selye, the paraventricular nucleus (PVN) of the hypothalamus releases the corticoid-releasing factor (CRF) and arginine vasopressin (AVP), which stimulate the pituitary gland to release adrenocorticotropic hormone (ACTH). ACTH prompts the synthesis and release of cortisol by the adrenal cortex on the kidneys. Later research has focused on the feedback loops that maintain hormone levels within a set level to achieve homeostasis (what Selye called 'resistance').

The secretion of CRF, AVP and ACTH is controlled by the level of cortisol in circulation through binding with receptors. There are two types of receptors for cortisol: mineralocorticoid (type-I) and glucocorticoid (type-II) receptors. Cortisol binds more readily with mineralocorticoid receptors (MRs) helping maintain the relatively low cortisol levels circulating in the blood normally. When cortisol levels are high, during a stressful situation, cortisol binds with glucocorticoid receptors (GRs). The activation of the GRs ends the stress response (Stephens & Wand, 2012).

Cortisol secretion is also affected by psychological factors. The extent of reaction to a stressor is impacted by the individual's perception, interpretation and feelings about a situation. Stress arises from uncertainty and control. That is, the less knowledge an individual has about a potentially threatening situation, the less control they experience over that situation, leading to greater levels of stress (Foy et al., 2005).

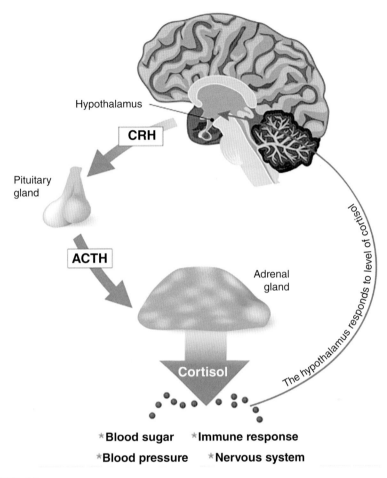

FIGURE 4.1

Adrenal stress response

Source: https://adrenalfatigue.org/what-is-stress-overdrive/

THE IMPACT OF THE STRESS RESPONSE

As a survival response, stress can be positive and assist the person to manage every-day encounters and potential dangers. When stress is at a manageable level the result is an increase in alertness and attention, increases in motivation and energy and productivity, including resourcefulness. This level of stress increases efficiency and output, whereas an absence of stress can result in lack of motivation, reduced efficiency and diminished productivity. Alternatively, when stress levels become too high our concentration and performance is impaired.

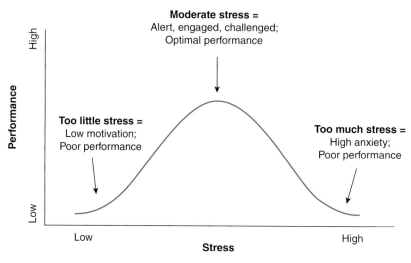

FIGURE 4.2

The Yerkes–Dodson Law

Source: Robert M. Yerkes and John D. Dodson, https://en.wikipedia.org/wiki/Yerkes-Dodson_law

The Yerkes–Dodson Law explains that there are optimal levels of stress to enhance performance.

If stress is chronic or exceeds our coping resources, the results on our health and wellbeing can be extremely damaging. Stephens and Wand (2012) identify three factors which may impact the level of cortisol an adult is exposed to: genetic background, early-childhood experiences, and current life stress. Chronic stress and its effects on the immune system increase an individual's propensity to develop a range of chronic medical ailments, including mental ill-health (Corbett, 2015). This occurs as exposure to chronic stress triggers a shift in the normal cortisol release as well as in stress-induced cortisol levels. An increase in baseline cortisol levels blunts the body's response to high levels of cortisol, and it takes longer to return to pre-stress levels. As a result, the HPA axis becomes more sensitive, leading to higher cortisol levels after each stressful event (Stephens & Wand, 2012).

Stress is unhelpful when we:
- can't switch off – feeling alert and anxious even when we want to be resting
- can't cope – even small things get us down, leave us exhausted
- withdraw from relationships, work or fun activities, or become irritable
- have difficulty concentrating
- have aches and pains unrelated to exercise or any medical condition
- have difficulty eating or sleeping properly.

Source: *https://www.lifeline.org.au/static/uploads/files/what-is-stress-wfvgiurqqawx.pdf*

CLINICAL AND BEHAVIOURAL MANIFESTATIONS OF STRESS (SIGNS AND SYMPTOMS)

There are many clinical signs and symptoms that may indicate that a patient is experiencing acute stress. An acute stress reaction can be understood as the variation of an output beyond its normal limits in response to an external stimuli or stressor. Acute stress can lead to increased heart rate, blood pressure and respiratory rate associated with the release of epinephrine and norepinephrine by the sympathetic nervous system. Cortisol release by the adrenal glands can also increase blood pressure by increasing constriction of blood vessels. When cortisol levels fall, blood vessels dilate, and hypotension occurs (Stephens & Wand, 2012). Acute stress is also associated with increases in blood sugar. Cortisol release increases blood glucose levels by promoting production of glucose molecules. It also modifies fat and protein metabolism to support the nutrient requirements of the central nervous system during stress (Stephens & Wand, 2012). The primary emotional responses to acute stress are arousal and hypervigilance. The triggering of the sympathetic nervous system readies the body for fight or flight through releasing epinephrine and norepinephrine, and the binding of cortisol with glucocorticoid receptors creates arousal. Fear responses support a range of defensive behaviours, such as freezing, fear-potentiated startle, aggression and avoidance.

People experiencing chronic stress or stress overload present with other symptoms. Amirikhan and colleagues (2018) identify a cluster of symptoms associated with stress overload. These may include body complaints, gastrointestinal disturbances, respiratory problems, moodiness, nervous habits and cognitive disruption. They surveyed people over two waves: the first wave involved completion of an on-site survey and the second wave was a follow-up survey a week later. They found that cognitive disruption was significantly associated with stress overload on both occasions. Cognitive disruption may include memory problems, loss of focus, inability to complete tasks, difficulty in making decisions, and disrupted sleep. Gastrointestinal disturbances and moodiness were significantly associated with stress overload in the first wave, and respiratory problems during follow-up. Difficulties with concentration and short-term memory arise from exposure to cortisol, which can block memory retrieval, with emotional memories most strongly affected (Roozendaal et al., 2008; Stephens & Wand, 2012). DeLongis and others (1988) found that the detrimental effects of ongoing stress on mood and body complaints is mediated by self-esteem and social support. That is, people with higher self-esteem and greater levels of social support are less likely to report negative emotions and body complaints when confronted with ongoing stress, whereas low self-esteem and limited social support leads to greater mood disturbance and more body complaints. Exposure to ongoing stress may also lead to lack of motivation. Lack of motivation may arise from depression and feelings of helplessness, but may also be adaptive. Animal studies demonstrate that exposure to extended periods of stress lead to weight loss and immobility may conserve energy (McKlveen et al., 2015).

CLINICAL AND BEHAVIOURAL MANIFESTATIONS OF STRESS

- Cardiovascular function – heart rate, BP and respiratory rate
- Lack of motivation
- Moodiness, increased or erratic emotions
- Increased irritability or frustration
- Inability to sleep or too much sleep
- Difficulty concentrating and impaired short-term memory storage
- Headaches
- Anxiousness or feeling overwhelmed
- Not coping with demands and responsibilities
- Reliance on alcohol or other substances to cope
- Increased eating, drinking or nervous habits

Source: *https://www.webmd.com/balance/stress-management/stress-symptoms-effects_of-stress-on-the-body#2*

Chronic stress and associated high cortisol levels can have an impact on mental health. Amirikhan and colleagues (2018) argue that it is important to discriminate between behaviours that arise from the stress reaction and behaviours that have been adopted as coping mechanisms for stress.

Stress is often associated with maladaptive coping mechanisms, such as avoidance behaviours, isolation and withdrawal, impaired interpersonal relationships, reduced help-seeking, excessive alcohol use, smoking, lack of exercise and poor diet (Finitsis et al. 2018). This can cause fatigue and anxiety, and leave us overwhelmed or completely burnt out. Other mental health changes arise from prolonged exposure to cortisol. Prolonged exposure to high levels of cortisol can result in structural and functional changes to the brain, such as atrophy of the hippocampal cells, reduction of the development of neural cells and interruption of synapses, which contribute to depression (Penninx, 2017).

Long-term exposure to stress can also contribute to physical ailments. Stress is associated with increased morbidity and mortality from cardiovascular disease (Sgiofo et al., 2017). It may also precipitate arrhythmias in those with pre-existing heart disease, increasing risk of cardiac arrest (Esler, 2017). Many reasons have been offered for this link. Some argue that stress triggers mental health issues, which are indirectly linked to cardiovascular disease. Penninx (2017) argues that stress contributes to depression, which is linked to cardiovascular morbidity and mortality. One mechanism may be through the adoption of unhealthy lifestyle behaviours, such as smoking, unhealthy diet and physical inactivity. Another hypothesis is that depression is associated with changes to the autonomic nervous system leading to greater sympathetic (e.g. adrenaline) release and reduced parasympathetic activity and noradrenaline release. A third mechanism may be through metabolic dysregulation. Depression has been associated with metabolic syndrome, which consists of a number of metabolic risk factors for cardiovascular disease, including abdominal obesity, hyperglycaemia, elevated blood pressure, increased triglycerides, and decreased high-density lipoprotein (HDL) cholesterol (Penninx, 2017).

Chronic stress has also been implicated in tumour growth in people diagnosed with cancer, and is correlated with poorer survival rates. One mechanism by which this occurs is through impacting the tumour's chemical environment, making it easier for tumours to metastasise. There is also evidence that stress hormones may reduce the effectiveness of chemotherapy for certain cancers, e.g. ovarian cancer. Undertaking stress-reduction techniques has been found to improve cancer outcomes. Random control studies of women with stage 0 to stage III breast cancer have found that women who received a 10-week cognitive behavioural stress-management intervention had better long-term survival rates and fewer recurrences of cancer (Finitsis et al., 2018).

CAUSES OF STRESS

Responses to stress are individual. That is, what might cause stress for one person may not cause stress for another person. Because of this, we cannot relate specific outcomes to specific types of stress (Piko, 2002). There are events, however, which are commonly known to cause stress. Early childhood experiences are a major precursor for chronic stress in adulthood. Fetal exposure to maternal stress is understood to impact later responses to stress, perhaps through altering neural circuits controlling neuroendocrine responses (Shonkoff et al., 2012). Adverse early childhood events such as child abuse, parental neglect, parental substance abuse, sexual abuse and maternal depression, and their associated stress for the child, are believed to impact the developing brain and metabolic systems, making that person more susceptible to stress in adulthood. Shonkoff and colleagues (2012) associate chronic stress with hypertrophy of the amygdala and loss of neurons and neural connections in the hippocampus. These changes, in turn, impair stress regulation, and the capacity to learn new skills and to adjust to adversity.

Work has also been identified as a major source of stress. Many features of the modern workplace, such as the casualisation of the workforce, increasing work demands, and new managerial techniques, all contribute to workplace stress (Wainright & Calnan, 2002). Workplace restructuring is also a major source of stress. Koukoulaki and others (2017) surveyed 1592 Greek employees in workplaces that were being restructured. They found that restructuring led to work intensification, job insecurity and greater emotional demands, all of which were associated with stress and emotional exhaustion. Other factors which have been identified as contributing to workplace stress include: being unhappy in your job; too much responsibility; working long hours; poor management and unclear work expectations; dangerous work conditions; and workplace bullying (WebMD, 2020). Consider the experiences of Josie in the case study at the beginning of the chapter. What aspects of Josie's workplace might contribute to her stress?

Grief and loss are also important sources of stress. Grief is a natural response to losing someone or something that is important to you. It can be a result of bereavement, but may also occur at the end of a relationship, or with job loss, chronic illness, or shifting home among other things. Dutch researchers studied the impact of bereavement on prolonged grief and post-traumatic stress disorder (PTSD). They found the respondents were more likely to experience prolonged grief and PTSD after loss of a child, loss of a partner or when the loss was due to violence. People with fewer years of education were also likely to experience more symptoms of prolonged grief and PTSD (Djelantik et al., 2017).

Stress may be associated with other life changes. Market research of 27,000 people in 22 countries in 2015 found that the five most commonly identified sources of stress were not having enough money (29%), pressure that people put upon themselves (27%), not getting enough sleep (23%), not having time for the things they want to do (22%), and workload (19%). Answers vary by age, with respondents under 30 placing greater emphasis on personal pressure, and those over 30 worrying more about finances. Health and workload became a greater concern with age, while those over 50 cite caring responsibilities as a source of stress (Canada News-Wire, 2015). Given the impact of life changes and events on stress, it is important to collect information about a patient's life history as part of an assessment of a patient demonstrating symptoms of stress.

LIFE EXPERIENCES THAT CONTRIBUTE TO STRESS RESPONSES

- Interpersonal relationship problems
- Personal or family illness
- Conflict, e.g. bullying, harassment
- Work pressures
- Traumatic events
- Financial problems
- Concerns about life direction
- Job loss
- Pressures from competing demands or a combination of the above

Source: *https://www.lifeline.org.au/static/uploads/files/overcoming-stress-wfrisntobpbj.pdf*

There are also populations at greater risk of experiencing chronic stress. The social determinants of health may moderate chronic stress contributing to poor physical and mental health outcomes. Socio-economic status has been tied to cardiovascular disease associated with chronic stress. There is a gradient of higher cardiovascular risk in those with lower social status, which Brunner (2017) argues can be associated with greater adoption of unhealthy lifestyles. There is also evidence that the health impact of exposure to chronic stress is greater for those populations who may be more vulnerable to the social and environmental factors (see above) that lead to chronic stress (Hébert et al., 2015). Hébert and colleagues (2015) argue that socially disadvantaged groups may have greater exposure to events beyond their control, such as financial problems and job losses, and may also adopt unhealthy behaviours, such as smoking, alcohol and drug abuse, poor diet/over-eating, and sedentary behaviour as coping mechanisms.

There are gender differences in the experience of chronic stress as well; however, there may be a biological component in these differences. Vaccario and Bremner (2017) argue that women may experience greater exposure to childhood trauma in the form of emotional, physical and sexual abuse, which can contribute to chronic stress. They also report higher rates of depression and anxiety. Exposure to childhood trauma can lead to stress-related neurobiological differences between men and women. Exposure to early life stress with associated depression can contribute to increased cortisol levels and/or blunted ACTH response to CRF. Men may experience greater cortisol release in relation to achievements, while women experience greater cortisol release associated with social rejection (Vaccario & Bremner, 2017). Gender differences in memory related to stress are also evident. Levels of the female hormone oestrogen can impact memory storage and capacity to learn in women experiencing stress, with higher oestrogen levels associated with improved memory storage and learning capacity (Foy et al., 2005).

Adolescence is also a time that has been associated with greater receptivity to stress. Romeo (2017) states that animal studies demonstrate that the adolescent brain is more receptive to glucocorticoids such as cortisol, and that adolescents experience prolonged hormonal responses to stress. Further, the amygdala is developing during adolescence, which may increase susceptibility to stress.

PARAMEDIC STRESS AND CARE OF 'SELF'

There is growing awareness that paramedics experience workplace stress related to the nature of their work. A recent review by Petrie and colleagues (2018) of 27 international studies which reported on 30,878 ambulance personnel, found estimated prevalence rates of 11% for post-traumatic stress injury (PTSI) and post-traumatic stress disorder (PTSD), 15% for depression, 15% for anxiety, and 27% for general psychological distress among ambulance personnel. Stress may have a negative impact on patient care because it reduces attention and decision-making skills, and may impair ability to connect with patients (Rudaz et al., 2017). A submission by Safe Work SA to the Australian Parliament Senate Inquiry into the high rates of mental health conditions experienced by first-responders, emergency service workers and volunteers stated that approximately 10% of claims from first-responders in the five years from 2011–12 to 2015–16 were for serious mental health issues, resulting in approximately 26 to 27 weeks off work (Safe Work Australia, 2020).

Factors that have been identified as contributing to stress in paramedics include: exposure to critical incidents (traumatic events that lead to emotional states that disrupt work performance) (Wiitavaaraa et al., 2007); the threat of violence and workplace bullying (Mayhew & Chappell, 2007); job demands; and the meeting of organisational expectations (Clompus & Albarran, 2016). Attending a 'scene' and the unpredictable nature of the pre-hospital environment also leads to stress for paramedics (Kleim & Westphal, 2011), as does repeated exposure to trauma (Walker et al., 2016).

Support for mental health can be obtained through the workplace. Most Australian states have work health and safety legislation which requires workplaces to protect employees from psychological risks (Safe Work Australia, 2020). One strategy is a formal peer-support program. Peer support is defined as 'a formal organisational structure through which trained colleagues offer support after a critical incident' (Gouweloos-Trines et al., 2017, p. 816). It provides a method of identifying and monitoring workers at risk of psychological problems. This approach is not without problems. Gouweloos-Trines and colleagues (2017), in a survey of pre-hospital service providers in eight industrialised nations, found that almost 40% of respondents were unaware that their service offered formal peer support. Secondly, workplace relations may prevent the sharing of information. Thirdly, what is identified as a critical incident by support services may not tally with individual experience. For example, bullying may be experienced as more detrimental than attending an accident scene. A second mechanism for workplace support is an Employee Assistance Program (EAP) which is a work-based intervention program designed to enhance the emotional, mental and general psychological wellbeing of employees. EAPs address workplace issues, but also personal problems that may impact work performance. The aim is to provide preventive and early detection services (Employee Assistance Professional Association of Australasia, 2009). Alternatively, support can be sought from a mental health website offering information about stress management. A list of recommended sites is provided at the end of this chapter.

Self-care strategies can be used to manage stress. Self-care has been defined as 'the practice of activities that individuals initiate and perform on their own behalf in maintaining life, health and well-being' (Grafton & Coyne, 2012, p. 19). Self-care is a conscious act undertaken to improve physical, mental and emotional health. Wise and colleagues (2012) identify four principles underpinning self-care. The first is to work towards flourishing rather than survival, as a focus on survival may involve preventing negative outcomes rather than promoting positive outcomes. A second principle is intentionality and a willingness to change approach and behaviours if they become unworkable. A third principle is reciprocity and willingness to share effective strategies. The fourth principle is integration. This principle recognises that changes are more likely to be made if they are integrated into current life rather than added to an already busy schedule.

Grafton and Coyne (2012) view self-awareness as a valuable component of self-care. Self-awareness allows people to reflect on their actions rather than acting on impulse and without thought to consequences. One strategy to improve self-awareness is mindfulness. Mindfulness can be defined as 'the quality of being present and fully engaged with whatever we're doing at the moment — free from distraction or judgment, and aware of our thoughts and feelings without getting caught up in them' (headspace 2020). Rudaz and others (2017) identify four components of mindfulness: (1) observation, which involves noticing internal and external experiences; (2) description or identification of the observed experiences; (3) purposeful action; and (4) acceptance of experiences without judgment.

Meditation is one means of increasing mindfulness. Strategies to increase mind-fulness during meditation include: focused attention, e.g. concentrating on your breathing to prevent your mind wandering; scanning your body from head to toe to identify discomfort or aches which may arise from stress; noting thoughts and feeling arising during meditation; focusing on the image of, and sending well wishes to, other people; focusing on a person you know, and paying attention to the sensations that arise; visualising an image that assists relaxation; allowing thoughts to arise and leave your mind; and focusing on a particular question and observing the thoughts and feelings that arise (headspace, 2020). Other self-care activities may involve: getting adequate sleep, a healthy diet and regular activity; face-to-face time with friends; activities to keep your mind engaged; positive self-talk; sharing problems; and establishing time for leisure activities (see Fig. 4.3).

REFLECTION

In our case study we were introduced to Josie, a paramedic experiencing chronic and acute stress. What strategies could Josie adopt to manage her stress?

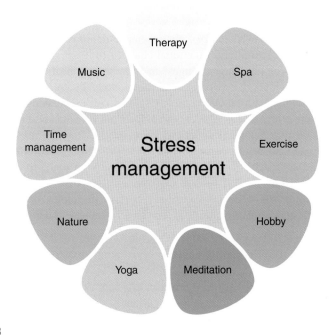

FIGURE 4.3

Stress management strategies

SELF-CARE ACTIVITIES FOR STRESS MANAGEMENT

- Exercise
- Guided imagery and meditation
- Progressive muscle relaxation
- Deep breathing
- Aromatherapy
- Creating artwork
- Eating a balanced diet
- Undertaking hobbies and leisure activities
- Positive self-talk
- Yoga
- Practising gratitude
- Reassessing your commitments
- Social support
- Removing things that create stress from your life
- Practising mindfulness

Source: *https://www.verywellmind.com/tips-to-reduce-stress-3145195*

MANAGEMENT OF STRESS: TRAUMA-INFORMED CARE

A trauma-informed care approach is recommended when caring for patients who are experiencing stress. As a concept, trauma-informed care (TIC) can be understood as both a philosophy of care and a set of guiding principles to inform clinical practice (Hamberger et al., 2019). Neuroscience demonstrates that exposure to trauma can lead to structural and functional changes to the brain that contribute to (mal)adaptive behaviours. These changes, in turn, may contribute to a cluster of symptoms and behaviours that impair social functioning. TIC recognises and makes allowances for the behavioural and neurological changes associated with trauma. It acknowledges the effect that negative experiences and previous and current social, interpersonal and psychological situations have on the way we respond and our neuropathology (Evans & Coccoma, 2014). This involves a paradigm shift from a pathology-based approach focused on 'What is wrong with you?' to one that asks, 'What has happened to you?' (Evans & Coccoma, 2014, p. 2).

In 2005, Elliott and colleagues outlined 10 key principles of TIC to guide the development and implementation of services in the healthcare setting. These include:

1. understanding the relationship between prior trauma experiences and present coping
2. identifying trauma recovery as a priority
3. designing interactions to empower the patient
4. providing the patient with options and choices
5. working collaboratively with the patient
6. creating an atmosphere of respect, safety and acceptance

7. emphasising patient strengths
8. working to minimise re-traumatisation
9. striving to be culturally competent and culturally humble
10. seeking consumer input in designing and evaluating services.

The principles of TIC are essential when clinicians interact with those they are caring for. For paramedics, the principles are key to how you approach and engage with all patients, but especially need to be recognised when dealing with those experiencing mental illness.

The application and implementation of TIC requires paramedics to recognise that everyone they attend may have experience with past trauma which has influenced how they perceive themselves, those around them, their circumstances, and how they have experienced previous interaction with the health system (particularly the mental health system). The individual's previous experience is going to be the lens through which they see paramedics and other health professionals. Past trauma leaves its mark in the way the brain develops and how the person responds to stress, which in turn, creates a challenge for how paramedics interpret and respond to a person's behaviour, the circumstances and whether the person is acting as 'expected' and is considered 'reasonable'.

Although paramedics may have only a brief time with the patient, if we approach every patient with the assumption that there is the potential of a history of past trauma, and a sense of loss or grief, we can then model our actions as a clinician so that not re-traumatising the person is our primary goal. For example, when attending a person who is displaying signs and symptoms of anxiety with increased sympathetic response, hypervigilance and hyper startle response, you would be conscious of your tone of voice (soft and clear), having small body movements with a slow approach and adopting an open non-threatening stance. The approach would require continual brief explanations of what you are doing and what is coming next, and gaining consent with each action. To include trauma-informed care, you would acknowledge and come from a stance that this individual has a past history and current circumstances that have led to their current behaviour and physiological response. You may not find out about the cause initially, but you can interact with the knowledge that this person may find encroachment in personal space, touch, sounds and new people and environments re-traumatising and uncomfortable. In approaching care, you would empower and collaborate with the patient by allowing them to dictate the pace of the interaction, the level of touch and when, through communicating to find out what has helped them in the past to manage and cope, and how you can best assist them reinstate positive coping mechanisms.

PRIORITIES OF CARE DURING STRESSFUL SITUATIONS
Scene awareness

1. **Scene awareness** as an observation, and assessment of risk and safety, is only part of the story. We approach the scene with potential hazards in mind and an

assessment of physical risk and safety, but we also need to observe, watch and assess how the individual interacts with others and their environment. The social control and reaction to space, and the dynamics that clinicians are walking in to, tell you vital information about how the individual may see themselves, those around them, their environment, and how they have constructed their interpersonal relationships. As we approach, we can watch family dynamics, and how the person is coping with their environment and those around them, from what they say, how they say it and how they react to what is around them. Paramedics often unconsciously watch and make assessments of 'what is going on' at a scene and then make a plan on how to proceed. Implementing a systematic way of observing and cataloguing behaviour (e.g. the mental state examination and initial assessment of behaviour) assists with not only an evaluation of risk, but allows us to assess whether there is past trauma that potentially influences their circumstances and behaviour. Recognition of past trauma reinforces skills to approach with compassion and empathy, and focuses all actions on the person's strengths, and the patient as collaborator and as inherently involved in their health decisions. It moves the clinician's role from directing the decisions to one of advocacy and education.

2. **Scene management** involves both physical and social management by paramedics. Physical scene management may involve removing hazards, clearing entry and egress around and from the scene, management of equipment, etc. Paramedics manage the scene socially by engaging family and bystanders as well as the patient; they will be aware of how a crowd is behaving and assess whether support is required. Social control also comes in the form of managing your own response and emotions to a given situation, e.g. remaining calm to assist a family member who is upset due to circumstances, or managing friends who want to help the patient but are actually making the provision of much-needed care more difficult. To manage these situations requires skills in communication (which were discussed in Chapter 3), and the recognition of how you respond and react in a given situation, and self-awareness of how you are coping emotionally and how that affects your ability to make clinical decisions.

Preparing and providing information

Another important aspect to our understanding of stress and the stress response is how it affects the way we process information. As outlined earlier in the chapter, stress affects how memories and information are retrieved, slows the ability to make decisions, and influences how we interpret sensory information. The delay and changes in perception and interpretation of information and sensory input means that we have to adapt the way we prepare for and provide information to our patients. When coming from a patient- or person-centred approach, we need to be aware of what we say, how we say it, and how it might be interpreted by the patient.

The information we provide needs to be relatable and understandable for the patient. This sounds obvious, but in practice, when someone is stressed, being able to gauge how they are receiving, processing and then using the information we provide may be challenging. In the case study, for example:

> *'Josie finds that she is unable to sleep through the night. She has trouble concentrating and is short-tempered with her children. She is becoming socially isolated and is drinking more in the evening. She is also starting to make excuses to call in sick for work.'*

All of these experiences will affect how Josie will manage complex information, as she needs to make decisions not only at work but in dealing with everyday circumstances. As outlined by Johansson and others (2009), mental fatigue is characterised 'by mental exhaustion and increased time needed for recovery following prolonged cognitive activity'. Studies have shown that increased mental fatigue alongside impaired performance with executive functioning and complex attention to tasks occur when prolonged stress is involved (Krabbe et al., 2017). The fatigue that stress induces creates slower recognition of changing environments, reduces the ability of the person to adapt, and decreases the person's tolerance to change. To mitigate the effects of fatigue and stress in our patients, we need to pace our information-sharing so that the person has time to process the information. The amount of information provided at one time needs to be modified to allow for the reduced capacity to process larger amounts of information. The information also needs to be provided in a concise, clear manner.

PROMOTING COMMUNICATION WITH PEOPLE EXPERIENCING STRESS

Do's

1. Observe how the person in stress responds to others and their environment.
2. Approach with open and inclusive body language.
3. Decrease environmental stimulus (make the environment feel safe for the person).
4. Take time to introduce yourself and explain why you are there.
5. Take time to allow the person to respond.
6. Try and decrease the 'cognitive load' for the person:
   a. Employ a measured tone and small body movements.
   b. Focus on one topic or task at a time with them.
   c. Slowly introduce questions and take time with history taking.
   d. Answer questions as simply as you can with minimal jargon or medical terminology.
   e. Construct all information in small sections so you are providing one bit of information at a time, especially if the information is complex – 'break it down!'
   f. Keep engaging the person, and realise they will be mentally fatigued so processing of information will take time.
   g. Be collaborative with decision making. Offer options, but only a few at a time so the person can understand and is not overwhelmed by the amount of options or decisions to be made. You might need to reiterate and repeat options and information.
   h. Don't get frustrated if they take time to process the information or make decisions.
   i. Gently 'ground' the person to the present – remind them of what they have said, acknowledge the emotions, and paraphrase what they are currently experiencing.

    j. Be aware of the effect of past experience – the concept of trauma-informed care. They may feel emotionally fragile and, hence, tolerance levels and irritability will increase.

    k. Keep calm, listen and watch.

Don'ts

1. Do not rush the person.
2. Do not overwhelm the person.
3. Do not override and try and dictate decisions for the person.
4. Do not discount the effect of past and current experience.
5. Do not create unnecessary sensory overload.

Accessing and engaging support networks

One of the challenges with chronic stress and the stress response is how it deceases the person's ability to engage with others. Electroencephalography (EEG) and neuro-imaging techniques demonstrate the increased activation of brain regions, i.e. the amygdala and medial PFC (pre-frontal cortex), which tend towards a negative formation of experience and emotions (Williams et al., 2009). Although studies have shown that acute stress has been associated with increased initial trust, sharing and prosocial behaviours (e.g. the relief and initial trust shown to paramedics when they arrive on scene), these behaviours change when stress becomes more chronic in nature or if the initial trust is broken (Vinkers et al., 2013). Typical patient experiences or history gained from others will recount deficits in social functioning, behaviours such as decreased motivation and willingness to socialise, social anxiety and avoidance, and high levels of anger, hostility or irritability and potential for violence. In the case study, the history of Josie increasingly socially isolating herself, and her increasing use of alcohol, increasing intolerance and shorter temper all point to the effect stress is having on her social functioning and her interpersonal life.

As paramedics, gathering the story of how the person has been functioning socially and interpersonally from the person themselves or from significant others allows you to tailor your approach and response to the individual. For example, as Josie has been increasingly withdrawing from social life, she has potentially lost an important part of her support network from family and friends. The effect of this loss of support might mean that your approach needs to consider:

a. her possible need for personal space

b. that her feelings of isolation may decrease her willingness to have you provide care and she may dismiss your attempts to build a rapport

c. that her withdrawal may influence how responsive she is to your questions

d. discussion of her increasing isolation may be a difficult topic for her to talk about, so she may become defensive to protect her own sense of self and her emotions.

In this case, how would we manage the sense of withdrawal and increasing loss of social functioning? A gentle approach with genuine interest in her story and not forcing questions conveys a willingness to listen and respect for her personal space. Start with finding 'common ground' or subjects of common interest with the person (non-threatening subjects are often easily observed when you enter their environment, e.g. local footy team, music, children, photographs). In this case, Josie allows you to gain trust before any challenging subjects are raised. Be aware that the person may be defensive and not answer your questions initially, but take time to gain their trust and focus on tasks or simple introductions and do not take any defensive behaviour personally. The person is trying to protect themselves and their emotions, and if you acknowledge that this is a normal response when someone loses their motivation for social and personal interaction with others, then as a clinician you will be less likely to lose patience with the person and be conscious of how you interpret what they say and how they say it.

One challenge you may face if you have gained information around the person's social and personal life from others is that the person may experience this as an invasion of their privacy. In this case, ask permission prior to talking to others if the situation allows, and be honest and assure the person you want to hear their story. Also, listen carefully to how they view themselves and their experience.

CONCLUSION

This chapter has outlined the physiology, causes and behavioural and clinical manifestations of stress. These may include increased cardiovascular function, hypervigilance, poor concentration, withdrawal, irritability, lack of motivation and the adoption of behaviours that may impair health, e.g. excessive alcohol use, use of other substances, poor diet, smoking. These behaviours may, in turn, impair physical and mental health. Many or all of these behaviours may be on display when a paramedic attends a scene in which the patient is experiencing stress. This chapter has promoted adopting trauma-informed care. Trauma-informed care recognises the psychological and physical impacts of negative experiences on the manner in which the patient reacts to the paramedic. This requires sensitivity to previous trauma and a willingness to negotiate interpersonal relationships with the patient, working with that person to establish and meet mutual goals. The chapter also recognises the impact of occupational stress on the paramedic and outlines strategies for self-care which may be used by the health professional or with patients.

LINKS AND RESOURCES

Lifeline's stress awareness and management tool kit: https://www.lifeline.org.au/static/uploads/files/overcoming-stress-wfrisntobpbj.pdf

Beyond Blue: https://www.beyondblue.org.au/home

Stressed about study during coronavirus? (resources for younger people): https://au.reachout.com/collections/stressed-about-study-during-coronavirus

Coping with Stress Course (free online course for stress management): https://thiswayup.org.au/courses/coping-with-stress-course/

2-Minute Neuroscience: HPA Axis (brief YouTube clip explaining the HPA Axis): https://www.youtube.com/watch?v=QAeBKRaNri0&vl=en

Understanding the stress response (Harvard Medical School): https://www.health.harvard.edu/staying-healthy/understanding-the-stress-response

Understanding Agitation: De-escalation (YouTube simulation for de-escalating stress): https://www.youtube.com/watch?v=6B9Kqg6jFeI

What is mindfulness? (headspace): https://www.headspace.com/mindfulness

REFERENCES

Amirikhan, J., Landa, I., Huff, S., 2018. Seeking signs of stress overload: symptoms and behaviors. Int. J. Stress Manag. 25 (3), 301–311.

Brunner, E.J., 2017. Social factors and cardiovascular morbidity. Neurosci. Biobehav. Rev. 74, 260–268

Canada NewsWire. 2015. Money and Self-Pressure are the Leading Major Causes of Stress Internationally. GfK, Nuremberg.

Clompus, S., Albarran, J., 2016. Exploring the nature of resilience in paramedic practice: a psycho-social study. Int. Emerg. Nurs. 28, 1–7.

Corbett, M., 2015. From law to folklore: work stress and the Yerkes–Dodson Law. J. Manag. Psychol. 30 (6), 741–752.

DeLongis, A., Folkman. S., Lazarus, R., 1988. The impact of daily stress on health and mood: psychological and social resources as mediators. J. Pers. Soc. Psychol. 54 (3), 486–495.

Djelantik, M., Smid, G., Kieber, R., Boelen, P. 2017. Symptoms of prolonged grief, post-traumatic stress, and depression after loss in a Dutch community sample: a latent class analysis. Pyschiatry Res. 247, 276–281.

Elliott, D.E., Bjelajac, P., Fallott, R.D., et al., 2005. Trauma-informed or trauma-denied: principles and implementation of trauma-informed services for women. J. Community Psychol. 33 (4), 461–477.

Employee Assistance Professional Association of Australasia, 2009. What is an employee assistance program? Online. Available: https://www.eapaa.org.au/site/.

Esler, M., 2017. Mental stress and human cardiovascular disease. Neurosci. Biobehav. Rev. 74, 267–276. http://dx.doi.org/10.1016/j.neubiorev.2016.10.011, pii: S0149-7634(16)30165-8.

Evans, A., Coccoma. P., 2014. Understanding trauma informed care. In: Evans, A., Coccoma, P. (Eds.), Trauma-Informed Care: How neuroscience influences practice. Taylor & Francis Group, ProQuest Ebook Central. http://ebookcentral.proquest.com/lib/flinders/detail.action?docID=1596855.

Faraday, M. 2006. Stress revisited: a methodological and conceptual history. In Yehuda, S., Mostofsky, D. (Eds.), Nutrients, Stress, and Medical Disorders Humana Press, Totowa, NJ, pp. 3–19.

Finitsis, D.J., Dornelas, E., Galleghar, J., Janis, H., 2018. Reducing stress to improve health. In Hilliard, M., Riekert, K., Ockene, J., Pbert, L. (Eds.), The Handbook of Health Behavior Change. Springer Publishing Company, New York, pp. 243–264.

Folkman, S., Lazarus, R., Dunkel-Schetter, C., et al., 1986. Dynamics of a stressful encounter: cognitive appraisal, coping, and encounter outcomes. J. Pers. Soc. Psychol. 50 (5), 992–1003.

Foy, M., Kim, J., Shors, T., Thompson, R. 2005. Neurobiological foundations of stress. In Yehuda, S., Mostofsky, D. (Eds.), Nutrients, Stress, and Medical Disorders Humana Press, Totowa, NJ, pp. 37–65.

Gouweloos-Trines, J., Tyler, M., Giummarra, M., et al., 2017. Perceived support at work after critical incidents and its relation to psychological distress: a survey among prehospital providers. Emerg. Med. J. 34 (12), 816–822.

Grafton, E., Coyne, E., 2012. Practical self-care and stress management for oncology nurses. Aust. J. Cancer Nurs. 13 (2), 17–20.

Hamberger, L.K., Barry, C., Franco, Z., 2019. Implementing trauma-informed care in primary medical settings: evidence-based rationale and approaches. J. Aggress. Maltreat. Trauma 28 (4), 425–444.

headspace, 2020. What is mindfulness? Online. Available: https://www.headspace.com/mindfulness.

Hébert, J., Braun, K., Keawe'aimoku Kaholokula, J., et al., 2015. Considering the role of stress in populations of high-risk, underserved community networks program centers. Prog. Community Health Partnersh. 9 (0), 71–82.

Johansson, B., Berglund, P., Ronnback, L., 2009. Mental fatigue and impaired information processing after mild and moderate traumatic brain injury. Brain Inj. 23 (13–14), 1027–1040.

Kleim, B., Westphal, M., 2011. Mental health in ESFR: a review and recommendation for prevention and intervention strategies. Traumatology 17 (4), 17–24.

Koukoulaki, T., Pinotsi, D., Georgiadou, P., et al., 2017. Restructuring seriously damages well-being of workers: the case of the restructuring programme in local administration in Greece. Saf. Sci. 100, 30–36.

Krabbe, D., Ellbin, S., Nilsson, M., et al., 2017. Executive function and attention in patients with stress-related exhaustion: perceived fatigue and effect of distraction. Stress, 20 (4), 333–340.

Lazarus, R. S., Folkman, S., 1984. Stress, Appraisal, and Coping. Springer, New York.

Martini, F.H., Nath, J., Bartholomew, E., 2015. The endocrine system. In Martini, F.H., Nath, J., Bartholomew, E. (Eds.), Fundamentals of Anatomy and Physiology. Pearson Education, London, pp. 656–701.

Mayhew, C., Chappell, D., 2007. Ambulance officers: the impact of exposure to occupational violence on mental and physical health. J. Occup. Health Saf. Aust. N. Z. 25 (1), 37.

McKlveen, J., Myers, B., Herman, J., 2015. The medial prefrontal cortex: coordinator of autonomic, neuroendocrine and behavioural responses to stress. J. Neuroendocrinol. 27 (6), 446–456.

Penninx, B.W., 2017. Depression and cardiovascular disease: epidemiological evidence on their linking mechanisms. Neurosci. Biobehav. Rev. 74, 277–286.

Petrie, K., Milligan-Saville, J., Gayed, A., et al., 2018. Prevalence of PTSD and common mental disorders amongst ambulance personnel: a systematic review and meta-analysis. Soc. Psychiatry Psychiatr. Epidemiol. 53 (9), 897–909.

Piko, B., 2002. Socio-cultural stress in modern societies and the myth of anxiety in Eastern Europe. Adm. Policy Ment Health 29 (3), 275–280.

Romeo, R., 2017. The impact of stress on the structure of the adolescent brain: implications for adolescent mental health. Brain Res. 1654, 185–191.

Roozendaal, B., Barsegyan, A., Lee, S., 2008. Adrenal stress hormones, amygdala activation, and memory for emotionally arousing experiences. Prog. Brain Res. 167, 79–97.

Rudaz, M., Twohig, M., Ong, C., Levin, M., 2017. Mindfulness and acceptance-based trainings for fostering self-care and reducing stress in mental health professionals: a systematic review. J. Contextual Behav. Sci. 6 (4), 380–390.

Safe Work Australia, 2020. Mental health. Online. Available: https://www.safeworkaustralia.gov.au/topic/mental-health.

Selye, H., 1956. The Stress of Life. McGraw Hill, New York.

Sgiofo, A., Montano, N., Esler, M., Vaccarino, V. 2017. Stress, behavior and the heart. Neurosci. Biobehav. Rev. 74, 257–259.

Shonkoff, J., Garner, A., Dobbins, M., et al., 2012. The lifelong effects of early childhood adversity and toxic stress. Pediatrics 129, e232.

Stephens, M.A.C., Wand, G., 2012. Stress and the HPA axis: role of glucocorticoids in alcohol dependence. Alcohol Res. 34 (4), 468–483.

Vaccario, V., Bremner, J.D., 2017. Behavioral, emotional and neurobiological determinants of coronary heart disease risk in women. Neurosci. Biobehav. Rev. 74, 297–309.

Vinkers, C.H., Zorn, J.V., Cornelisse, S., et al., 2013. Time-dependent changes in altruistic punishment following stress. Psychoneuroendocrinology 38 (9), 1467–1475.

Wainright, D., Calnan, M., 2002. Work Stress: The making of a modern epidemic. Open University Press, Buckingham.

Walker, A., McKune, A., Ferguson, S., et al., 2016. Chronic occupational exposures can influence the rate of PTSD and depressive disorders in ESFR and military personnel. Extreme Physiol. Med. 5, 8.

WebMD, 2020. Causes of stress. Online. Available: https://www.webmd.com/balance/guide/causes-of-stress#1.

Wiitavaaraa, B., Lundmana, B., Barnekow-Bergkvist, M., Brulin, C. 2007. Striking a balance—health experiences of male ambulance personnel with musculoskeletal symptoms: a grounded theory. Int. J. Nurs. Stud. 44 (8), 770–779.

Williams, L.M., Gatt, J.M., Schofield, P.R., et al., 2009. 'Negativity bias' in risk for depression and anxiety: brain-body fear circuitry correlates, 5-HTT-LPR and early life stress. Neuroimage 47 (3), 804–814.

Wise, E., Hersh, M., Gibson, C., 2012. Ethics, self-care and well-being for psychologists: re-envisioning the stress-distress continuum. Prof. Psychol. Res. Pr. 43 (5), 487–494.

Assessment: history taking and the mental state examination

Blair Hobbs

LEARNING OUTCOMES

By the end of this chapter, you should be able to:

* understand the components of a comprehensive biopsychosocial assessment
* understand the components of a mental state examination
* recognise characteristic symptoms of mental illness
* recognise the relationship between mental state and risk
* begin to identify factors influencing risk and safety
* develop an understanding of urgency of care.

INTRODUCTION

Paramedics encounter individuals with complicated biopsychosocial issues on a daily basis. Conducting a mental health assessment may be viewed as time-consuming and complicated. However, with increasing demand for ambulance services by people experiencing mental health problems there is an obvious expectation that paramedics are appropriately skilled and trained to conduct a mental health assessment. Furthermore, the overlap between medical and psychiatric symptoms is often difficult to assess or understand. Under time constraints, pressures of competing demands, and responding to individuals in distress, the paramedic is expected to make an accurate and skilled assessment of a person's physical and mental state. Assessment of risk, making complex decisions based on urgency, and often in an unpredictable environment, add to the challenge of paramedic work. Paramedics are in the position of often being a first responder to a mental health crisis, and have the opportunity to assess people in their own environment, perhaps during the worst moments of their lives. Paramedics are perfectly placed to observe the scene and assess relevant contributing or consequential factors. Potentially paramedics need to contend with highly distressed patients, as well as with families or bystanders who are emotionally distraught.

Other emergency-based assessments tend to focus only on symptoms and problems, whereas the mental health assessment needs to consider all of the biopsychosocial aspects of a person, including an assessment of strengths and supports. Traditional psychiatric models of care, often paternalistic in their approach with the aim primarily at alleviating symptoms, have partly made way in recent years for recovery-orientated models of care. Recovery-orientated approaches promote self-advocacy, empowerment of individuals to make decisions about their treatment, and a collaborative approach to identify desired health outcomes. Increasingly, advanced care directives or statements are becoming a relevant consideration in decisions about treatment. Delivery of mental health services has been geared towards community-based models, and (with varying success) to rely less on bed-based hospital resources. Given the challenges with access to in-patient beds, and the focus on community-based care, emergency department (ED) clinicians have a reasonable expectation that paramedics demonstrate sound decision making when bringing patients to hospital.

Growing demand and pressures on EDs, in conjunction with improved legislation and protection of human rights, means that paramedics need to be judicious and considered in their decision making, particularly when transporting someone who is resistive to going to hospital or who may be at risk. Bearing all of this in mind, conducting a mental health assessment in an effective and safe manner within appropriate ethical and legal parameters is a challenging aspect of paramedic work.

WHAT IS A MENTAL HEALTH ASSESSMENT AND WHY DO WE DO IT?

Mental health assessment forms the foundation of clinical practice in hospital and pre-hospital settings. Conducting an assessment serves to identify the presence of a possible mental illness, any potential dangers or risks, and the urgency of care required. Decisions about patient care, including whether to transport a person to the ED, is based on the outcome of the assessment. Non-psychiatric clinicians often feel overwhelmed or out of their depth when undertaking mental health assessments. Having a lack of confidence and knowledge gap in understanding mental illness can be a barrier to the effective assessment and treatment of people experiencing these problems. Developing the competency and capability to effectively elicit the signs and symptoms of mental illness and psychiatric-related risks is therefore imperative to paramedic work.

The goal of a mental health assessment for the paramedic is not to definitively diagnose a mental illness. However, it is reasonable to expect you are familiar with common mental health presentations, can identify the presence of possible mental illness, and are able to formulate differential diagnoses. The paramedic must be vigilant of any risks that may be associated with the person's mental state, and the degree of urgency for the person to access help. Determining the urgency of more expert care or transportation to an ED can by guided via the descriptors in the Mental Health Triage Tool (see Table 5.1).

Table 5.1 Mental Health Triage Tool

Triage Code	Description	Presentation	Management
1	Definite danger to life (self or others) Severe behavioural disturbance with immediate risk of violence	**Observed** • Violent behaviour • Possession of a weapon • Extreme agitation (psychomotor movement) or restlessness • Bizarre/disorientated behaviour **Reported** • Recent violent behaviour • Command hallucinations to harm self or others and person unable to resist	**Supervision** • Continuous visual observation **Action** • Call for support (police, clinical support, duress alarm) • Use planned exits • Notify Operational Communications for support • Provide safe environment for person, colleagues, others • Notify ED triage • Medication **Consider** • Potential causes, comorbidities, intoxication • Use of Mental Health Act • Physical and mechanical restraint, but only as a last resort
2	Probable risk to self or others AND/OR Is already physically restrained by police AND/OR Severe behavioural disturbance or threats of violence	**Observed** • Extreme agitation/restlessness • Physically/verbally aggressive • Confused/unable to cooperate • Hallucinations/delusions/paranoia • Requires containment • High risk AND likely to not remain/cooperate for treatment **Reported** • Attempt/threat of self-harm • Threats to others • Unable/unwilling to wait	**Supervision** • Continuous visual observation **Action** • Call for support (police, clinical support) • Notify Operational Communications support • Provide safe environment for person, colleagues, others • Attempt to de-escalate the situation • Medication **Consider** • Potential causes, comorbidities, intoxication • Use of sedation • Use of Mental Health Act • Physical and mechanical restraint only as a last resort

Continued

Table 5.1 Mental Health Triage Tool *continued*

Triage Code	Description	Presentation	Management
3	Possible danger to self or others Moderate behavioural disturbance Severe distress	**Observed** • Agitation/restlessness • Intrusive behaviour • Confused • Hallucinations/delusions/paranoia • Ambivalence about treatment • Drug and/or alcohol intoxication • Not likely to remain/cooperate for treatment **Reported** • Suicidal ideation • Situational crisis • Unable/unwilling to wait • Psychotic symptoms: hallucinations, delusions, paranoia, thought disorder, bizarre thoughts/behaviour • Mood disturbance: severe symptoms of depression, withdrawn, uncommunicative, elevated or irritable mood, highly anxious or distressed	**Supervision** • Close observation **Action** • Provide safe environment for person, colleagues, others • Decrease stimulation and engage de-escalation and communication techniques • Provide or arrange support (e.g. carers) **Consider** • Re-triage if increasing risk, distress, aggression • Existing support structures • Medication
4	Semi-urgent mental health problem No immediate risk to self or others May have supports present	**Observed** • No agitation/restlessness • Irritable without aggression • Cooperative • Coherent • Not intoxicated **Reported** • Pre-existing mental illness • Situational crisis • Willing to follow direction, wait, get treatment	**Supervision** • Follow operational safety structures **Action** • Provide safe environment for person, colleagues, others • Decrease stimulation • Provide or arrange support (e.g. carers) **Consider** May not require hospital transfer, consider alternatives: • Remain at home with support

Table 5.1 Mental Health Triage Tool *continued*

Triage Code	Description	Presentation	Management
			• Referral to community mental health team, GP or other service • Discuss with clinical support or mental health supports for background history
5	No danger to self or others No acute distress No behavioural disturbance Known person with chronic symptoms Social crisis, clinically well	**Observed** • Cooperative • Coherent • Engaging in developing management plan **Reported** • Pre-existing mental illness, chronic symptoms • Requests for medication only • Minor adverse effects of medication • Financial, social, accommodation or relationship problem • Situational crisis	**Supervision** • General observation **Action** • Discuss with current support (e.g. carers, mental health team, GP) **Consider** May not require hospital transfer, consider alternatives: • Remain at home with or without support • Non-urgent referral to community mental health team, GP, or other service • Discuss with clinical support

Adapted from: Australian Government Department of Health, 2013

HOW TO CONDUCT A MENTAL HEALTH ASSESSMENT

The central components to any mental health assessment are the patient history and the mental state examination (MSE). The mental health assessment follows a similar process of assessment to those of other specialty areas, i.e. taking a patient history, conducting an examination, investigations, formulating differential diagnosis, managing acute risk and planning treatment. A thorough biopsychosocial assessment of the person and consideration of the risks associated with any identified mental illness will then inform treatment. The mental health assessment carefully considers the biopsychosocial history of a person, including previous medical or psychiatric illness, drug and alcohol use, developmental and social history, family history, aspects of culture, spirituality or religion.

Arguably the most pertinent aspect of assessment is the interview or interaction with the patient. Having a good interview technique is essential in establishing rapport to enable the effective gathering of information while ensuring a therapeutic effect. Establishing trust, providing comfort to the distressed person and attempts to put them at ease can go a long way to ensuring an effective assessment and plan for the patient. Strategies for this will depend on the circumstances and the paramedic's personal set of skills and attributes. Being genuine, authentic, curious and demonstrating empathy are all necessary ingredients to develop trust with a person. It is important not to make any false assurances or to appear authoritarian in your approach, as this may undermine the development of rapport and any attempts to ensure the safe transportation of the person to hospital if necessary.

In most circumstances it is helpful to commence the assessment by personal introduction and explaining the purpose of the assessment. The interviewer can begin by asking a series of non-threatening questions, such as demographic information, who they identify as supports, or what they think would help at this time. Where possible, attempt to ensure privacy when conducting the assessment.

ENVIRONMENTAL ASSESSMENT

The environment in which the paramedic conducts a mental health assessment is an important consideration. Behaviorally disturbed people are often fearful, overwhelmed and may find the presence of emergency services either reassuring or threatening.

Try to ensure a quiet, private space that makes the patient feel safe. Ensure you have clear access to exit the scene if necessary. Attempt to identify any potential environment risks such as weapons in the immediate area, and remove if possible. Paramedics may need to remove from the area other people who are disruptive, or conversely invite a family member who has a reassuring presence to be with the patient.

The paramedic is in a position of being able to assess the living environment and many aspects of the social situation, and then provide this information to the treating team. This would include an initial and ongoing assessment of:

- how the person interacts with their environment and others
- the family and household structure (who lives there), the social dynamics (e.g. significant relationships, whether family are supportive, abusive or hostile) or whether the person lives alone, social inclusion and supports
- the living environment, including standard of living, cleanliness, presence of food, etc.
- insight to financial or legal problems
- evidence of substance abuse
- factors contributing to risk, or to be considered as part of a risk assessment (e.g. co-residents using drugs or aggressive dogs).

OBSERVATION AND HISTORY-GATHERING SKILLS

The paramedic is often the first clinician to observe the scene and the person's mental state. This initial information is vitally important to all clinicians in the patient's journey to recovery. The patient's presentation is likely to change or evolve over time, and so a detailed paramedic assessment accompanied by informative documentation is helpful to all those across the continuum of care. For example, when a paramedic arrives on scene the person may be very distressed or behaving in a bizarre manner, but by the time the person arrives in the ED they are calmer and appropriate in demeanour. This is often the case when sedation has been administered by paramedics, and so must be considered by the assessing hospital-based clinicians. The paramedic should inform ED clinicians of observations made about the living environment and other factors that may inform a more comprehensive assessment of the person's condition and risk. Without the benefit of paramedic assessment and other sources of collateral information, the ED clinician is gaining only a limited insight into the person's mental state and behaviour. Cross-sectional and time-limited mental health assessment in an ED can be challenging. Invaluable information gained from paramedics, and other sources – family, friends, bystanders or other healthcare providers – leads to a more comprehensive and accurate assessment. The paramedic should not underestimate how invaluable a comprehensive psychosocial history is for ED clinicians and, more importantly, for patient care.

Use of open-ended questions

This style of questioning is most useful at the commencement of the assessment to ascertain the most immediate and concerning problem. During the initial minutes of interview, the clinician can ascertain the presence of symptoms and begin to put together the MSE. Time for 'free talk' allows the opportunity to identify whether the person has thought disorder, is expressing any paranoid or unusual themes, and whether they are speaking in an appropriate tone/rate or volume. Identifying the main problem/s and themes in the first few minutes of the interview allows the paramedic to identify clues into possible diagnosis and risks, and then to focus their questioning to explore this further. Additionally, when the person is afforded time to speak freely for a few minutes, this allows the opportunity to identify what the most immediate concern for the patient is and enable the paramedic to listen empathically and build rapport. Use of open-ended questions and allowing the person time to tell their story can also help them to calm their emotions or behaviour. Frame a question using validation and acknowledgement of how the person is feeling. For example, *'I see that what you're going through is very distressing … Can you tell me more about what has been happening for you?'*

Use of closed-ended questions

After ascertaining details about the patient's problem, it then becomes pertinent to focus the enquiry on aspects of the patient presentation that may lead to a more concise understanding of the problem and inform decision making. Closed-ended questions are used to clarify specific points. This technique is also useful for the patient who is over-talkative or has difficulty getting to the point. An example might include asking a patient to tell you exactly what medications they have taken.

In the event of exploring a person's suicide risk, it is also important to recognise when someone may be skirting around the question. Be explicit in your questioning about suicidal thoughts; for example, *'It sounds like you are feeling horrible at the moment, are you thinking about harming or killing yourself?'*

CONTEXT OF MENTAL STATE AND PSYCHOSOCIAL FACTORS

Presence of symptoms needs to be considered in reference to their duration, context and the level of distress or impairment they cause. A person's mental state (including mood, emotions, thinking) is dynamic and changeable according to a range of factors. Mental state may alter according to the presence of mental or physical illness, how well symptoms are controlled, the use of medication, drug and/ or alcohol use, psychosocial stressors and supportive interventions. For example, a person may feel highly anxious and distressed after a relationship break-up, then feel reassured and composed as supportive family and friends rally around them. Likewise, a person's level of risk may alter rapidly depending on mental state and ever-changing circumstances in their life.

THE BIOPSYCHOSOCIAL ASSESSMENT

Although the cause of mental illness is not entirely known, it is understood that there is a complex interplay between various factors that determine the development (or not) of mental illness in any particular person. These factors are unique to every individual and include, but are not limited to, genetic, biological, psychological, social and environmental determinants. There are many theories on why people develop a mental illness, the most contemporary of which is the stress-vulnerability model (Goh & Agius, 2010). This theory postulates that people have a predisposition to a certain illness, such as family heredity, and combined with the right (or wrong!) environmental factors (e.g. trauma, drug use, injury) result in a person developing a mental illness. Conversely, there are biopsychosocial factors that help to protect a person against the development of a mental illness; for example, a loving and nurturing home environment. As the reasons that contribute to the cause and recovery of mental illness are multifactorial, it is vital that these aspects are incorporated into the mental health assessment. Hence, the typical psychiatric or mental health assessment considers in detail all the components of a person's biopsychosocial history.

The 'bio' (biological) aspect of assessment considers the presence of any biological or genetic factors; for example, family history, head injury, history of medical and psychiatric illness, substance use history, and the effects of medication, including herbal remedies.

The 'psycho' (psychological) aspect of an assessment tends to be a bit more complex, and paramedics may be able to glean only relatively superficial detail of a person's 'psychology'. This may include an understanding of the patient's usual coping methods and personality style. The paramedic may be able to enquire from the patient or significant others what they are usually like; for example, happy-go-lucky, bubbly, perfectionistic, intense, shy.

This would consider the development of the person throughout life stages, especially critical years of infancy, childhood and adolescence. Any history of abuse, trauma, bullying or other significant life events needs to be identified in the psychosocial history. Other considerations include a person's temperament and how they coped previously with stressful situations.

The 'social' aspect includes an examination of the lifestyle, relationships, support structures and understanding of family and social dynamics. It includes factors such as housing, employment, education, family, friends, hobbies, social activities, and cultural, religious and spiritual beliefs or practices.

Gathering a thorough psychosocial and environmental assessment helps to inform effective treatment options and the viability and safety of home-based care. Table 5.2 provides paramedics with some suggested questions when undertaking a patient history and mental state examination.

Text continued on p. 5-14

Table 5.2 Mental Health Assessment

Area of Enquiry	Questions(s)	Rationale
Reason for call/ referral	What does the dispatch information say? Can you obtain any other information from the referrer?	The referrer (if not the patient) can provide vital history and a different perspective than the patient may provide.
Patient's response to referral (if referral was from someone else)	Does the patient agree that they need help?	You need to know the patient's perspective; especially whether they agree there is a problem.
Presenting problem	• What is happening? • What can we do to help? • Why now?	These questions help clarify the presenting problem as the patient sees it. They also help clarify the patient's expectations.
History of presenting problem	• How long has this been happening? Have you had problems like this before? • Have you found any way of dealing with the problem? • Have you ever had problems such as very low mood, very high mood, anxiety, sleep problems, difficulty coping with everyday problems?	• This helps establish the duration of the problem, any fluctuation in severity and any strategies that might be helpful. • The presenting problem may be part of a pattern. Establish whether the problem is new or may represent a worsening of a long-term problem.

Continued

Table 5.2 Mental Health Assessment *continued*

Area of Enquiry	Questions(s)	Rationale
Mental health history	• Have you ever sought professional help or counselling for mental-health-related problems? • Have you ever heard voices when there was no one there? • Have you had any unusual thoughts or perceptions (give examples, such as thoughts of being controlled, receiving messages from the television, etc.)? • Have you ever had thoughts that you would like to be dead? Or of ending your life? • Have you had any hospital admissions for mental health problems? • What treatment have you had, and did it help? Ask for names of medications, doses taken, benefits and side effects, and reasons for discontinuation. Where possible, obtain medications and bring them with the patient.	• The person may have had previous mental health problems that influence their response to the current problem. • Exploring previous help-seeking will help understand attitudes to health professionals, degree of trust, and strategies that have been useful in the past. • Direct questions such as thoughts of self-harm should be raised naturally if possible. Try to give a brief explanation of why you are asking (e.g. *'Some people who feel depressed have thoughts about ending their life'*). • Understanding the patient's experience of medication is important in considering the role of medication for the current problem.
Family history	• Has anyone in your family been diagnosed with a mental illness? • Has anyone in your family been admitted to a mental health unit? • Has anyone in your family or close to you died by suicide?	• A family history of mental illness is known to be a predisposing factor. • The person's experience of a family member's mental illness may influence their expectations. • Suicide of a family member is a risk factor for other family members.
Substance use history	• Have you had any drugs and/or alcohol today? (If so, how much and when?) • Do you usually drink alcohol? What is your drinking and drug use pattern? • Has your drinking or drug use increased recently?	An assessment needs to consider the patient's short- and long-term pattern of alcohol and drug use. Brief screening has been shown to increase the possibility of help seeking and behaviour change.

Table 5.2 Mental Health Assessment *continued*

Area of Enquiry	Questions(s)	Rationale
	• Do you use methamphetamine, cannabis, cocaine, MDMA, GHB, synthetic drugs? • Do you smoke cigarettes? How many per day? Have you tried quitting?	
Medical history	• Use a question-and-answer format to ask about illnesses, hospitalisations, injuries (especially head injuries), past and current treatment. • Consider a systems review. • Ask whether the person has a general practitioner and when was the last visit.	• Physical health is sometimes overlooked in mental healthcare. • People with mental illness have higher rates of physical comorbidity and mortality. • Physical health problems may contribute to mental health presentations and increase the risk of mental illness; for example, hyperthyroidism may cause anxiety; hypothyroidism may cause depressive symptoms.
Social history	• Ascertain number and order of siblings, relationships with family members, friendships, peers and intimate relationships. • For students, enquire about study program, achievement, stress associated with study and future plans. • What is your area of employment? How long have you been in your current job? Do you enjoy your work? What are your future employment plans? • Explore patterns of sexual relationships, including gender identification and gender preference. • Information on marital status may already be known, but explore the quality of relationships and whether there have been recent changes or stressors.	• Understanding family and personal relationships can help in identifying sources of stress as well as support systems. • Study and employment can be both a source of stress and a protective factor in helping to build a sense of worth and hope for the future. Areas such as sexuality are quite sensitive, so any discussion needs to consider the degree of rapport established and whether the assessment situation is an appropriate one in which to explore these issues.

Continued

Table 5.2 Mental Health Assessment *continued*

Area of Enquiry	Questions(s)	Rationale
Trauma	• Have you ever experienced any form of interpersonal violence or sexual assault? • Have you ever been bullied at school/at work/at university? • Have you ever been bullied on social media?	• If there is current violence, consider the vulnerability of children. For older adults, consider their vulnerability from caregivers or family members. • Trauma is known to contribute to mental illness and to limit patients' willingness to engage with professionals. • Experiences of trauma may be discussed without the need for specific questioning. • Most people expect to be asked about trauma, even if they find it difficult to talk about it. • Making an enquiry about trauma is an opportunity to validate the consumer's experience and to offer intervention.
Cultural/spiritual needs	• What culture/s do you identify with? • Do you have any specific cultural needs or preferences? • Are you religious or a spiritual person? How would you describe your spiritual beliefs or practices?	• Cultural and spiritual beliefs can impact on the expression of mental distress and illness. • Cultural and spiritual beliefs can also offer an opportunity for the paramedic and consumer to engage in dialogue about what interventions are helpful and appropriate.
Forensic history	Have you ever been involved with the police? Do you have any current charges?	It is not uncommon for people with mental illness to have had contact with the police, either in response to a mental health emergency or due to criminal charges. For some, contact with the police is a pathway into mental healthcare.
Mental state assessment	See pages 107–114	Mental state assessment provides a snapshot of the person's emotional and cognitive functioning at the time of the assessment. It provides an important baseline for assessing the response to intervention.

Table 5.2 Mental Health Assessment *Continued*

Area of Enquiry	Questions(s)	Rationale
Clinical formulation/ summary	See pages 114–116	This is a summary of the significant information from the assessment, presented in narrative form. More than a list, it is an attempt to show the relationship between various past and current factors, and how they influence the likely course of the person's mental health treatment.
Risk assessment	Risk assessment draws on the information discussed above, but might include a risk formulation, a narrative statement of the risks identified and the factors thought to contain risk or that might exacerbate risk. See page 115 for a discussion of risk assessment.	• Risk is just one area of assessment and should not be the only factor considered in developing an understanding of the person and a plan of care.
Differential diagnosis/ problem list	A list of the major problems the person is experiencing in prioritised order; for example, suicidal thoughts, homelessness, alcohol abuse. List possible mental illness (e.g. depression, psychosis).	Problems can include symptoms of mental illness, physical health problems, issues of risk and safety, relationship problems, and social problems such as employment, housing and finances. The problem list is an attempt to focus on the main issues. It does not include every problem the consumer has – only those that can benefit the most from mental healthcare or from referral to another agency.
Plan	• A statement of the intended actions to be taken by the paramedic and the consumer. • Where possible, the plan should be negotiated with the consumer.	Both the paramedic and the consumer need to have a considered strategy for actions to be taken to address identified problems.

Adapted from: O'Brien & Allman, 2017

REFERRAL DETAILS/PATIENT COMPLAINT

Paramedics should firstly try to ascertain the nature of the emergency and reason for responding to scene at that particular time. It is worth considering who made the call to the ambulance service, who is present at the scene, what their relationship is to the patient, and what others have seen or heard that may assist you in your assessment. Gathering information from collateral sources helps to inform you about what circumstances and clinical factors to consider when making an assessment. It is often useful to get the patient to recall the previous 48–72 hours leading up to the event in an attempt to establish what has precipitated the presentation at this time. Be curious and invite the person to share their story about how things have led to this predicament. This usually leads to cues that prompt further questioning regarding current difficulties. For example, are there any psychosocial stressors, other contributing factors, and are drugs and/or alcohol involved?

HISTORY

Taking a patient history and identifying the primary problem requires succinctly gathering all the relevant details pertaining to the patient's presentation. A good patient history includes a description of the primary problem, as well as the course of onset, the duration, and the nature and severity of any symptoms. Identifying how the onset of symptoms developed, and the period of time over which this occurred, will inform clinicians whether the presentation is an acute or a chronic clinical picture, and assist diagnostic reasoning and treatment. For example, the previously well adult who has a sudden onset of paranoia, hallucinations or confusion over a 24-hour period needs to be investigated for delirium and organic aetiology, including substance abuse. The treatment approach for delirium, for example, differs substantially to the person who has a history of schizophrenia and experiences a gradual re-emergence of psychotic symptoms. Delirium is an often missed clinical syndrome mistaken for psychiatric illness. Be vigilant for sudden changes in mental state and cognitive impairment. Also have a high index of suspicion for organic causes of mental disturbance when a person is of older age and has no history of psychiatric illness. Clues about previous diagnosis can be ascertained by asking about any current medical or psychiatric treatment or whether they take any medications. Ask if they have a doctor, counsellor or other types of health or social agencies involved. Often sources of information such as housing workers can provide invaluable history.

Taking into account that the time available to paramedics to conduct an assessment is limited, it is worthwhile to explore the biopsychosocial history in as much detail as possible in an attempt to understand the person as a whole. Having as much information as possible allows paramedics and other clinicians a greater opportunity to make reliable diagnostic formulations and treatment plans. In the event decisions are made to rapidly transport a person to hospital, there may be further opportunity during transportation to explore the patient's history in more detail. As long as the clinician is engaged in conversation with the patient, there remains an opportunity to build rapport and work within a collaborative process of assessment and treatment. Mental health assessment is a continuous process using skills of observation, listening and enquiry. Time allowing, the paramedic may be able to elicit other useful clinical information, such as what previous attempts they made to address their problems, whether they are receiving any treatment, if they have ever seen a doctor or counsellor about their situation, and what effect this has had. If the person takes any medication, it is worthwhile assessing what effect, if any, the medication has had, the duration of being on medicine, what dose they are on, and if there have been any recent changes to dose or agent. For example, an antidepressant may take 4–6 weeks to take effect, but during this time the person may experience several adverse effects and a worsening of their depression.

Sleep pattern and dietary intake are reliable and important indicators of mental ill-health. Sleep disturbance in particular is often one of the first symptoms to appear in the development of mental illness, including depression, mania or psychosis. Sleep disturbance may manifest in many ways, commonly as initial insomnia (difficulty getting to sleep), early morning waking, waking repeatedly through the night, and nightmares. Lack of sleep or a person feeling like they do not need to sleep may be suggestive of mania.

Ask the person whether there has been anything that has made things worse; for example, drugs, lack of sleep, stress, housing issues, or relationship or financial problems. It is equally important to ask what has been helpful, positive or important to the person to manage or cope thus far, and to acknowledge the positive steps and resilience they have already demonstrated.

PHYSICAL EXAMINATION

People with mental illness have premature mortality and significantly poorer physical health compared with the population who do not have a mental illness. It has been estimated people with chronic mental illness die up to 25 years earlier than the rest of the population (Australian Institute of Health and Welfare, 2016). People with mental illness have higher rates of smoking, substance use, obesity and metabolic syndrome due to socio-economic disadvantage, lifestyle factors and medication. They are less likely to access specialised medical treatment.

Physical examination of the patient is necessary to identify or exclude organic causes that may be contributing to the presenting complaint and to detect comorbid physical health conditions. In terms of diagnostic hierarchy, organic aetiology of symptoms must be excluded before a psychiatric diagnosis can be made. For example, when a person first presents to emergency services with chest pain or tachycardia, a cardiac event or metabolic disturbance needs to be excluded before considering a panic attack.

Paramedics should complete a set of vital signs including oximetry, and conduct a brief cognitive examination to determine level of consciousness, orientation, memory and attentivenesss. In some circumstances the paramedic should conduct a head-to-toe examination of the person, observing for signs of physical trauma or injury, infection and inflammation. Take a history of medical problems and surgical procedures.

Once in the emergency department investigations are used in psychiatric practice to establish or exclude a diagnosis, to aid in the choice of treatment, or to monitor treatment effects or side effects. Common investigations include full blood count, urea and electrolytes, inflammatory markers, liver function test, thyroid function test, blood toxicology, serum drug levels, urine drug screen and radiological scans.

STRENGTHS, SUPPORTS, SOCIAL FACTORS (INCLUDING CULTURAL AND SPIRITUAL NEEDS)

It is important when working with any person who is mentally ill to identify positive aspects of how they are able to live and cope in the face of adversity. Despite enduring possibly torturous symptoms of mental illness or a sense of hopelessness, the person no doubt possesses strengths that have enabled them to cope so far. A curious approach of enquiry, seeking to understand how the person 'survives', can help the person to unlock or identify their personal strengths and abilities.

Exploring cultural, religious or spiritual beliefs helps to not only demonstrate respect for the person, but to understand how their particular beliefs may influence their expression of mental health. Consider whether in fact their beliefs are in keeping within the norm of their religion/culture; and how their beliefs may influence treatment or access to health services. For the paramedic, reflecting on your own personal set of beliefs and values is important when considering how these interplay with the patient. For some cultures, mental illness can represent shame or contribute to being an outcast within their cultural group. For others, their culture, religion or spirituality may provide a source of strength, comfort and protection. It is valuable for the paramedic to seek insight into how aspects of culture and religion or other beliefs influence the person. Health services need to ensure the dignity of a person by ensuring their needs are provided for with respect to their beliefs and customs.

COLLATERAL HISTORY

Gathering collateral history from sources other than the patient is vital to ensure the clinician is obtaining an accurate assessment of the person's mental state and risk. Sources of collateral history include other health professionals, emergency services and social welfare agencies. By far the most important source of information is family, or others close to the person who spend a lot with them or know their pattern of behaviour best. Families can help to fill gaps of enquiry when the person may not be able or willing to provide a complete account of their situation. For example, the person reluctant to engage with clinicians may minimise concerns about their welfare, and state that they feel fine, whereas the person's family may describe how they spend all night pacing the house, anxious and crying, unable to leave the house and searching on the internet for ways to suicide.

Family or carer involvement in treatment and decisions about care is often pivotal when it comes to determining what course of action to take. Paramedics may feel reassured to leave a person at home in the care of supportive and informed family. On the other hand, despite best efforts, families may feel unable to continue to safely care for their loved one at home.

THE MENTAL STATE EXAMINATION (MSE)

The MSE is a significant component of a psychiatric assessment. Mental health clinicians use the MSE analogous to neurologists who undertake a neurological examination. In itself it is not diagnostic, however when taken into account with the patient history and other investigations the MSE will contribute to clinical formulation and diagnosis. The MSE helps clinicians identify signs and symptoms of behaviour, appearance, thinking, mood or cognition that enable them to conclude whether a person is experiencing a mental illness.

Paramedics may have traditionally thought it was too complicated or time consuming to conduct an MSE (Roberts & Henderson, 2009) when in fact a lot of the content of an MSE can be gained relatively quickly, within five minutes or so, by observing and listening to the patient. Within several minutes the clinician can readily ascertain from the patient's verbal responses the existence of any unusual thoughts or beliefs, or whether the person can communicate in a logical and coherent manner. This information is gathered by skilful questioning of history and current experience, taking note of prompts and themes to guide questions that may elicit symptoms, whilet at the same time maintaining a therapeutic relationship with the person. The MSE is not conducted by working systematically through a list of question and answers. Clinicians engage in observation of the person and environment, and converse with them, to then be able to pull out the elements of the MSE. Direct questions about specific symptoms or to tease out the person's degree of risk will be required using open and closed questioning techniques.

The components of an MSE are outlined below (see Table 5.3); however, there are also numerous mnemonics that can assist the paramedic to remember more easily, for example BAC-PAC (see Table 5.4).

APPEARANCE

Observation and description of a person's appearance offers many clues to their mental state and level of functioning, including an individual's ability to self-care. For example, is the person clean, tidy, well dressed and groomed, or do they appear dishevelled, dirty and neglectful of their hygiene? Note whether the person is dressed appropriately or congruently for the weather or conditions. People with schizophrenia have been known to dress incongruently to the climate; for example,

Table 5.3 Components of the Mental State Examination (MSE)

- Appearance
- Behaviour
- Conversation/speech
- Affect and mood
- Perception
- Thought form
- Thought content
- Cognition
- Insight and judgment
- Rapport

Table 5.4 Mental State Assessment BAC-PAC

- **B**ehaviour
- **A**ppearance
- **C**onversation
- **P**erception (including hallucinations and thoughts)
- **A**ffect (and mood)
- **C**ognition

wearing multiple layers of warm clothing on a hot day. The paranoid person may appear unusual by placing objects in their ears to block out voices, or fashion an object to defend themselves from lasers or surveillance devices. Alternatively, a manic person may wear skimpy, revealing clothing, apply heavy, bright make-up or wear unusual ensembles of garments.

Extremely depressed or psychotic people may be so unwell that they neglect to wash, consume adequate food and fluid, or clean their hair and nails. The paramedic may observe a person who is self-neglecting to be underweight, malnourished, dehydrated and malodorous.

Observe for signs the person has any visible injuries, rashes, inflammation or other illness.

Observe for visible scars indicating self-harm behaviour. Observation of the scars can inform the paramedic whether these are new, old or chronic wounds. Bear in mind the scars/wounds may be covered by clothing or tattoos.

The paramedic is often placed to observe the living environment of the person, so can note the state of living, considering whether it appears tidy, clean or otherwise. The living environment often reveals evidence of any substance use such as empty liquor bottles or drug paraphernalia, or the use of medications that may offer additional clues.

In worst-case scenarios the paramedic may observe extreme squalor and hoarding conditions that often indicate an untreated mental illness and evidence of risks such as fire and poor physical health.

BEHAVIOUR

Observing a person's behavior or demeanour is an important aspect of MSE, particularly with regard to risk assessment and how the paramedic may initially approach the person. For example, a patient who appears highly agitated and hostile needs to be approached with caution. Increasing signs of aggression and agitation may be evidenced by motor restlessness, pacing, hand wringing or clinching fists. If the person (or bystanders) is hostile and confrontational in their demeanour, this may suggest the need for police assistance.

Without effective engagement, tension may escalate rapidly, so steps to diffuse the situation need to be taken early. Conversely, people who appear calm and co-operative can be assessed as being less of a risk to the paramedic. Bear in mind this also needs to be considered in the context of how and why the patient came to the attention of emergency services. Even though a patient appears calm at that moment, it may be that just prior to ambulance arrival they were sitting on the edge of a bridge, or perhaps they were in a fight. Maintain vigilance of a person's potential to rapidly change demeanour. The person who appears anxious, panicky or distressed needs assessment of their level of impulsivity versus how able they are to engage and de-escalate. For example, does the distressed person with suicidal thoughts have the urge to run off?

Bizarre behaviour, abnormal posturing, unusual or repetitive behaviours should be noted. This may indicate unpredictable behaviour in the psychotic patient, particularly in the setting of thought disorder or a lack of communication. The paramedic should note how appropriately the person engages in conversation, whether they make eye contact, appear interested, distracted, avoidant or aloof.

CONVERSATION/SPEECH

The paramedic should note the rate, volume and rhythm of the person's speech. This can range from completely mute, through monosyllabic answers, to rapid, loud speech indicative of pressure of speech. Pressured speech is a symptom of mania. The tone, inflection, content and structure of speech should be noted. Determine if the speech is fluent, if the thoughts behind it are logical, and whether it flows appropriately for the situation.

AFFECT AND MOOD

Affect and mood are the objective and subjective description of a person's emotional and feeling state. Affect refers to the external expression of one's mood, or how it appears to another person. Mood refers to the subjective experience of the person.

Mood is assessed by asking people to subjectively describe it – for example, the person may say they feel sad, happy or angry – the paramedic should document verbatim how the person describes this. On occasions, it may be helpful to ask the depressed person to offer a subjective rating of their mood out of 10 (0 being the most depressed and 10 the happiest).

After asking the person about their mood (internal feelings), the paramedic should then consider whether this is congruent or in keeping with affect (external expression). For example, an incongruent affect can be noted in the person who is describing a traumatic or distressing situation but is smiling or appears to be happy. A person with a labile affect swings wildly between extremes of emotion, such as anger, crying and laughing, all within minutes.

PERCEPTION

Hallucinations are disturbances in the five senses of hearing (auditory), seeing (visual), touch (tactile), smell (olfactory) and taste (gustatory). Auditory hallucinations are the most common form of hallucinations in mental disorders, and are more likely associated in psychotic disorders such as schizophrenia. Visual and tactile hallucinations are rare in chronic psychotic conditions, and are more commonly associated with organic pathology or drug-related presentations. Common hallucinatory content may be themed as persecutory, paranoid, derogatory, religious, grandiose, controlling, guilty, somatoform and suicidal.

Observe for signs that the patient appears distracted or their eyes dart about for no apparent reason or they appear to be listening to a voice. A patient may be actively hallucinating despite denying this on questioning, particularly if they are guarded about their mental state or afraid of being taken to hospital. Signs that someone is hallucinating can be quite subtle and easily missed. Often you may have been speaking to the person and then realise they have not heard or noticed what you said. Even in the event you suspect someone is hallucinating, you may not be able to conclude this with any certainty. Some people experiencing hallucinations may deny their existence due to commands or instructions from the source of voice (e.g. God), fearing possible catastrophe if they do not obey the voice.

If the person feels able to tell you about the hallucinations, ask about the content and nature of the hallucinations; for example, type of voice being heard, what they sound like and what they say. Enquire how the voices make them feel. For some people hearing voices may make them feel frightened or threatened, irritable or angry if they are derogatory in nature, while for some people they are a comforting presence that they like to live with. Identify whether the person is experiencing command hallucinations, and if so ask the patient whether they feel compelled to act on a specific instruction that could lead to dangerous actions. Ask about the patient's capacity to resist or control any commands from the voices.

THOUGHT FORM

Thought disorder is characteristic of psychosis. It is conversation that is illogical or lacks cohesion, sequence or connection of ideas. It varies in severity from milder forms of circumstantiality to derailment and word salad at the severe end of the spectrum. Flight of ideas (characterised by jumping swiftly from topic to topic) is a common feature of mania; while a slowed stream of thought, poverty of thought or thought blocking can occur in schizophrenia, severe depressive states and catatonia.

THOUGHT CONTENT

The paramedic should listen and identify the prominent themes being expressed by the patient. These may revolve around feelings of hopelessness or helplessness, worthlessness, suicide, grief, loss, guilt and shame, suggestive of a possible depressive illness.

Delusions, hallucinations and formal thought disorder are features of psychotic disorders, and are known collectively as positive symptoms of schizophrenia. Delusions and hallucinations may manifest in a range of disorders or syndromes aside from schizophrenia or mental disorders. In its most simple definition, a delusion can be described as a fixed false belief. Delusions are not determined by religious, cultural, spiritual, sexual and political ideology or preferences. For some people, the presence of delusions and hallucinations may be readily evident and obvious to the paramedic. Other people may be more guarded or reluctant to disclose intimate thoughts and beliefs, especially if they are suspicious or mistrustful as a result of a psychotic illness.

Themes of persecution and paranoia, being controlled or under surveillance, uncharacteristic or overzealous religious ideas, grandiosity, delusions of poverty or nihilism (the belief that part of the self does not exist, or is dead or decaying), are suggestive of a psychotic illness.

Note how often or intense the person is expressing these ideas or thinking about these themes. Does the person obsess and ruminate over specific ideas, or are they passing thoughts that do not cause any particular distress or impairment? Are they consumed by a particular idea, quest or injustice that they are pursuing relentlessly? This may involve the person spending long periods on computers or awake all night, interfering with daily life activities.

The paramedic may also note an absence of symptoms or types of ideas, in any of the above to assist in determining severity of symptoms, or exclusion of symptoms for diagnostic reasoning. For example, the patient reports feeling like people are talking about him or watching him but denies the belief he is in danger or in the presence of surveillance devices in his home.

COGNITION

Screening of cognitive function is a necessary part of the psychiatric assessment. The paramedic should assess whether the patient has a delirium or other organic aetiology that may account for psychiatric-like symptoms or behavioural disturbance.

Observe the person's level of consciousness and alertness, whether this fluctuates or remains in a steady state. Assess the person's ability to maintain attention or not, and whether they are orientated to day/date/time, place and person.

Delirium is a medical emergency diagnosed according to the patient history and examination, not via diagnostic investigations. The onset is mostly acute and the cause is often multifactorial, though investigations may later help to identify the cause of the delirium and inform treatment. Generally speaking, delirium is demonstrated by fluctuating consciousness, usually with disorientation and inattentiveness. Psychotic symptoms such as paranoid beliefs or visual hallucinations may be a presenting clinical feature of delirium also.

People with depression may demonstrate reduced concentration and problems with short-term memory. The patient's ability to concentrate may also diminish with mood disturbance, psychosis and other acute stress states, reflected by the ability to perform normal work or home duties, read, study or watch TV. Memory problems may also be indicative of depression, dementia or delirium.

A number of tools are available to assess cognitive functioning. These comprise assessments of orientation, concentration, attention, memory, language and abstraction.

The Folstein Mini Mental State Examination (MMSE) (Folstein et al., 1975) is a validated, reliable and frequently used tool to screen for cognitive impairment. While used in isolation the MMSE is not diagnostic, however it will inform clinicians about the need for further diagnostic investigations. The MMSE is a relatively quick and easy test of cognition to administer, usually taking no more than 5 minutes and providing a score out of 30. A score of <25 reliably indicates significant impairment. The MMSE does not take into account the person who has an intellectual disability, is intoxicated with prescribed or illicit drugs, or is non-English speaking.

Another reliable and evidence-based screening tool for delirium which may be easier to use in the pre-hospital setting is the Confusion Assessment Method (CAM). The CAM (Inouye et al., 1990) comprises four clinical features of consideration to assist with the identification of delirium:

1. Acute onset and fluctuating course
   Is there evidence of acute change in mental status from baseline?
   Does the behaviour change fluctuate over the course of the day?
2. Inattention
   Does the person have difficulty focusing attention or have difficulty keeping track of what is said?
3. Disorganised thinking
   Is the person's thinking incoherent, illogical or irrelevant rambling?
4. Altered level of consciousness
   Is the person's level of consciousness alert (normal), vigilant, lethargic, difficult or unable to rouse?

A diagnosis of delirium is likely if the answers to all of questions from 1 and 2 are yes, and if the answer is yes to either question 3 or 4.

The presence of impaired cognitive function or an intellectual disability will influence decisions about diagnosis and appropriate treatment and disposition.

INSIGHT AND JUDGMENT

It is important to gain an understanding of the patient's attitudes, views and understanding in relation to their illness and possible treatments. Insight involves the person's view and understanding of what is happening and why. This may include the following:

- denial of illness
- awareness of being ill and needing help but denying it at the same time
- awareness of being ill but blaming it on external factors
- awareness that illness is due to something unknown within the patient
- intellectual insight – understanding of illness, but reluctance to apply this to personal circumstances
- insightful – good awareness of motives and feelings, illness, treatment and implications of decisions.

To assess insight, the paramedic should ask the patient about their beliefs and views of their health and what needs or problem areas they identify from their perspective. Determining a person's insight and judgment will influence decisions about patient care and treatment, including the level of supervision required or likelihood of adherence to a treatment plan. Judgment involves forming an understanding about the person's decision-making capacity and what they are likely to do in a given situation. This not about predicting a person's behaviour, but gaining an understanding about how reasonably a person is likely to approach a problem in the context of their mental state and circumstances.

Considering the concept of capacity and competence to make decisions about medical treatment is an integral though often challenging aspect of practice. In the first instance, clinicians must always take a stance of presuming a person has the capacity to make decisions about their health. When the notion of incompetence or lack of capacity to make decisions arises, the onus is on the clinician to demonstrate the rationale for this. When assessing whether a person has the capacity to make a decision, the clinician has to determine whether the person is able to:

- understand the information relevant to the decision and the effect of the decision
- retain that information to the extent necessary to make the decision
- use or weigh that information as part of the process of making the decision, and
- communicate the decision and the person's views and needs as to the decision in some way, including by speech, gestures or other means (Office of the Public Advocate, n.d.).

RAPPORT

The paramedic needs to be self-aware and sensitive to how their interaction or questions are affecting the person. Consider how your approach may be perceived; for example, being too 'pushy' with questions, or authoritarian with instructions. An effective paramedic needs to have a flexible approach that can respond accordingly to changing circumstances or individuals. In principle, always look to offer reassurance, and be engaged, genuine and interested in what the person is telling you.

The person who is difficult to engage or is not speaking may require a gentler approach. Offers of reassurance or validation of their distress may help to impart empathy and a sense they feel understood. Gaining some level of 'connection' with the person may help in developing a sense of trust and comfort in disclosing their thoughts or feelings. *'I can see that you are really struggling right now, and you must be terrified … I'm here to help … can you tell me about what has happened?'* It is important to clarify what is being communicated and ask the person to elaborate on broad statements such as 'I don't want to be here anymore' or 'I'm paranoid'. Ask them to talk more about this and elaborate on what they mean, if possible, asking for a specific example. Rapport can be both changeable and variable between different people.

RECOGNISING RISK: THE RELATIONSHIP BETWEEN MENTAL STATE, SUBSTANCE USE AND RISK

Assessment of risk and its association with mental state is complex, and even for the most skilled clinician can be a challenging task. It is important to gain an understanding of how symptoms of mental illness can contribute to various at-risk behaviours. Following chapters will discuss in more detail how the paramedic can recognise and assess various risks in relation to mental illness. However, it is worth mentioning here the relevance of mental health assessment, and the interplay between mental state, substance use and risk.

Though substantial risks may present for many people who experience mental illness, it must be emphasised that the vast majority of people with mental illness are not a danger to other people. Considerable work has been done over the years to reduce the stigma of mental illness and the false perception that people with mental illness are dangerous, yet we still have a way to go to educate the public and allay fears perpetuated by negative media portrayal.

At the forefront of a clinician's thinking are often thoughts that relate to the patient's risk of suicide, self-harm and violence. Understandably these are critical risks to consider during every patient assessment. It is also vital to consider some of the less obvious though potentially destructive risks the acutely unwell person may manifest. When assessing a person's risk, the paramedic must think beyond the usual realms of suicide and violence. Other broad domains of risk to consider include a person's vulnerability, risk of absconding (leaving without permission when under a legal order), refusing or not following recommended/prescribed treatment, misadventure or unintentionally coming to harm, inadvertently harming others, deteriorating further in mental or physical health, and losses or damage to employment, relationships, finances and reputation.

With regard to risk in specific clinical conditions, for example mania, the paramedic would consider in the manic person whether they may be spending excessively or engaging in foolish investments, regarding themselves as being royalty or aristocratic, behaving in a disinhibited or promiscuous way, potentially exposing themselves or others to sexually related harm, or turning up to work and behaving inappropriately, compromising their employment, damaging interpersonal relationships or their reputation.

Grandiose people can present with significant variability in the nature of their beliefs. Some may feel invincible or believe they have the ability to fly – a particular worry, especially in the event the person lives in a high-rise apartment. Experiencing grandiose beliefs of special powers may expose the manic patient to a range of dangers. They may drive erratically or at high speed, believing they have special abilities and feeling invincible. A sense of great power or invincibility can expose a person with mania to myriad risks. The grandiose person may feel euphoric and elated, and believe they are a famous rock star or possess intelligence beyond the understanding of clinicians. Others may be convinced they are of such importance that they should not be hindered in their mission or plans. Understandably, efforts to provide psychiatric treatment or facilitate the person into hospital can be met with resistance or hostility.

Psychosis manifests in myriad ways. Although there can be commonalities of symptoms, the experience and the way a person behaves or responds to symptoms is unique to the individual. For example, the presence of paranoid ideas in one person may have relatively benign effects, whereas in another individual they may result in a highly distressing experience and expose the person to a range of possible risks. Risks associated with paranoid beliefs may include the person falsely accusing or confronting others and being frankly aggressive to perceived persecutors. The identified persecutor could potentially be an innocent bystander, unaware that the psychosis sufferer is misinterpreting their behaviour or experiencing phenomena suggesting they are sinister or a threat. Other behaviours of the paranoid person may include dismantling electronic equipment, disposing of phones or devices, or fearing they are under surveillance or in danger. They may be unusually hostile or accusatory, suspicious of conspiracy or plots against them. The highly fearful or distressed paranoid person may be at risk of suicide if they believe their demise is imminent, or that suicide is a less painful option than that of being harmed via the delusional existence of persecutors.

Religious beliefs may result in fairly harmless behaviours, such as preaching or public displays of prayer; but could be as harmful as the person maiming themselves in an act of religious sacrifice, to ward off evil spirits, or shockingly ridding themselves of a sinful body part by self-amputation. Similarly, delusions related to physical ill-health, or the belief there is an object implanted in the body or an infestation, could result in horrific acts towards their own body in an attempt to remove whatever they wrongly believe is implanted or compromising their health; for example, insects, worms or a surveillance device.

Substance use is a common comorbidity with mental health problems, and often complicates assessment and treatment approaches. Intoxication with drugs or alcohol has the potential to exacerbate or mask psychiatric symptoms and can imitate symptoms of mental illness. Similarly, individuals in acute withdrawal can be mistaken for being psychotic or behaving in a deliberately uncooperative manner. Intoxication of substances increases the risk of impulsivity and behavioural disturbance, and impairs insight and judgment. Intoxication of alcohol or other drugs is a common contributing factor in acts of violence, self-harm and suicide. Paramedics must show particular caution to the substance-affected person, both in terms of personal safety and the risk the person poses to themselves.

Depression, like psychosis and other types of mental illness, can manifest in many varying ways. Some people can become profoundly suicidal, while this is not a problem for others. Risk of suicide must always be assessed in the depressed or psychotic person. Ask direct questions regarding future outlook and thoughts of suicide. It is important to be direct in asking the patient about suicide and whether there is a formulated plan. A well-thought-out plan with clear means of carrying out suicide requires immediate intervention.

For other acutely unwell people there may be other vulnerabilities to consider, such as whether they are wandering off or walking at night, going missing and not communicating their activities to loved ones, absconding from care facilities, putting themselves at risk of exploitation or abuse, using substances excessively, neglecting their physical health or nutritional state, have medical comorbidities, whether they are taking necessary medication, or living in squalor.

CLINICAL FORMULATION

Formulation is a way of bringing all the assessment information together in a way to understand what is happening for the patient and why. It is a method of summarising events or symptoms leading up to presentation, contributing factors, possible diagnoses, risk formulation, and factors that may influence safety, resolution of symptoms and recovery.

A formulation provides a more detailed understanding of the patient experience compared with a diagnosis alone. As well as providing an introduction to the patient, a description of the issues and pertinent mental health findings, the clinician forms a hypothesis of causative and contributing factors, and identifies factors that mediate or ameliorate symptoms and risk. A formulation can be structured by using the information gained from the biopsychosocial assessment and cross-referencing the 'bio', the 'psycho' and the 'social' data with the four components to a formulation (Selzer & Ellen, 2010):

• Predisposing factors
• Precipitating factors
• Perpetuating factors
• Protective factors

(Think the 4 Ps.)

DIFFERENTIAL DIAGNOSIS

A diagnosis is a useful way for clinicians (and patients) to communicate to others in brief terms about a health condition. Diagnosis can be a helpful way for people to gain an understanding of their experience, and for some it may even serve as a relief. For others, diagnosis is not so important and may feel stigmatising or represent a misleading 'label' or a reductionist way of understanding a patient. For this reason, a clinical formulation is often preferred and felt to be more informative and useful. Paramedics can ask a person about their diagnosis and whether it is something they agree/disagree with, and whether there are aspects of the diagnosis that they identify with or represent meaning for them.

For most clinicians undertaking a mental health assessment, formulating a list of possible diagnoses is important to help determine what course of action or treatment is necessary. There are two diagnostic manuals accepted universally for the provision of psychiatric diagnosis – the *Diagnostic and Statistical Manual of Mental Disorders*, generally referred to as the *DSM*, currently in its fifth edition; and the International Classification of Diseases, currently in its eleventh revision. The *DSM* is produced by the American Psychiatric Association and is widely used in Australia, while the ICD is published by the World Health Organization (WHO). Paramedics should gain some understanding of diagnostic hierarchy, or which of the key psychiatric diagnoses take precedence over another (see Selzer & Ellen, 2010).

DOCUMENTING THE MENTAL HEALTH ASSESSMENT

Documentation of the assessment and mental state involves a gathering of objective and subjective information based on your observations and what is reported by the patient and other key informants. The key to accurate and informative documentation is to keep the data objective. Avoid making judgments based on personal values or emotions. Terms to describe a person's behaviour such as 'manipulative', 'behavioural' or 'attention-seeking', for example, are judgmental and ill-informed, and potentially compromise necessary treatment. The risk in making subjective judgments is that you may get it wrong, which can have a flow-on effect to other clinicians. It is important to document clear statements of observation, history gathering and subjective patient reports. It is vital to state the source of information that is documented. For example, it is not helpful to document 'the patient is suicidal' without providing further details on how you know this, such as direct patient quotes or reports from collateral sources. Accurate documentation is also vital to ensure effective communication about symptoms for emergency department staff. For example, noting a person is 'delusional' without any substantiating documentation is vague and unhelpful. It is much more useful to document examples from direct sources; for example, the patient reports believing that his mother is an imposter sent by the government to kill him.

CASE STUDY
Helen

The following documentation and other notes focus primarily on the MSE. Other parts of the comprehensive assessment are not covered here; for example, the medical/physical assessment, risk assessment, formulation and plan.

Dispatch and initial assessment

The ambulance dispatch is to a residential address for a 41-year-old female who is suspected of taking an overdose. The daughter has arrived to check on her mother and found her sitting in the corner of the lounge with a blanket over her head stating she doesn't want help. She has told her daughter that she has taken temazepam and paracetamol and has been steadily drinking since early morning.

Before documenting Helen's mental state or doing other observations, assess how safe it is to approach and enter the environment that you find her in. Maintaining entry and exit points, watching and observing how Helen is interacting with her physical environment and with others at the scene is essential to understanding potential risks, and will give clues to how Helen is viewing your presence and others. Your approach and patient engagement needs to be documented to provide context for the presentation, for example:

On arrival paramedics were greeted by the patient's daughter who gives a brief history of her mother's past difficulties with depression, self-harm, alcohol use and inpatient mental healthcare (approximately 2 weeks ago). Clear entry and exit to house, which appears to be clean, but with surfaces cluttered with 8 empty cider bottles on the kitchen sink. The patient was found sitting in the corner of her lounge wrapped in a blanket. GCS 13.

History

Document any allergies, past history, the current presenting complaint and medications, and any physical and vital sign observations that are able to be obtained. Given that the call is for a suspected overdose, it is important to try to determine how much, what type of substances and what time Helen may have ingested these as soon as possible. Establishing a strong rapport will assist in gaining a comprehensive history and the details you need to assess the potential overdose.

Helen has seen her general practitioner about a week and a half ago because she felt that she was losing control of her suicidal and self-harm feelings. The GP has placed her on Zyprexa (olanzapine) which she has been taking over the last seven days, and he has been working with the mental health services to coordinate her long-term care. Diagnosed with depression approximately 15 years ago.

Appearance and behaviour – Helen, a 41-year-old female, was found sitting on the lounge room floor wrapped in a blanket, wearing faded blue cotton pyjamas with a flower design. She has shoulder-length brown hair, glasses, with a tattoo on her right wrist and a nose piercing. She is holding the blanket tightly around her, she is not engaging in eye contact with either the paramedics or her daughter, and is crying. She is slowly rocking back and forth, but is responsive to paramedic presence and questions. No visible signs of recent self-harm (later admitted to having old scars from previous self-inflicted injuries to upper legs).

Conversation and speech – Helen's speech is slightly slurred but coherent. Hesitant and slow to respond to questions and quietly spoken. Her volume increases when asked about the amount of alcohol she has consumed, and she appears to become more distressed when talking to her daughter.

Perception – Helen states she has tried to pull herself together but just cannot seem to manage. She feels as though she doesn't want to try to manage any more, wants to sleep and feels she is a burden to her daughter. She has tried help and was in the 'unit' not that long ago, but she seems to 'lose it' every time she has to try to manage on her own. She has been taking Zyprexa (olanzapine) over the last seven days. Helen states that this makes her feel worse, more disconnected and less controlled.

Affect and mood – Helen has tears falling down her cheeks and downcast facial expressions which remain throughout our care. She states she has been feeling increasingly despondent, thinking about self-harm and feeling so sad she doesn't want to try and fight it any more.

Cognition – Helen is orientated to her surroundings, her daughter, and paramedic presence. She is able to follow the conversation and her statements appear logical and in context to her current situation. She is aware of the day, date and the approximate time.

CONCLUSION

Conducting a thorough and well-informed mental health assessment is essential to ensuring patient safety and provision of further care. Utilising effective skills of engaging and communicating with the mentally unwell patient while undertaking an assessment leads to gathering better information and a better assessment. The better the assessment, the better the decision-making and overall experience for the person. Do not underestimate the value of good communication skills within the mental health assessment, and the impact this may have during every interaction with an unwell or distressed person.

Paramedics undertake an essential aspect of clinical practice when conducting the mental health assessment of a person. Being a first-responder allows a valuable assessment of the patient's setting, usually their home environment. The process of assessment affords the paramedic the opportunity to gather information about a person, and to intervene therapeutically with a distressed or unwell person. Paramedics demonstrating genuineness and empathy utilise valuable interpersonal skills to provide comfort and reassurance to distressed persons. A paramedic's role extends to one of advocate for a patient. Person-centred therapeutic care is essential to demonstrate beyond the pre-hospital setting to the ED (or elsewhere) to help ensure a smooth transition of care.

LINKS AND RESOURCES

- Mental Health and Drug and Alcohol Office, Mental Health for Emergency Departments – A Reference Guide 2015. NSW Ministry of Health, Sydney. Available: https://www.health.nsw.gov.au/mentalhealth/resources/Publications/mental-health-ed-guide.pdf. November 2019.
- Department of Health and Ageing, 2009. Emergency triage education kit (ETEK). Australian Government, Canberra; 37–48. Available: http://www.health.gov.au/internet/main/publishing.nsf/content/casemix-ed-triage+review+fact+sheet+documents (updated 2013) This resource was specifically developed for the emergency department triage, but has relevance in both the pre-hospital setting and for handover from the paramedic to triage staff.

Risk assessment

- https://www.square.org.au/risk-assessment/
- https://www.square.org.au/wp-content/uploads/sites/10/2013/05/Risk-Assessment_Black-and-White_May2013_Handout1.pdf

While this is considered a somewhat outdated risk assessment in hospital/mental health services, the headings used here would be applicable and simple for a paramedic in pre-hospital care.

Understanding the mental state examination (MSE): a basic training guide:

https://tnicholson2013.files.wordpress.com/2014/01/msedvdbookletoct2011highresolution.pdf

These videos relate to this document:

Lisa: https://www.youtube.com/watch?v=83i2MWMqph8&t=3s

Glen: https://www.youtube.com/watch?v=ktEUiCLu_9s&t=3s

Barry: https://www.youtube.com/watch?v=6ss827LbbtA&t=4s

Cognitive screening including the mini mental state examination (MMSE)

https://www.dementia.org.au/information/for-health-professionals/clinical-resources/cognitive-screening-and-assessment

Cultural aspects of mental health

http://www.vtmh-culturalassesmentformulation.online/overview

REFERENCES

Australian Government Department of Health, 2013. Mental Health Triage Tool (last updated January 2013). Online. Available: http://www.health.gov.au/internet/publications/publishing.nsf/Content/triageqrg~triageqrg-mh. November 2019.

Australian Institute of Health and Welfare (AIHW), 2016. Australian burden of disease study: impact and causes of illness and death in Australia 2011 (updated May 2016). Australian Burden of Disease Study series no. 3. BOD 4. AIHW, Canberra. Online. Available: https://www.aihw.gov.au/reports/burden-of-disease/abds-impact-and-causes-of-illness-death-2011/contents/highlights. November 2019.

Folstein, M., Folstein, S., McHugh, P., 1975. A practical method for grading the cognitive state of patients for the clinician. J. Psychiatr. Res. 12 (3), 189–198.

Goh, C., Agius, M., 2010. The stress-vulnerability model: how does stress impact on mental illness at the level of the brain and what are the consequences? Psychiatr. Danub. 22 (2), 198–202.

Inouye, S., van Dyck, C., Alessi, C., 1990. Clarifying confusion: the confusion assessment method: a new method for detecting delirium. Ann. Intern. Med. 113 (12), 941–948.

O'Brien, A., Allman, M., 2017. Assessment in mental health nursing. In: Evans, K., Nizette, D., O'Brien, A. (Eds.), Psychiatric and Mental Health Nursing, fourth ed. Elsevier, Sydney.

Office of the Public Advocate Victoria, n.d. Assessing whether a person has decision making capacity. Online. Available: https://www.publicadvocate.vic.gov.au/assessing-whether-a-person-has-decision-making-capacity. November 2019.

Roberts, L., Henderson, J., 2009. Paramedic perceptions of their role, education, training and working relationships when attending cases of mental illness. J. Emerg. Primary Health Care 7, 3.

Selzer, R., Ellen, S., 2010. Psych-Lite: Psychiatry that's easy to read. McGraw-Hill Australia, Sydney.

Legal and ethical issues in pre-hospital mental healthcare

6

Dr Ruth Townsend

LEARNING OUTCOMES

The aim of this chapter is to introduce:

- the key legal and ethical principles in mental healthcare
- the structure of mental health legislation
- key common features across national jurisdictions
- how legal and ethical principles inform practice for paramedics in the pre-hospital setting.

INTRODUCTION[1]

Paramedics will encounter patients with mental health issues on a regular basis. Every state and territory in Australia has its own legislation with respect to the care and treatment of the mentally ill. The overall purpose of the law is to ensure that a mentally ill person will receive the best possible care and treatment in the least restrictive environment. This includes limiting any restriction or interference with their civil liberties, rights, dignity and self-respect to the minimum necessary to effectively provide care and treatment.

This chapter will set out the legal and ethical issues most commonly experienced in pre-hospital mental healthcare. It is by no means exhaustive and readers are advised to supplement this chapter with a reading of the laws of the state in which they practise. The Mental Health Acts in general are very prescriptive, which means that they contain a lot of detail about what lawfully can and should be done to care for people who come under the protection of the Act.

---

[1]Some elements of this chapter have been extracted from Townsend, R., Luck, M., 2019. Mental illness and the law in the pre-hospital emergency care setting. In: Applied Paramedic Law, Ethics and Professionalism: Australia and New Zealand, second edn. Elsevier, Sydney.

MENTAL HEALTH LAW IN AUSTRALIA

Mental health law in Australia has been developed at a state level. That means that each state and territory has its own laws with respect to the management of mental healthcare and treatment. There are many similarities between the various jurisdictions, but it is advisable that you familiarise yourself with the particular law that applies in your state to ensure that you comply with any state-specific particularities. In addition, most states have developed other resources, including plain language guides and codes of practice, which can be found in the resource section at the end of the chapter. Mental health laws are fairly prescriptive, which means that they set out in detail, step-by-step, what is required to be done to comply with the law. The laws that apply in each state are:

- Mental Health Act 2007 (NSW)
- Mental Health Act 2014 (Vic)
- Mental Health Act 2015 (ACT)
- Mental Health Act 2013 (Tas)
- Mental Health Act 2016 (Qld)
- Mental Health Act 1996 (WA)
- Mental Health Act 2009 (SA)
- Mental and Related Services Act 2009 (NT)
- Mental Health (Compulsory Assessment and Treatment) Act 1992 (NZ).

CASE STUDY

Catherine

You are dispatched to a home address in a residential suburb at 10.35 am for a 32-year-old female who has called 000 with suicidal ideation. Catherine has told the emergency dispatcher over the phone that she wants to kill herself because she has been arguing with her partner/carer within the house and she just wants an ambulance.

This is the third time in four days that you have personally been dispatched to Catherine for similar situations. You understand that Catherine has a diagnosis of schizophrenia that has been poorly managed over the years. Catherine grew up in a dysfunctional home where she suffered both physical and sexual abuse, spent many years in foster care, and was not diagnosed, and therefore not treated early for her illness. With the complications of long-term intravenous drug abuse, no social support, and poor engagement with mental health services, Catherine has deteriorated mentally and physically over the past few years. She has attempted suicide multiple times by prescription drug overdose, and there has been a recent diagnosis of hepatitis C. She now lives with an abusive partner who is also her carer.

When you arrive on the scene, you find Catherine outside the front of her house in the driveway smoking a cigarette and the partner is in the house. She has a shuffling gait, mumbles her words in recognition of your arrival and does not appear to be aggressive.

Vital signs
- Glasgow Coma Score: 15
- Oxygen saturations: 100%
- Respiratory rate: 18

- Heart rate: 85 strong / regular
- Blood pressure: 130/85
- Electrocardiograph: Sinus rhythm
- Blood sugar level: 6.3 mmol
- Pain score: 2/10

CRITICAL REFLECTION

- When thinking about the social determinants of health, what factors have played a significant role in the deterioration of Catherine's mental and physical health?
- Why do you feel that Catherine has called the ambulance so many times in such a short timeframe?
- Your colleague says that Catherine is a time waster and that this is an abuse of the ambulance service. How would you reply?
- What questions would you like to ask Catherine, and why would these particular questions be relevant to her treatment/care today?

Further information

When you question Catherine, it becomes apparent that she is unable to give you a coherent story of the past few days, the facts change often and she can't remember what she said previously. She says that she has not been using heroin, but you can see recent track marks on her arms which seem to contradict this. While Catherine avoids answering any direct questions about suicidal ideation, she only says that her suicidal thoughts are 'no more than usual' and the only reason she called an ambulance was to get away from her partner who has been mean to her.

After a few more minutes of questioning Catherine, she suddenly becomes quite verbally aggressive and violently throws her cigarette lighter on the ground and shouts, 'Well if you're not going to help me then you can just get lost!' Catherine then runs into the house and slams the front door.

CRITICAL REFLECTION

- What would be your next actions to manage the situation?
- From the information presented, does this patient fit the Mental Health Act for possible involuntary care by paramedics?
- What sort of power does the law provide paramedics in this situation?
- What is the objective of the Mental Health Act in cases like Catherine's?
- How would you go about assessing Catherine's capacity to make decisions?
- What rights does Catherine have?

Further information

The police arrive on scene and peacefully facilitate Catherine exiting the house, and she resumes communicating with you. Catherine apologises for her outburst and says she is just under lots of stress, but everything is fine now and she just wants to go back inside and watch TV.

CRITICAL REFLECTION

- Under what circumstances would you feel comfortable leaving Catherine at home?
- Under your current legislation are you able to transport Catherine involuntarily to hospital?
- Are there any other community or organisational services that could be provided for Catherine during this acute episode, or is hospital the only option?

LEGAL CONTEXT OF MENTAL HEALTHCARE

Mental health law is a special area of law, and sits in what is called the protective jurisdiction alongside other areas of law that protect vulnerable people; for example, child protection and guardianship laws. As such, you will find that the overriding principles of the law make specific reference to the need to uphold the guiding principles of the legislation which protect the vulnerable patient from harm. The key principles of the protective jurisdiction are essentially human rights principles, including the right for people to be self-determining; that is, to make decisions about themselves for themselves. These rights apply to all people regardless of their ability to advocate for themselves, so even when a patient is unable to tell you what they would like to do, the right for them to do so remains. In these cases, often a person who knows the patient well will act as a proxy for the patient. The reason for this is to recognise that people who know the patient well, while maybe not knowing everything about the patient, certainly know them better than the paramedic treating the patient. The protective jurisdiction of the law recognises that there are people within particular groups that may sometimes be unable to advocate for themselves – children and the mentally ill or disordered – and that there is therefore a need to have provisions within the law that allows someone else to act as if they were the person in that person's stead and in that person's best interest. This affords the person human worth and dignity and supports the human rights principles that inform the law.

OBJECTIVES AND HISTORY OF MENTAL HEALTH LAW

It is important for context to understand the history of the development of mental health legislation (see Townsend & Luck, 2009). In short, the history is that mentally ill or disordered patients are particularly vulnerable to abuse and historically they have been abused. They have had limitations placed on their rights because society has, in the past, wrongly believed that patients were not capable of making decisions for themselves and so has taken a paternalistic approach to managing these patients. This has been done with good intentions, but the intention is, in and of itself, not enough to justify the limitation of a patient's rights to make decisions for themselves where they have the capacity to do so. There have also been examples where society, and individuals responsible for the care of these vulnerable people, have not acted with good intentions, or have acted out of fear or ignorance or prejudice, and in so doing have harmed these patients.

A number of reports into the abusive care that many people have received, combined with a growing understanding of mental health and its treatment, has led to changes to the provision of mental healthcare and the guiding principles that govern the management of these patients. The essence of these principles, and a recognition of the flawed history of the way in which we have treated mental health patients, have been codified in law.

The guiding principles follow that mental healthcare is about upholding the rights of the individual to ensure that they are involved in decision making regarding their care and treatment, that they have access to care, that care be provided in the least restrictive environment possible to maintain the wellbeing of the patient and others, and that persons who fall under the provisions of the law are provided access to treatment to prevent harm to themselves or others. These guiding principles are captured well in the various state and territory Mental Health Acts. As an example, section 3 of the NSW Mental Health Act clearly sets out the objectives of the Act and reflects these guiding principles, and paramedics are required to apply these principles in practice when caring for those with mental illness.

The objectives of the NSW Act are as follows:

'a) *to provide for the care and treatment of, and to promote the recovery of, persons who are mentally ill or mentally disordered, and*

b) *to facilitate the care and treatment of those persons through community care facilities, and*

c) *to facilitate the provision of hospital care for those persons on a voluntary basis where appropriate and, in a limited number of situations, on an involuntary basis, and*

d) *while protecting the civil rights of those persons, to give an opportunity for those persons to have access to appropriate care and, where necessary, to provide for treatment for their own protection or the protection of others, and*

e) *to facilitate the involvement of those persons, and persons caring for them, in decisions involving appropriate care treatment and control.'*

(Mental Health Act 2007 (NSW), s3)

The state and territory Mental Health Acts set out a set of 'exclusion' criteria, which outline when a person is not considered to have mental illness by reason only of any one or more of the following 'conditions':

- political activity or orientation
- religious activity or orientation
- philosophical orientation
- sexual preference, gender identity, sexual orientation or sexual promiscuity
- cultural identification or background
- immoral conduct
- illegal conduct or antisocial behaviour
- intellectual disability
- intoxication with drugs or alcohol
- economic or social status
- on the basis of previous treatment for mental illness.

This list, which may have variations in each jurisdiction, reflects some of the history and reasons why some people were wrongly treated as being mentally ill in the past. The presence of elements of this list does not exclude somebody from having a mental illness, but they must be seen in the context of their history and mental state examination. Furthermore, acute intoxication alone does not mean that a person does or does not have a mental illness; however, it could well mask or contribute to other potential 'symptoms' such as depression or suicidal ideation. The similarity of the criteria of what is not, on its own, to be considered a mental illness reflects the broader national view that the definitions and understanding of what constitutes mental illness have moved on and are more standardised than they may have been in the past.

GUIDING PRINCIPLES FOR CARE AND TREATMENT

The guiding principles for the care and treatment of mental health patients are generally standardised across all jurisdictions. The principles, as exemplified in section 68 of the NSW Act, include that people with a mental illness or disorder should, as far as practicable, be provided with the best possible care and treatment in the least restrictive environment that enables the effective provision of that care and treatment (Mental Health Act 2007 (NSW) s68(a)). Other guiding principles include:

'(b) *people with a mental illness or mental disorder should be provided with timely and high quality treatment and care in accordance with professionally accepted standards,*

(c) *the provision of care and treatment should be designed to assist people with a mental illness or mental disorder, wherever possible, to live, work and participate in the community,*

(d) *the prescription of medicine to a person with a mental illness or mental disorder should meet the health needs of the person and should be given only for therapeutic or diagnostic needs and not as a punishment or for the convenience of others,*

(e) *people with a mental illness or mental disorder should be provided with appropriate information about treatment, treatment alternatives and the effects of treatment and be supported to pursue their own recovery,*

(f) *any restriction on the liberty of patients and other people with a mental illness or mental disorder and any interference with their rights, dignity and self-respect is to be kept to the minimum necessary in the circumstances,*

(g) *any special needs of people with a mental illness or mental disorder should be recognised, including needs related to age, gender, religion, culture, language, disability or sexuality,*

(g1) *people under the age of 18 years with a mental illness or mental disorder should receive developmentally appropriate services,*

(g2) *the cultural and spiritual beliefs and practices of people with a mental illness or mental disorder who are Aboriginal persons or Torres Strait Islanders should be recognised,*

(h) *every effort that is reasonably practicable should be made to involve persons with a mental illness or mental disorder in the development of treatment plans and recovery plans and to consider their views and expressed wishes in that development,*

(h1) every effort that is reasonably practicable should be made to obtain the consent of people with a mental illness or mental disorder when developing treatment plans and recovery plans for their care, to monitor their capacity to consent and to support people who lack that capacity to understand treatment plans and recovery plans,

(i) people with a mental illness or mental disorder should be informed of their legal rights and other entitlements under this Act and all reasonable efforts should be made to ensure the information is given in the language, mode of communication or terms that they are most likely to understand,

(j) the role of carers for people with a mental illness or mental disorder and their rights under this Act to be kept informed, to be involved and to have information provided by them considered, should be given effect.'

(Mental Health Act 2007 (NSW), s68)

LEGAL DEFINITIONS OF MENTAL ILLNESS

The clinical definition of mental illness is best summarised in the *DSM-5* (American Psychiatric Association, 2013), which defines a mental disorder as:

'... a syndrome characterized by clinically significant disturbance in an individual's cognition, emotion regulation, or behaviour that reflects a dysfunction in the psychological, biological, or developmental processes underlying mental functioning. Mental disorders are usually associated with significant distress in social, occupational, or other important activities. An expectable or culturally approved response to a common stressor or loss, such as the death of a loved one, is not a mental disorder. Socially deviant behaviour (e.g. political, religious, or sexual) and conflicts that are primarily between the individual and society are not mental disorders unless the deviance or conflict results from a dysfunction in the individual, as described above.'

(American Psychiatric Association, 2013)

This clinical definition is not the same as a legal definition. There are a variety of legal definitions for mental illness. The important distinction between the legal and the clinical definitions for the purpose of applying the law by paramedics is that in order for the legal definition of mental illness or disorder to apply, a person must be symptomatic as per the symptoms set out in the Act. If a person does not meet the legal definition of someone who falls under the provisions of the Act, then the power that paramedics have to act that is granted to them by the Act will not apply. In other words, the paramedic could be acting unlawfully if they attempt to use their powers of sedation or restraint found in the Mental Health Act when a patient does not fit the definition of mentally ill or disordered as stated in the relevant Act.

All jurisdictions have slight variations on the definition of mental illness, but all have the following key components within their definitions (see Fig. 6.1):

1. Impairment, which prevents the person being able to function within their work, social, personal or physical environment.
2. A significant change in capacity (which will be further discussed later in the chapter).
3. Assessment.
4. Risk to self or others.
5. The determination of the need for further care.
6. The prospect of mental and physical deterioration.

In NSW the definition is:

'*"**mental illness**" means a condition that seriously impairs, either temporarily or permanently, the mental functioning of a person and is characterised by the presence in the person of any one or more of the **following symptoms**:*

(a) delusions,

(b) hallucinations,

(c) serious disorder of thought form,

(d) a severe disturbance of mood,

(e) sustained or repeated irrational behaviour indicating the presence of any one or more of the symptoms referred to in paragraphs (a)–(d)'

(Mental Health Act 2007 (NSW), s4(1))

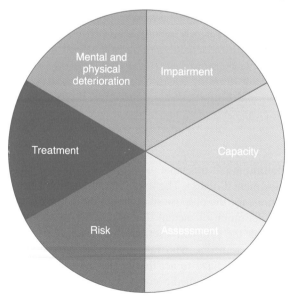

FIGURE 6.1

Key components of the definition of mental illness within a Mental Health Act

NSW also differentiates mental illness from mentally disordered. It defines mental disorder as:

> '*A person (whether or not the person is suffering from mental illness) is a mentally disordered person if the person's behaviour for the time being is so irrational as to justify a conclusion on reasonable grounds that temporary care, treatment or control of the person is necessary:*
>
> *(a) for the person's own protection from serious physical harm, or*
> *(b) for the protection of others from serious physical harm.'*
>
> (Mental Health Act 2007 (NSW), s15)

This piece of law provides an opportunity for a patient who is experiencing an acute episode of illness that may pose a risk to their own safety or the safety of others, to be treated under the provisions of the Act without necessarily having to be diagnosed with a mental illness first or, indeed, at all.

In the Victorian Mental Health Act 2014, mental illness is defined as a 'medical condition that is characterised by a significant disturbance of thought, mood, perception or memory' (s4). This is similar to Tasmania's definition which is: 'For the purposes of this Act – (a) a person is taken to have a mental illness if he or she experiences, temporarily, repeatedly or continually – (i) a serious impairment of thought (which may include delusions); or (ii) a serous impairment of mood, volition, perception or cognition; and (b) nothing prevents the serious or permanent physiological, biochemical or psychological effects of alcohol use or drug-taking from being regarded as an indication that a person has a mental illness.' (Mental Health Act 2013 (Tas), s4(1)).

The Northern Territory puts elements of both NSW and Tasmania's definitions together. In this Act:

> '*A **mental illness** is a condition that seriously impairs, either temporarily or permanently, the mental functioning of a person in one or more of the areas of thought, mood, volition, perception, orientation or memory and is characterised:*
>
> *(a) by the presence of at least one of the following symptoms:*
>   *(i)   delusions;*
>   *(ii) hallucinations;*
>   *(iii) serious disorders of the stream of thought;*
>   *(iv) serious disorders of thought form;*
>   *(v)   serious disturbances of mood; or*
> *(b) by sustained or repeated irrational behaviour that may be taken to indicate the presence of at least one of the symptoms referred to in paragraph (a)'*
>
> (Mental Health and Related Services Act 1998 (NT), s6)

In South Australia, mental illness is defined as 'any illness or disorder of the mind' (Mental Health Act 2009 (SA), s3) with potential exclusions (relating to conduct) found within Schedule 1. While this definition may be considered vague, the intent of this was for the Act to be less exclusive; that is, not to exclude acute organic illness (e.g. delirium) simply because it was not *psychiatry*. Although the benefits of the broad definition of mental illness allows for other causes of changes in mood, perception and behaviour to be considered, it may also allow for potential misuse and abuse of the Act.

CONSENT AND CAPACITY

There is a large amount of information to be aware of with regards to the legal understanding of consent, but for the purposes of this chapter this will be a brief outline of the key elements. In short, capacity is the ability of a person to understand the nature, purpose and consequences of a decision. The term 'capacity' is often used interchangeably with 'competence'. For the purpose of this chapter, the two terms will mean the same thing.

Patients have a right to make decisions about their medical treatment. The High Court of Australia has said that 'except in cases of emergency or necessity, all medical treatment is preceded by the patient's choice to undergo it'.[2] This right exists even if the patient has a mental illness or disorder. It is possible in the case of a patient with a mental illness or disorder that they may move in and out of capacity to consent to or refuse treatment. It is critical that paramedics undertake good clinical assessments of the patient's capacity to consent or refuse consent for treatment which is a competent adult's right.

There is a presumption in law that anyone over the age of 18 has capacity, and it is up to the paramedics who may doubt the capacity of their patient to consent or refuse consent to treatment to assess and provide evidence to support any claim suggesting that a patient has lost capacity to make decisions for themselves. Those under the age of 18 are presumed to be not competent to consent or refuse consent for treatment. Therefore, if a paramedic makes an assessment that a person under 18 is in need of treatment and the person is refusing, the onus is on the person to demonstrate that they have the capacity to refuse. New South Wales, South Australia and the Northern Territory have laws that allow medical practitioners to provide emergency treatment to children without consent for a broad range of emergency care, but again, it is likely that a person providing treatment to a person without capacity may be authorised to do so under the principle of necessity, or, in the case of New South Wales and Tasmania, under legislation, if that treatment is necessary to save a person's life, prevent serious damage to the patient's health, or to prevent the patient from suffering or continuing to suffer significant pain or distress.

It is common for paramedics to treat patients who do not have capacity. An example is an unconscious patient. In the case of an unconscious patient, the paramedic may look to see if there is a surrogate decision maker authorised to make

---

[2]*Rogers v Whitaker* (1992) HCA 58 175 CLR 479.

decisions on behalf of the incompetent patient. In the case *Re F*,[3] the judge, Lord Goff, discussed which legal principle could apply to medical treatment given without consent. He did not find 'implied consent' – which is a common misunderstanding among paramedics. He instead found the principle of necessity. The necessity principle is one that can be used to attempt to justify behaviour if the behaviour would otherwise be a breach of the law. For example, if someone is speeding to get a patient to hospital urgently because of a life-threatening condition and breaks the law to do so, then this may be justified on the basis of necessity – that it was necessary to break the law in order to save the person's life. This same principle is applied to almost all paramedic work where there is a patient requiring immediate life-saving interventions and the patient cannot give consent and there is no one else who is legally able to give or refuse consent on the patient's behalf.

Often with elderly patients who may suffer from confusion that is transient – that is, it comes and goes – they may have a health guardian appointed who is authorised to make decisions on the patient's behalf when the patient is not competent to do so. The overarching principle of guardianship law is that the guardian is to act as if they were the patient. Mental health runs on the same principles and, as stated earlier, falls into the same protective jurisdiction of the law. If the patient is not competent to make decisions for themselves, it may be that there is a guardian who is authorised to do so. If not, and the treatment is necessary to be administered in order to prevent a further harm from occurring to the patient, then paramedics may rely on the principle of necessity. This offers them a defence against any charge of assaulting the patient (i.e. touching the patient without consent). There have been no cases in Australia of a paramedic having been charged with assault for treating an incompetent patient under the principle of necessity.

Often mental health patients do not realise they are in need of care and treatment. They may or may not be competent to make their own decisions about their care. It is necessary for a paramedic to assess the patient's capacity to do so carefully, and it should not be assumed that just because the patient has a mental illness or disorder that they are lacking in capacity. A good example is a patient who has bi-polar disorder, a recognised mental illness, but is well managed with medication and is perfectly capable of making decisions about their own life and wellbeing.

PRESUMPTION OF COMPETENCE

As mentioned above, there is a presumption at law that anyone over the age of 18 is competent to consent or refuse consent for treatment. If the patient is unconscious and treatment is necessary to save further harm to the patient, then the paramedic can act without consent unless there is an advanced care directive that

---

[3] *re F (mental patient: sterilisation)* [1990] 2 AC 1.

specifically refuses consent for treatment. Often in mental health cases, if a paramedic is required to assess a mental health patient for involuntary transport to a mental health facility, it is likely that the patient either cannot consent or is refusing consent for treatment. If the paramedic suspects that the person is not competent, the onus is on the paramedic to show it.

A way to check this is to ask: was the patient free of 'undue influence' at the time of refusing treatment? Does the refusal cover the action that is being planned? Was the person competent at the time they made the decision? In determining competence, the paramedic will establish if the person has comprehended and retained the relevant information, believed it and weighed up the information before communicating a decision.[4]

SAFEGUARDS WITHIN MENTAL HEALTH LEGISLATION

There are a number of safeguards within the mental health law beyond just the list of the things at the beginning of the Act that are not mental illnesses. The ACT and Victoria are areas that are referred to as human rights jurisdictions, and this is because, although human rights are the rights that humans have just by virtue of the fact they are human, these two jurisdictions have chosen to explicitly consider and include references to human rights in their law making. In section 15 of the Mental Health Act 2014 (Vic), for example, this inclusion is reflected in the right of the patient to communicate with any person for the purpose of seeking legal advice or legal representation. Under the law, staff of a mental health service are required to ensure that reasonable steps are taken to assist an inpatient to communicate lawfully with any person. This is because, historically for example, patients have been placed in locked mental health facilities with no way for them to make contact with those on the outside for often extensive periods of time.

Another example of a protection that is provided to patients is a statement of rights which sets out a person's rights under the Mental Health Act. Further, as well as a written statement, there is a legal requirement that an oral explanation of this statement of rights be given as soon as the patient is capable of understanding the information (Mental Health Act 2014 (Vic), s13).

PARAMEDICS AND MENTAL HEALTH LEGISLATION ROLES AND POWERS

Paramedics are referenced in almost all Mental Health Acts, but not necessarily using the term 'paramedic'. The terms 'ambulance officer', 'authorised officer' and

---

[4]*re C Adult; refusal of medical treatment* [1994] 1 WLR 290.

'prescribed persons' are examples of the terminology within the Acts that include or refer to paramedics.

In New South Wales, paramedics are still referred to in the Act as 'ambulance officers'. 'Ambulance officer' means a member of staff of the NSW Health Service who is authorised by the Secretary to exercise the functions of an ambulance officer under this Act. It is likely that this term will be amended to paramedic at some later time. Until it is amended, there is a potential for the term 'ambulance officer' to extend to any other ambulance employee of New South Wales that may be referred to as an 'ambulance officer.'

PARAMEDIC POWERS AUTHORISED BY LAW

The powers of an 'ambulance officer' under the Mental Health Act in New South Wales include the transport of a patient to a declared mental health facility, on an involuntary basis, 'if the officer believes on reasonable grounds that the person appears to be mentally ill or mentally disturbed and that it would be beneficial to the person's welfare to be dealt with in accordance with this Act' (Mental Health Act 2007 (NSW), s20).

This power is also found in Mental Health Acts in the Northern Territory (s31), South Australia (s56) (where a paramedic is referred to as 'an authorised officer'), Tasmania (s212) and the ACT (s80). This piece of law places a great deal of power in the hands of paramedics. It authorises paramedics to detain and transport someone against their will. An individual's liberty is as prized by many as their life, so having the power to remove an individual's freedom should be taken very seriously. Remember, these people have not broken any laws. They are not like criminals who have been tried, convicted and sentenced to jail, and thus have lost their liberty as a price for committing crime. Mental health patients are the only other members of our adult society who have legal limits placed on their freedom. Paramedics have to use a two-stage test to exercise this power. They should be sure that they have 'reasonable' grounds for making the decision. 'Reasonable grounds' requires more conviction from the paramedic than mere suspicion or 'gut instinct,' but less evidence than conclusive proof[5] that (1) the person 'appears' to be mentally ill or 'mentally disturbed' and (2) that it would be 'beneficial to the person's welfare to be dealt with in accordance with this Act'. This assessment is essentially subjective, but it would be recommended that paramedics make this assessment in accordance with their clinical guidelines and provide supportive evidence for their assessment. In other words, this determination should not be made purely on the basis of a 'gut instinct'.

It should also be noted that the Act itself reminds paramedics of the criteria for assessing whether a patient should be transported to a mental health facility on an involuntary basis; that is, the patient has not asked or consented to be transported.

---

[5]*George v Rockett* (1990) HCA 26 170 CLR104.

The criteria include an assessment that the patient is in fact mentally ill or mentally disordered as defined in the Act (see above) and:

> *'(2) In considering whether a person is a mentally ill person, the continuing condition of the person, including any likely deterioration in the person's condition and the likely effects of any such deterioration, are to be taken into account.'*
>
> (Mental Health Act 2007 (NSW), s14(2))

In making this determination paramedics can gather information

> *'... personally/by audio visual link examining or observing the person, account may be taken of other matters not so ascertained where those matters:*
>
> *(a) arise from a previous examination of the person, or*
> *(b) are communicated by a reasonably credible informant.'*
>
> (Mental Health Act 2007 (NSW), Sch 1)

There is a further power that allows ambulance officers to request police assistance 'if they are of the opinion' that there are *serious* concerns about the safety of the person or other persons if they were to take the person to a mental health facility without the help of a police officer (Mental Health Act 2007 (NSW), s20(2)). This provision is designed to allow paramedics to seek police help when necessary, but places the decision in the hands of health professionals rather than of law enforcement. Consider the following case:

CASE STUDY

Anne

You are called to a patient who is partially clothed and crying outside the front of their house. The caller reports that the patient had appeared to be dancing. On arrival, you find a middle-aged woman who is topless and wearing only a skirt on the lawn of her house in a suburban street. The woman tells you that she has recently been divorced and her ex-husband has been given custody of the children. You ask her if she thinks she needs help and whether she would like to go to the hospital. She says no. The woman tells you that she is from one of the Pacific Islands, and in her culture a part of grieving is to dance and sing in traditional dress. You know that you need to assess whether the patient is mentally ill or disordered to the point that she poses a risk to herself and others BEFORE you can consider transporting her to a mental health facility and certainly before any force can be applied to her.

In terms of the force that may be used to exercise the powers set out in the Act, it is noted at section 81(2) that a person authorised under the Act to take a person to a mental health facility (which therefore includes paramedics as noted above), may:

> *'(a) use reasonable force in exercising functions under this section or any other provision of this Act applying this section, and*
> *(b) restrain the person in any way that is reasonably necessary in the circumstances.'*
>
> (Mental Health Act 2007 (NSW), s81(2))

Restraint does extend to sedation, but again this should be considered in conjunction with the paramedic's clinical guidelines. In South Australia, a paramedic may administer a drug for restraint only if they are authorised to do so under the Controlled Substances Act 1984 (Mental Health Act 2009 (SA), s56(6)). In New South Wales, the law stipulates that the person may be sedated for the purpose of being taken to (or from) a mental health facility or other health facility 'if it is necessary to do so to enable the person to be taken safely to or from the facility' (Mental Health Act 2007 (NSW), s81(3)). There are similar laws authorising restraint, apprehension, search and transportation in most other jurisdictions.

Reasonable force means force that is proportionate to the exercise of the function. It does not mean excessive force, but nor does it mean no force. In the ACT law the limit of force that can be used is the 'minimum amount of force necessary to apprehend the person and remove them to a mental health facility' (Mental Health Act 2015 (ACT), s263). This way of thinking about the force that can be used may be more useful and safer for paramedics than the term 'reasonable' force.

It should be noted that this provision of the law provides paramedics with even more power to limit a person's liberty but authorising them to 'restrain' a person 'in any way' that is 'reasonably necessary'. Again, the key for paramedics here in terms of working inside the law is to refer to professional clinical guidelines, and exercise professional judgement about the most legal and ethical way to exercise the powers that paramedics are given to work in the best interest of the patient. The principles of the law must be kept in mind – that the patient is to be treated in the least restrictive way possible to provide the patient with the care and treatment they need.

Included in the powers provided to paramedics in a number of jurisdictions is the ability to search person and property, remain in place, and remove or make safe objects that may be considered dangerous or pose a risk to the individual or others. A further power that the NSW Mental Health Act authorises for paramedics is the power to carry out a frisk search. A 'frisk search' means:

'(a) *a search of a person conducted by quickly running the hands over the person's outer clothing or by passing an electronic metal detection device over or in close proximity to the person's outer clothing, or*

(b) *an examination of anything worn or carried by the person that is conveniently and voluntarily removed by the person, including an examination conducted by passing an electronic metal detection device over or in close proximity to that thing.'*

(Mental Health Act 2007 (NSW), s81(4))

Again, this places an enormous degree of power in the hands of paramedics that can be used and potentially abused against vulnerable patients. The appropriate exercise of these powers requires paramedics to act, at all times, with the utmost professionalism. At law an individual has a right to bodily inviolability. That is, the individual controls who can touch them, when and how. Any unauthorised touching of an individual can amount to an assault. An example of authorised touching includes when the person gives consent to be touched, but there are also examples where the person does not give consent; for example, when a person is arrested. Paramedics are among the most trusted professionals in our society, and it is essential that paramedics maintain that trust in order for them to be able to do their job. Paramedics are frequently required to act in the best interest of vulnerable patients, commonly when the patient is unable to give or refuse consent to touch. The treatment of mental health patients is a further example of the role of the paramedic acting to place the patient's interests first, and to protect the trustworthy position they have been given. The power given to paramedics to conduct frisk searches is an example of power given to someone other than the individual to infringe on that individual's right to bodily inviolability. This responsibility should be taken extremely seriously.

This is a responsibility that presents as a concern among paramedics when they are dealing with suicidal patients. The law is clear that a person who expresses suicidal thoughts or ideation is not necessarily mentally ill[6] so the expression of suicidal thoughts is not enough on its own to justify a paramedic transporting a patient to hospital to protect them from themselves. In order for the paramedic to be authorised under, for example, the ACT law to apprehend and transport a person involuntarily to a mental health facility, the paramedic must have formed a 'reasonable' belief that the person has a mental disorder or mental illness AND the person has attempted or is likely to attempt suicide, or poses a risk to others (Mental Health Act 2015 (ACT), s80(1)(a), (b)(i)). In order to safely assess the patient and form this belief, the paramedic should be adequately trained and have an understanding of the person's engagement with others, their environment, internal and external resources, help seeking, as well as the physical risks to self and others.

If paramedics transport a patient directly to a mental health facility in the ACT, they are required to provide a written statement containing a description of the action taken under that section of the Act and specifically include the following:

'(a) the name and address (if known) of the person taken to the facility;

(b) the date and time when the person was taken to the facility;

(c) detailed reasons for taking the action;

(d) the nature and extent of the force or assistance used to enter any premises, or to apprehend the person and take the person to the facility;

(e) the nature and extent of any restraint, involuntary seclusion or forcible giving of medication used when apprehending the person or taking the person to the facility;

(f) anything else that happened when the person was being apprehended and taken to the facility that may have an effect on the person's physical or mental health.'

(Mental Health Act 2015 (ACT), s83(1))

---

[6]*Stuart v Kirkland-Veenstra* (2009) 237 CLR 215.

Variations of this information may be required by all states with regard to report writing, but it is an example of best practice from a legal perspective.

CROSS-BORDER ARRANGEMENTS

From time to time paramedics may be required to work across borders, and the state by state nature of mental health laws mean that there may be confusion about specific provisions of the respective Acts of each state. The state in which you are treating the patient is the law that generally applies. However, it is likely that there will exist an agreement between the border states that addresses which law should apply. For example, there is an agreement in place between Victoria and New South Wales on the transfer of patients between states (Eburn, 2018).

CONFIDENTIALITY AND PRIVACY

There is a legal and ethical requirement for paramedics to work to preserve the confidentiality and privacy of their patients. This means that paramedics should not engage in the promotion of patient information in any public forum, be it television or social media. The rule to remember is that the information you collect as a part of the privileged position of being a trusted professional paramedic is not your information to share. There are rare public health exceptions under the respective privacy laws of each state that allow for the sharing of patient information to health authorities if it is necessary to prevent harms to other persons, but this sharing of information should be considered carefully. It is critical that paramedics place the interests of their patient ahead of any other interest including that of their employer.

PRACTITIONER MENTAL HEALTH AND THE LAW

Now that paramedics are registered health practitioners regulated under the Health Practitioner Regulation National Law Act 2009 (Qld) ('the National Law'), there are some extra legal and ethical requirements that will apply to paramedics with regard to the management of their own and fellow health practitioners' mental health. The legislation is primarily designed to protect patients and, as such, there are particular provisions within the law that mandate the reporting of either self or other health practitioners who may pose a risk to themselves or others because they are suffering from a notifiable condition. This condition could be a mental health condition, including, for example, anxiety, that is so serious that it is affecting the way in which the practitioner is working to such an extent that they pose a risk to their patients.

Under the National Law, the Paramedicine Board has the power to develop and implement a registration standard with regard to the physical and mental health requirements for registration of practitioners and the suitability of individuals to competently and safely practise. The Board has established mandatory notification requirements (see the 'Guidelines for Mandatory Notifications March 2020').

A mandatory notification to the Australian Health Practitioner Regulation Agency must be made by any registered health practitioner if they form a reasonable belief that they or another registered health practitioner has behaved in a way that constitutes notifiable conduct. Notifiable conduct by registered health practitioners is defined as:

- practising while intoxicated by alcohol or drugs;
- sexual misconduct in the practice of the profession;
- placing the public at risk of substantial harm because of an impairment (health issue); or
- placing the public at risk because of a significant departure from accepted professional standards.

In terms of the type of impairment related to health that is of concern, it 'means the person has a physical or mental impairment, disability, condition or disorder (including substance abuse or dependence) that detrimentally affects or is likely to detrimentally affect the person's capacity to practise the profession or for a student, the student's capacity to undertake clinical training'. Once the regulator becomes aware, they are then able to ask the practitioner to undertake a health assessment to determine whether the person has an impairment. This 'includes a medical, physical, psychiatric or psychological examination or test of the person' (Health Practitioner Regulation National Law Act 2009 (NSW), s5). This action is designed to not only protect the public but to protect the practitioner, who, if diagnosed with an impairment, can be treated as a patient with the same rights and opportunities as any other. The Paramedicine Board has the power to place limits on the practitioner's practice until such time as they believe the practitioner is well enough, for their own sake and that of their patients, to return to full duties.

Awareness of this provision of the National Law is especially relevant to paramedics as a registered health practitioner group because of the very high levels of mental health conditions experienced by paramedics (Dawson, 2018). The mandatory reporting requirement should not be considered as 'dobbing' in a fellow healthcare practitioner, but rather helping that practitioner to get the support they need to get well and not risk any harm coming to them or their patients, the result of which could be much more serious outcomes for both.

CONCLUSION

In short, paramedics hold a position of power over their patients, and mental health patients are particularly vulnerable to abuse and exploitation. As such it is essential that paramedics practise with the utmost professionalism and comply with the requirements of the law in caring, treating and advocating for this group of people.

All healthcare professionals have the responsibility of being aware of their local legislation, as well as policy and procedures, to ensure that their patients are provided with the best care within a legal and ethical framework.

LINKS AND RESOURCES

Australian Capital Territory
Charter of Rights for people who experience mental health issues: https://health.act.gov.au/services-and-programs/mental-health/charter-rights

Mental Health Act plain language guide: https://www.health.act.gov.au/sites/default/files/2018-09/Plain%20Language%20Guide_MH%20ACT.pdf

New South Wales
Mental Health Act 2007 guide book: https://www.health.nsw.gov.au/mentalhealth/resources/Pages/mhact-guidebook-2007.aspx

Northern Territory
Mental health information for health professionals: https://health.nt.gov.au/professionals/mental-health-information-for-health-professional

Queensland
A guide to the Mental Health Act 2016: https://www.health.qld.gov.au/__data/assets/pdf_file/0031/444856/guide-to-mha.pdf

South Australia
Mental Health Act 'plain language guide': https://www.chiefpsychiatrist.sa.gov.au/legislation/mental-health-act/guides

Mental Health Act clinician's guide and code of practice: https://www.sahealth.sa.gov.au/wps/wcm/connect/e76b440043346e90a64cfe15eab6e6ef/clinicians-guide-and-code-of-practice-mha-mhsb-02130320.pdf?MOD=AJPERES&CACHEID=e76b440043346e90a64cfe15eab6e6ef

Mental Health and Emergency Services memorandum of understanding: https://www.chiefpsychiatrist.sa.gov.au/legislation/mental-health-act/mental-health-and-emergency-services-memorandum-of-agreement

Tasmania
An overview of the Mental Health Act 2013: https://www.dhhs.tas.gov.au/mentalhealth/mental_health_act/mental_health_act_2013_new_mental_health_act/information_for_consumers,_carers_and_the_community_sector/fact_sheets/an_overview_of_the_mental_health_act_2013

Victoria
Mental Health Act 2014 handbook: https://www2.health.vic.gov.au/mental-health/practice-and-service-quality/mental-health-act-2014-handbook

Western Australia
Consumer handbook to the Mental Health Act 2014: https://www.mhc.wa.gov.au/media/1437/consumer-handbook-to-the-mental-health-act-2014-version-2-1.pdf

REFERENCES

American Psychiatric Association, 2013. Diagnostic and Statistical Manual of Mental Disorders, fifth ed. DSM-5™. APA, Washington.

Australian Health Practitioner Regulation Authority (AHPRA), 2020. Guidelines for mandatory notifications March 2020. Online. Available: https://www.paramedicineboard.gov.au/professional-standards/codes-guidelines-and-policies/guidelines-for-mandatory-notifications.aspx.

Controlled Substances Act 1984 (SA). Online. Available: https://www.legislation.sa.gov.au/LZ/C/A/CONTROLLED%20SUBSTANCES%20ACT%201984/CURRENT/1984.52.AUTH.PDF.

Dawson, D., 2018. Ambulance paramedic psychosocial health study. Unpublished doctoral dissertation. Victoria University, Melbourne.

Eburn, M., 2018. Mental health services by paramedics across the NSW/Victoria border. Emergency Law Blog. Online. Available: https://emergencylaw.wordpress.com/2018/10/25/mental-health-services-by-paramedics-across-the-nsw-victoria-border/.

Health Practitioner Regulation National Law Act 2009 (Qld). Online. Available: https://www.legislation.qld.gov.au/view/pdf/inforce/current/act-2009-045.

Mental and Related Services Act 2009 (NT). Online. Available: https://legislation.nt.gov.au/en/Legislation/MENTAL-HEALTH-AND-RELATED-SERVICES-ACT-1998.

Mental Health and Related Services Act 1998 (NT). Online. Available: https://legislation.nt.gov.au/Legislation/MENTAL-HEALTH-AND-RELATED-SERVICES-ACT-1998.

Mental Health Act 2015 (ACT). Online. Available: https://www.legislation.act.gov.au/a/2015-38/.

Mental Health Act 2007 (NSW). Online. Available: https://www.legislation.nsw.gov.au/#/view/act/2007/8.

Mental Health Act 2016 (Qld). Online. Available: https://www.legislation.qld.gov.au/view/pdf/asmade/act-2016-005.

Mental Health Act 2009 (SA). Online. Available: https://www.legislation.sa.gov.au/LZ/C/A/MENTAL%20HEALTH%20ACT%202009.aspx.

Mental Health Act 2013 (Tas). Online. Available: https://www.legislation.tas.gov.au/view/html/inforce/current/act-2013-002#GS4@EN.

Mental Health Act 2014 (Vic). Online. Available: https://content.legislation.vic.gov.au/sites/default/files/2020-02/14-26aa022%20authorised.pdf.

Mental Health Act 1996 (WA). Online. Available: https://www.legislation.wa.gov.au/legislation/statutes.nsf/law_a491.html.

Mental Health (Compulsory Assessment and Treatment) Act 1992 (NZ). Online. Available: https://www.legislation.govt.nz/act/public/1992/0046/latest/DLM262176.html.

Townsend, R., Luck, M., 2009. Protective jurisdiction, patient autonomy and paramedics: the challenges of applying the NSW Mental Health Act. Aust. J. Paramed. 7 (4).

Physical health and mental health

David Lawrence

INTRODUCTION

Mental disorders are among the most common, persistent and disabling chronic health conditions in developed countries (Whiteford et al., 2013). As well as suffering the direct symptoms of their mental illness, people with mental illness have substantially poorer physical health than the rest of the community. People with mental illness have substantially reduced life expectancy, and higher rates of most common health conditions, including cardiovascular diseases, respiratory diseases and metabolic conditions such as diabetes and obesity. However, they are less likely to receive appropriate healthcare for these conditions.

Life expectancy of people with persistent mental illness is substantially reduced by 12–16 years, and up to 25 years for some specific mental illnesses (Chang et al., 2011; Lawrence et al., 2013). While this life expectancy gap is greatest for people with schizophrenia and other psychoses, substantial gaps also exist for people with depression and anxiety disorders (Erlangsen et al., 2017; Lawrence et al., 2013). When considered in the context that the gap in life expectancy between Aboriginal and Torres Strait Islander Australians and other Australians is approximately 10 years, and considering the high proportion of Australians who have a mental illness, this represents a substantial gap and should be a major health priority. That such a high degree of health burden does not attract wider attention is perhaps a measure of the stigma that mental illness still carries today.

There are many types of mental illness, just as there are many types of physical illness. Recognising the type of disorder, the nature and persistence of the symptoms, and the degree of functional impairment are important factors. People with persistent disorders with severe functional impairment have the highest rates of comorbid physical health conditions and the poorest outcomes.

The majority of excess deaths or premature deaths among people with mental illness is due to physical health conditions, with cardiovascular disease, respiratory diseases and cancers being the major causes of excess death. Many of these deaths are preventable with appropriate primary prevention, screening, intervention and treatment. People with mental illness who have a physical health condition are less likely to have it detected, more likely to have it detected at a later stage, and less likely to receive standard interventions. For most interventions there is no evidence to suggest they are any less effective for people with mental illness, and these inequalities in healthcare are linked to systemic issues associated with stigma, the way health services are organised, and the impact that mental illness has on patients' abilities to seek and manage their own healthcare needs.

With increasingly specialised medical care, greater effort is required to coordinate and deliver holistic healthcare for people with multiple health conditions or issues. It is human nature to try to simplify complex problems, and there is a natural tendency to identify the most pressing issue and resolve it first. While this may be the most urgent concern, it may not be the most important concern in the longer term. Failure to deliver holistic healthcare when patients interact with the health system can result in delays in diagnosing and appropriately treating chronic conditions that ultimately impact on quality of life and life expectancy.

Multiple factors contribute to the high rate of physical health conditions in people who have mental illness. These include the side effects of medications, risk behaviours including smoking, alcohol and drug use, diet and exercise, levels of family and social support, cognitive impairments and communications impairments that are often associated with symptoms of mental illness, stigma in the healthcare system, and in general a lack of coordinated care for more complex cases with multiple comorbid conditions (De Hert, Cohen et al., 2013; Rethink Mental Illness, 2013).

Traditionally, the primary role of paramedics has been seen as responding to medical- and trauma-related emergencies. There is increasing recognition that chronic health conditions, both physical and mental, represent a significant part of paramedic case load (Eastwood et al., 2018; McKetin et al., 2018). Moreover, the care of people with mental illness who have comorbid physical health conditions is as important in emergency care as in other healthcare settings because:

- people with mental illness are over-represented in emergency care settings and are less likely to receive primary care – paramedics may be the first, and, in some instances, the only health professionals to provide healthcare to some individuals
- in cases of medical or psychiatric emergency, responding to the immediate presenting issue may be the most urgent priority; however, failure to detect and respond to the underlying chronic physical and mental health issues a patient faces may result in repeat emergency call-outs

- while transporting a patient, paramedics may have time to take a more comprehensive history of the patient and screen for chronic physical conditions that subsequent treating practitioners may not have time to undertake
- being able to recognise, assess and manage all common aspects of mental illness in everyday practice is important to improve the quality of care provided to people with mental illness (Shaban, 2006).

The Australian National Mental Health Commission has produced the Equally Well consensus statement on improving the physical health and wellbeing of people living with mental illness in Australia (National Mental Health Commission, 2016). The consensus statement outlines six essential elements:

1. *A holistic, person-centred approach to physical and mental health and wellbeing*
2. *Effective promotion, prevention and early intervention*
3. *Equity of access to all services*
4. *Improving quality of health care*
5. *Care coordination and regional integration across health, mental health and other services and sectors which enable a contributing life*
6. *Monitoring of progress towards improved physical health and wellbeing.*

Each of these elements is relevant to the paramedic context. To improve the physical health of people with mental illness, it has been recommended that all health professionals are educated in the issues affecting the poor physical health of people with mental illness (Van Hasselt et al., 2015).

Australian governments have committed to implementing the principles of Equally Well through the fifth National Mental Health and Suicide Prevention Plan, which has identified a priority area of 'Improving the physical health of people living with mental illness and reducing early mortality' (Council of Australian Governments, 2017).

CASE STUDY
Anthony

You have been dispatched to a residential care facility for a 38-year-old male with behavioural disturbance. The facility's manager has called the ambulance service. Upon your arrival, the manager takes you to the rear courtyard where Anthony is pacing. You see some upended (but not broken) garden furniture and pot plants. The manager informs you that Anthony has never been violent, but she has never seen him this agitated before. Furthermore, Anthony has always been polite and takes direction from staff, but she had been unable to get him inside after almost three hours of pacing.

Anthony has a diagnosis of schizophrenia. You have been provided with a packet of medication which is prescribed by a GP (olanzapine 10 mg). The manager gives Anthony his medication each evening and she had thought he was taking it; however, the manager hands you two tablets which the cleaner found in his bedroom that morning.

Anthony continues to pace around the garden. He does not appear to be distressed by your presence, but he does not respond to your questions and he initially refuses to sit for you to take a set of observations. He appears dishevelled, wearing dirty old clothes – you are told that this is normal for him. His hair is shoulder length and uncombed, he has a long full-faced beard, and, you notice, heavily nicotine-stained fingers on his right hand. He is moderately obese.

The manager offers Anthony one of her cigarettes only under the condition that he sits down and allows you to take his observations. He agrees and cooperates. You notice that he has a productive cough with used tissues, sputum and other evidence scattered around.

Vital signs
- Glasgow Coma Score: 14
- Oxygen saturations: 91%
- Respiratory rate: 25
- Heart rate: 122
- Blood pressure: 187/105
- 12 lead ECG: prolonged QT complex
- Pain score: States it is 10/10 although he has a blunted affect and no visual impression of experiencing pain
- Blood sugar level: 11 mmol
- Skin: cold, clammy
- Pupils: PEARL

CRITICAL REFLECTION

- At this stage, are you more concerned about Anthony's mental health or physical health? Why?
- What are your priorities at this time?
- What further information would you like to know about Anthony? As there is limited communication from Anthony, where and how would you get this information?

The manager tells you that the community mental health team stopped seeing Anthony about two years ago, advising he can go to his GP for medication. Anthony smokes 30 cigarettes a day. He would smoke more but they are rationed by the manager. He does not take illicit substances.

CRITICAL REFLECTION

- Your partner advises that he has met people like Anthony before and thinks that he is having a relapse of schizophrenia due to medication non-adherence. You tend to agree, but what other potential differential diagnosis might you consider?
- List the risk factors in an otherwise healthy person who smokes 30 cigarettes a day.
- Now list the additional risk factors of someone with schizophrenia who smokes 30 cigarettes a day.
- Consider the Recovery Model (from Chapter 2), and list all of the biopsychosocial factors that should be considered in Anthony's case. Identify who may assist Anthony in each of these areas (include clinicians, non-clinicians and other supports).

Anthony denies medication non-adherence, but admits to having missed one or two doses because he fell asleep before taking them. He agrees to take an olanzapine tablet in front of you, and after a short time he sits with you and talks about his history. He says that his main concern at the moment is his cough and the pains he is getting through his chest and abdomen.

Based on your examination, you have significant concerns for Anthony's physical health, especially in regard to having chest pain and an abnormal electrocardiograph. You talk to Anthony about your concerns, and suggest he should come with you to hospital to get checked out. Anthony declines this offer, saying he wants to stay home and go to bed. You have now assessed Anthony to be alert and orientated, GCS 15, he has no acute psychotic symptoms, and he has stated that he has no thoughts of hurting himself or anyone else. Your partner says that you can force him to come to hospital for assessment and treatment of the chest pain because he has schizophrenia and therefore has no capacity to refuse.

CRITICAL REFLECTION

- Under what circumstances can Anthony refuse to go to hospital?
- Under what circumstances can you force Anthony to come with you to hospital?
- If you do not think that you have the right or ability to bring Anthony in an involuntary capacity, what else could you do to assist him?

Anthony refuses to come with you to hospital. The manager assures you that she will speak with the GP who is scheduled to visit the facility next week.

ACTIVITY

- Complete a clinical handover document for Anthony to be given to the GP.

Five months later the manager again calls the ambulance service requesting urgent help for Anthony as part of their standard procedures for responding to suspected acute myocardial infarction.

THE RELATIONSHIP BETWEEN PHYSICAL AND MENTAL HEALTH

The high rates of most physical conditions among people with mental illness have been known for many years (Baldwin, 1971). There are an estimated 13 million premature deaths in people with mental and substance use disorders each year (Charlson et al., 2015). There is some evidence that the gap in life expectancy between people with and without mental illness is actually increasing in Australia (Lawrence et al., 2013; Saha et al., 2007). Eating disorders have among the highest mortality rates of all mental illnesses and significantly impact physical health (Arcelus et al., 2011). While physical health is poorest among people with severe mental disorders, including psychoses and eating disorders, people with mood, anxiety, substance use or impulse control disorders, whether receiving treatment for these conditions or not, are also at high risk for common chronic physical health conditions (Scott et al., 2016).

While there has been some academic interest in whether mental disorders and physical disorders are related through some common genetic or hormonal link, little evidence has accrued to support this theory to date. Instead, most of the evidence supports this association being primarily due to well-known pragmatic and public health issues, such as exposure to health risk factors, in particular smoking, and inequities in access to and quality of healthcare (Mental Health Commission of New South Wales, 2016). While these issues would appear readily addressable with current knowledge, they have proved very difficult to modify in practice, with wide disparities in health outcomes continuing to be observed across developed countries (De Hert, Correll et al., 2013).

THE PERSON AS A WHOLE

As emphasised in the first essential element of the Equally Well consensus statement 'a holistic, person centred approach to physical and mental health and wellbeing' is key to improving both physical and mental health outcomes for people with mental illness. With the increasing specialisation of healthcare, there are fewer organisations and individual healthcare providers who have the knowledge and skills to be able to provide holistic care for people who have multiple health conditions. People with multiple conditions often have greater degree of disability and persistence of their health problems and, as a fundamental principle of equity in healthcare delivery, may need higher levels of care. The siloed and compartmentalised healthcare system often fails to identify and treat all relevant aspects of a person's health. This often compromises the success of the treatment for the condition that is identified (Naylor et al., 2016). As in the case of 'Anthony', who was only seeing his GP after his mental health team stopped seeing him two years previously, people with mental illness are often initially seen in mental health settings with potentially less involvement of mental health practitioners over time, and the responsibility tends to be left to general practitioners with constraints to the holistic provision of care in the primary setting.

In being the first to respond to a medical or psychiatric emergency, and having some control over the clinical handover to other healthcare providers, paramedics have the opportunity to use their broad knowledge across medical specialties to obtain a history of multiple presenting conditions and to provide this information to subsequent healthcare providers.

THE EFFECTS OF MENTAL HEALTH ON HELP SEEKING AND HEALTHCARE

With the exception of dementia and eating disorders, there are no biological models or research evidence to suggest that mental illness is directly linked to poorer physical health and early death. One of the contributing factors is the impact that common symptoms of mental illness can have on help seeking and receipt of healthcare when needed (Thornicroft, 2013). Mental illness can be associated with cognitive impairments. These impairments may affect memory, and they may affect decision making. In Australia and New Zealand the primary responsibility for seeking and coordinating healthcare is primarily left with the individual. Cognitive impairments associated with mental illness may impair people's efforts to seek help when needed.

More fundamental, though, is the impact that symptoms of mental illness often have on communications ability, and the ability to form and maintain relationships. This can be particularly challenging in healthcare settings, where most healthcare providers are time poor. One of the most valuable things paramedics and healthcare providers can offer people with mental illness is time – sufficient time to demonstrate a level of empathy, and sufficient time to develop an understanding of the relevant history of the patient.

While attitudes towards mental health issues have been changing, and the stigma associated with mental illness has lessened, it is not uncommon for people with mental illness to have a history of experiencing negative or stigmatising reactions, which may also affect their communication.

THE NEGLECT OF PHYSICAL HEALTH IN THE MENTAL HEALTH SYSTEM

Historically, there were documented reports of the terrible general health and high mortality rates of people with mental illness in the 'asylum' era (Farr, 1841). As our knowledge of mental health has improved, many new treatments have been established and many historical myths concerning mental health and illness have been discredited. From the 1960s and 1970s, throughout the developed world, there was a large-scale movement to close or dramatically reduce the size of inpatient facilities in favour of providing care in the community. While this movement had undoubtedly improved the freedom and lives of many people with mental illness, it has presented some challenges. One of these has been the provision of adequate levels of care in community-based settings. Another consequence has been an increased presence of people with mental illness in emergency care settings (Hiscock et al., 2018; Perera et al., 2018). People with mental illness should be afforded the opportunity to live in the least restrictive setting appropriate to their needs, and to have the greatest ability to participate in work, family and community activities. Nevertheless, a greater emphasis on community-based living and community-based care may lead to a higher incidence of emergency events that require paramedic attendance.

PHYSICAL HEALTH CONSIDERATIONS AND HISTORY TAKING FOR PARAMEDICS

The profile of health service use for people with mental illness varies from the general population, particularly for people with severe mental illness, who are more likely to be seen in specialist services, emergency care and emergency departments than in primary care. In recent years there has been an increase in the proportion of people with mental illness presenting to emergency departments, and for some the emergency department is their first contact or their only contact with the health system (Hiscock et al., 2018; Perera et al., 2018). There is ongoing debate about the appropriate role of paramedics and emergency care, and whether this role should be focused solely on responding to acute emergencies, or whether it could contribute to addressing health inequalities and preventing chronic disease (Allen et al., 2013; Ford-Jones & Chaufan, 2017). Some argue that the resources devoted to non-life-threatening emergencies can restrict the availability of resources for those emergencies that are life-threatening. There is a larger argument as to how to most appropriately address inequalities in access to and use of healthcare that adversely affect people with mental illness. If primary healthcare were equitably available and used by all in proportion to need, and if all people with mental illness received regular screening and monitoring of their physical health, this may significantly improve the health of people with mental illness. In the absence of such fundamental reforms, any policies that try to divert or turn away non-critical calls may cause more harm (Ford-Jones & Chaufan, 2017). For people who have more complex health needs, with multiple comorbid conditions, which often include comorbid mental health conditions, responding to the urgent need without identifying and resolving the underlying issues can result in multiple call-outs. People with mental illness are over-represented among frequent callers to ambulance services (Thompson et al., 2011).

Preventing rather than resolving crises is ultimately in the best interest of the patient, and would lead to reduced overall demand for emergency services. The advent of extended-care paramedics, who are able to treat patients in their home environment and refer patients to GPs or other health providers as appropriate, recognises the increasing role paramedics play as primary carers and in the management of chronic conditions. To this end, while a focus on response times as a key performance indicator for ambulance services may be a useful measure of the provision of emergency medical care, it may be counter-productive in relation to patients with more complex needs or for the provision of primary care in the pre-hospital setting. When paramedics have the time to do so, taking that time to develop a rapport with the patient and undertaking a comprehensive health assessment can be very valuable to the patient and to other primary and specialist physicians, often time poor themselves, who will be involved in the care of the patient.

Patients with mental illness often benefit when healthcare professionals are able to take more time with them. Mental illness is often associated with impacts on cognitive processing, decision making, personality, communications ability and style, and fundamental processes of establishing and maintaining relationships with others. These factors can significantly impact what can be communicated in a short encounter with a health professional. While it is human nature to assume that the speed and intensity of how someone communicates their health issues is related to how much they are affected, this sense may be misleading if the impact of mental illness is impairing the person's communication abilities. The impact of mental illness on personality and communications skills is a fundamental component of the pervasive stigma of mental illness (Stuart, 2008). This stigma is also common among health professionals, and has been recognised as a contributing factor to the inequalities in healthcare delivery to people with mental illness (Sartorius, 2002). The recent position statement from the Royal College of Psychiatrists in the United Kingdom identified addressing stigma among health service providers as one of the keys to achieving parity between mental and physical health (Bailey et al., 2013).

If there is time while transporting a patient to develop a rapport, take a comprehensive history and perform some basic screening and metabolic monitoring. While basic screening is relatively straightforward, it is not consistently undertaken in practice (De Hert, Cohen et al., 2013). Screening and a comprehensive history may be valuable, particularly if full details are conveyed to subsequent treating professionals. Where patients do communicate other health issues and concerns, it is important to honour the fact that they have entrusted their health history to you by ensuring the information is passed on during clinical handover.

The majority of people with mental illness also have physical health conditions, and these often go undetected. As not all patients are good at communicating their symptoms succinctly in a way that facilitates diagnosis, where there is opportunity to take a history and identify the possibility of underlying chronic conditions it should be taken.

The following are some of the most common physical health conditions affecting people with mental illness.

METABOLIC SYNDROME

Metabolic syndrome is very common in people with serious mental illness, and has been the focus of much research attention in recent years (Morgan et al., 2014). Metabolic syndrome is a cluster of symptoms that occur together, including unhealthy cholesterol (high LDL cholesterol, low HDH cholesterol, and high triglycerides), high blood sugar, high blood pressure and obesity. These symptoms are commonly associated with lifestyle factors, including poor diet, lack of exercise, smoking and alcohol consumption. They are also associated with sleep disturbances (Kritharides et al., 2017). Additionally, there is growing evidence that they are linked to common antipsychotic drugs. Second-generation antipsychotics in particular can cause significant weight gain, and there is emerging evidence that some antidepressants and lithium, which is used to treat bipolar disorder, are also associated with metabolic syndrome (Ho et al., 2014). Antipsychotics, antidepressants and mood stabilisers have been associated with metabolic conditions including obesity, dyslipidaemia and diabetes, as well as cardiovascular disease, gastrointestinal disorders, thyroid disorders, and movement and seizure disorders (Correll et al., 2015). In patients with severe mental illness such as schizophrenia, bipolar disorder or major depressive disorder, a combination of the direct metabolic effects of their medications, unhealthy lifestyles and lack of monitoring can compound the risk. Significant weight gain and disturbance of metabolism can be associated with significant fatigue and lack of motivation, which can decrease the likelihood of the patient modifying their lifestyle by increasing their exercise or modifying their diet. It can also lead to reduced social interaction or participation in daily events, leading to further social isolation and increasing depression.

Metabolic syndrome is recognised as a precursor to, and significant risk factor for, the development of cardiovascular disease and diabetes. People with mental illness who are taking psychotropic drugs should be regularly monitored, including monitoring blood pressure, body mass index (BMI), blood sugar and lipids (Stanley

& Laugharne, 2010). While metabolic monitoring is most appropriately undertaken in primary care, or by the prescribing physician, people with mental illness are known to have reduced access to primary care, and are less likely to have a regular GP. While recent guidelines from the Royal Australian and New Zealand College of Psychiatry (RANZCP, 2015; Lambert et al., 2017) identify psychiatrists as having a primary role in monitoring and managing the physical health of their patients, acceptance of this position is not uniform among psychiatrists (Mitchell & Hardy, 2013). Treatment of metabolic syndrome in people with mental illness can include lifestyle modifications, changing antipsychotics or prescribing metformin.

DIABETES

The prevalence of diabetes mellitus is two to three times higher in people with severe mental illness (Holt & Mitchell, 2015). People with severe mental illness who also have diabetes mellitus are more likely to have complications associated with their diabetes, and are at greater mortality risk. Despite this, people with severe mental illness receive less and lower-quality diabetes care (Mitchell et al., 2012). Screening for metabolic disorder and diabetes is important to reduce the rate of undiagnosed diabetes in people with mental illness.

In people with schizophrenia, bipolar disorder or major depressive disorder, the prevalence of Type 2 diabetes mellitus has been estimated at 3% in patients never exposed to antipsychotics, and 11% in those taking antipsychotic medications (Vancampfort et al., 2016). People with serious mental illness have been identified as a high-risk group requiring proactive screening for diabetes (Vancampfort et al., 2016).

CARDIOVASCULAR DISEASE

Cardiovascular disease is the main cause of premature mortality in people with mental illness (Lawrence et al., 2013). There are multiple contributing factors. All of the common lifestyle risk factors for cardiovascular disease – including smoking, substance use, poor diet and lack of exercise – are more common in people with mental illness. As noted above, psychotropic drugs have been linked to metabolic dysregulation and metabolic syndrome, and cardiovascular events may also be side effects of psychotropic drugs. Despite being at high risk of cardiovascular disease, the quality of cardiovascular healthcare is lower in people with mental illness, who are less likely to receive screening for cardiovascular risk (Mangurian et al., 2016), and less likely to receive healthcare interventions, including pharmaceutical or surgical treatments (Lawrence & Kisely, 2010; Mitchell & Hardy, 2013). As seen in the case study with 'Anthony', patients whose primary contact with the health system is with a mental health service may not receive active management of physical health issues. Not all people with serious mental illness are in regular contact with a GP, and among those who do have a regular GP the focus of care may still be on managing mental health issues.

EXERCISE AND DIET

Poor diet and exercise are both important risk factors for metabolic syndrome, diabetes and cardiovascular disease. People with schizophrenia often have a poor diet high in refined carbohydrates, saturated fat and salt, and low in fibre and fruit (Dipasquale et al., 2013). While this is often considered a result of poor lifestyle choices, a number of factors have been identified in the literature associated with poorer dietary patterns. These include socio-economic factors and reduced efficacy in cooking and food preparation leading to higher consumption of cheaper prepared foods, the metabolic effects of antipsychotic medications, which can affect taste and dietary preference, as well as regulation of the amount of food consumed, and exposure to traumatic environments in childhood, through a posited pathway of stress, hormonal imbalance and dietary impact (Dipasquale et al., 2013). Exposure to stress has been linked to higher consumption of sugar and fat and reduced consumption of protein and fibre (Rutters et al., 2009).

Lack of regular exercise is also a problem for people with mental illness. Among people with schizophrenia, lack of exercise has been associated with social isolation, low self-efficacy, side effects of antipsychotics, and low levels of motivation (Vancampfort et al 2012, Vancampfort et al 2015). People with schizophrenia, bipolar disorder and major depressive disorder are estimated to spend an average eight hours per day being sedentary during waking hours, and to have an average of 40 minutes of moderate or vigorous activity per day, which is significantly lower than population averages (Vancampfort et al., 2017). Additional factors identified as linked to lower levels of exercise and physical activity in people with mental illness include lower levels of fitness and greater difficulty undertaking physical activity, and higher BMI and levels of obesity.

While healthy levels of exercise are encouraged to improve physical health, exercise is also beneficial in improving mental health, particularly decreasing depression (Knapen et al., 2014). When undertaken in the context of group sports or other group activities, it can also have the positive benefits of increasing social connection and engagement.

TOBACCO USE

Tobacco use is a well-known risk factor for common physical illnesses, including cardiovascular disease, respiratory diseases and cancer. While there has been significant progress in reducing smoking rates in the general population, smoking rates remain high among people with mental illness (Britton, 2015). In the 2010 Australian Survey of Psychosis, two-thirds of people with psychotic illness were current smokers (Cooper et al., 2012). While smoking rates are highest in people with psychotic illness, smoking rates in people with depression and anxiety disorders, even mild anxiety disorders, are well above the population average rates, and make a significant contribution to the reduced life expectancy and excess mortality of people with mental illness (Lawrence et al., 2009; Lawrence et al., 2010). People with mental illness account for about 40% of tobacco-attributable deaths in the

United States (Prochaska et al., 2017). Despite the high prevalence of smoking and the clear detrimental impact of tobacco use on people with mental illness, the issue of smoking and mental illness has not been given significant attention in public health or healthcare (Prochaska, 2011; Prochaska et al., 2017).

Despite significant evidence that quitting smoking enhances both mental health and physical health (Ziedonis et al., 2008), there are widespread beliefs that addressing smoking in people with mental illness is a lower priority than more immediate problems associated with symptoms of mental illness, and that self-medication with nicotine is helpful for mental illness (Association of American Medical Colleges, 2007; Britton, 2015; Sheals et al., 2016). While many health professionals believe that people with mental illness are less interested in quitting smoking, research studies consistently show that people with mental illness are interested in quitting, but find it more challenging to do so. Nevertheless, healthcare professionals are less likely to talk about smoking with people with mental illness. It is now recommended that people with mental illness be routinely asked whether they smoke, and be offered brief advice and encouragement to quit smoking if they do (Nursing, Midwifery and Allied Health Professions Policy Unit, 2016). As can be seen in the case study with 'Anthony', cigarettes have historically been used in mental health settings to facilitate therapeutic relationships and to seek cooperation from patients.

SLEEP AND SLEEP DISTURBANCE

Sleep problems are common symptoms of many mental health conditions, and are listed as part of the diagnostic criteria for major depressive disorder, generalised anxiety disorder, post-traumatic disorder, bipolar disorder and many others in the *Diagnostic and Statistical Manual of Mental Disorders*, fifth edition (*DSM-5*; American Psychiatric Association, 2013). Disturbed sleep can also be a side effect of psychiatric medications. However, there is growing evidence that sleep problems can be both a contributing cause and a symptom of mental illness (Krystal, 2012). Longitudinal studies have shown that sleep disorders such as insomnia are risk factors for the development of depressive and anxiety disorders, as well as suicidal ideation (McCall et al., 2010).

EATING DISORDERS

Eating disorders are among the few mental illnesses where there are direct biological models linking the mental illness with poor physical health outcomes. In severe cases, the substantial weight loss and malnutrition can be life-threatening. People with eating disorders are also at risk of poor physical health outcomes related to the same mechanisms that affect other mental illnesses, including not seeking or receiving treatment due to the stigma associated with the condition, and being treated in a siloed or specialist facility that doesn't provide holistic care. Eating disorders can affect multiple organ systems and are associated with a high risk of premature death (Arcelus et al., 2011; Mitchell & Crow, 2006).

Malnutrition associated with eating disorders can affect muscle mass, including the heart muscle, and can present as cardiac symptoms or chest pain. Malnutrition and associated dehydration can also impact liver function, and lead to osteoporosis. Frequent purging can result in gastric acid reflux and associated gastrointestinal complaints (Mascolo et al., 2012). As people with eating disorders may actively hide their behaviour or may not recognise their problem, screening for possible eating disorders should be undertaken if warning signs are detected, including evidence of weight change, concern about body shape or weight, evidence of vomiting, cold sensitivity or dizziness (Trent et al., 2013).

As a paramedic it is important to understand the various physiological factors at play and what to include in an assessment of someone with an eating disorder. The initial dispatch may be related to dizziness, fatigue, dehydration, palpitations, syncope or seizures, but these may be secondary to complications from malnutrition (Mascolo et al., 2012). While there may be various psychological factors involved, assessment should primarily focus on the physiological factors first, and include vital signs including lying and standing BP and pulse, temperature and ECG. The paramedic should be concerned about cardiac arrhythmias, including prolonged QTc, hypotension and postural changes, bradycardia, postural tachycardia, hypothermia and hypoglycaemia. In addition, starvation, severe weight loss, dehydration, hypoglycaemia and electrolyte abnormalities can lead to cognitive impairment, impacting on a person's capacity for decision making.

ORAL HEALTH

People with severe mental illness have poor oral health (Kisely et al., 2011), with substantially higher rates of decayed and missing teeth, and a higher risk of edentulousness (total tooth loss). Poor oral health is also associated with eating disorders (Kisely et al., 2015b). While rarely life-threatening, poor oral health can be associated with significant pain. A simple oral health assessment can be completed using standard checklists by non-dental personnel (Kisely et al., 2015a). Self-induced vomiting in patients with eating disorders is associated with poor oral health. Other risk factors include dry mouth as a side effect of psychotropic medications, poor diets that are highly acidic or high in sugars and refined carbohydrates, and poor self-care and oral hygiene. Both internationally and in Australia, poverty and access to dental care have been identified as major issues associated with poor oral health in people with serious mental illness (Happell et al., 2015; McKibbin et al., 2015).

THE EFFECTS OF CHRONIC ILLNESS ON MENTAL HEALTH

While mental illness is associated with increased risk of chronic physical health conditions, poor physical health can also negatively impact on mental health, and can be cyclically reinforcing if patients are not treated in a holistic way. Chronic pain and functional limitations can increase anxiety, stress and depressive symptoms.

Chronic physical conditions can impact on people's ability to work and participate in daily activities, reducing social connection and support, and impacting on self-esteem (Naylor et al., 2012).

CASE STUDY
Hannah

You have been dispatched to a residential address for a 21-year-old female with acute abdominal pain. The patient's mother has called the ambulance service. On arrival you are met by her mother and directed to the lounge room where Hannah is sitting. Hannah states that she is in a lot of pain and needs help. Her mother informs you that Hannah suffers from Crohn's disease.

Hannah has been experiencing increasing abdominal pain and diarrhoea over the past two months, and the previous night had very little sleep, as it was interrupted by pain and the need to get up to the toilet constantly. She is currently seeing a gastroenterologist who has been working with her on a management plan and treatment options. Hannah has been on steroids previously to reduce the inflammation. The course of steroids worked well, but made Hannah feel disoriented and manic. They had to slowly reduce the dose so they could try other longer-term medication.

Vital signs
- Glasgow Coma Score: 14 (distracted by the pain)
- Oxygen saturations: 99%
- Respiratory rate: 22 shallow
- Heart rate: 85
- Blood pressure: 115/75
- Electrocardiograph: sinus tachycardia
- Pain score: 8/10 (abdominal pain)
- Blood sugar level: 17 mmol
- Skin: flushed, sweaty
- Pupils: PEARL

Hannah appears to have a supportive mother, but on questioning, her mother appears to be one of her few social contacts. Hannah's father left the family when Hannah was 10 years old, and she has no siblings. Hannah has virtually no contact with friends, and rarely leaves the house as she is concerned about having 'an attack'. Most of her social contacts are through an online group of fellow suffers. She has never had a romantic relationship. Hannah is worried about going on long-term steroids or the prospect of a colostomy bag, which she has heard about even though her doctor is not suggesting this.

CRITICAL REFLECTION
- What biopsychosocial factors place Hannah at increased risk of developing a mental illness?
- In what ways do chronic physical illnesses such as inflammatory bowel disease lead to a mental illness? List and discuss.
- List the various healthcare professionals currently (and potentially) involved with Hannah's care, including paramedics. What are their potential roles in assisting to prevent, diagnose or treat a mental illness that stems from a chronic physical illness?
- As a paramedic how would you communicate with Hannah? Discuss what influence age and her current circumstance would have on how you communicate with her and her mum.
- How would you manage Hannah's pain levels and the associated emotional and psychological stress she is experiencing?

Mum tells you that Hannah was previously an outgoing young woman with a large group of friends, and she was studying environmental science until her symptoms first started about a year ago. She now has a full range of symptoms for depression, i.e.:

- poor sleep
- low appetite
- weight loss
- low energy
- poor motivation
- low mood.

CRITICAL REFLECTION

- How would you assess/differentiate whether the above symptoms are due to Hannah's physical illness or a potential mental illness (depression)?
- List and discuss any known or potential risk factors for Hannah, both short term and long term.

CONCLUSION

Physical and mental health conditions often co-occur. The majority of early and excess deaths in people with mental illness are due to physical conditions, particularly cardiovascular and respiratory disease and cancer. Many of these deaths are preventable with appropriate primary prevention, screening, intervention and treatment. Higher rates of unhealthy lifestyle risk factors – including smoking, alcohol and drug use, poor diet and lack of exercise – contribute to these poorer outcomes. Also contributing is poorer access to and use of healthcare, and lack of coordinated and ongoing care. Many people with mental health conditions, and particularly those who frequently come in contact with paramedics and emergency departments, have complex health problems with multiple contributing factors. Attention to the most urgent presenting issue in an emergency context may not identify underlying chronic health conditions that contribute to longer-term health outcomes.

Australia's fifth National Mental Health and Suicide Prevention Plan commits to improving the physical health of people living with mental illness through improving quality and equity of access to healthcare and taking a holistic, person-centred approach to physical and mental health. Paramedics can contribute to achieving this goal by using their broad knowledge across medical specialties to take a holistic approach, including comprehensive history taking and assessment of physical health where possible in patients presenting with mental health issues, and communicating case complexities effectively with subsequent healthcare providers. Understanding how mental illness can affect cognition, behaviour and communication skills is also important in developing effective rapport and therapeutic relationships with people with mental illness.

LINKS AND RESOURCES

- Equally Well – National Mental Health Commission's consensus statement: https://equallywell.org.au/
- Equally Well: Physical Health – Equally Well New Zealand has compiled a thorough evidence review of the poor physical health of people with mental health conditions or substance use addictions: https://www.tepou.co.nz/initiatives/equally-well-physical-health/37
- Butterfly Foundation – support for eating disorders and body image issues: https://thebutterflyfoundation.org.au/

REFERENCES

Allen, M., Allen, J., Hogarth, S., et al., 2013. Working for Health Equity: The role of health professionals. UCL Institute of Health Equity, London.

American Psychiatric Association (APA), 2013. Diagnostic and Statistical Manual of Mental Disorders, fifth ed. APA, Washington, DC. (DSM-5).

Arcelus, J., Mitchell, A.J., Wales, J., et al., 2011. Mortality rates in patients with anorexia nervosa and other eating disorders: a meta-analysis of 36 studies. JAMA Psychiatry 68, 724–731.

Association of American Medical Colleges (AAMC), 2007. Physician behavior and practice patterns related to smoking cessation. AAMC, Washington, DC.

Bailey, S., Thorpe, L., Smith, G., 2013. Whole-Person Care: From rhetoric to reality: Achieving parity between mental and physical health. Royal College of Psychiatrists, London.

Baldwin, J.A., 1971. Aspects of the Epidemiology of Mental Illness: Studies in record linkage. Little, Brown, Boston.

Britton, J., 2015. Treating smoking in mental health settings. Lancet Psychiatry 2, 364–365.

Chang, C.K., Hayes, R.D., Perera, G., et al., 2011. Life expectancy at birth for people with serious mental illness and other major disorders from a secondary mental health care case register in London. PLoS ONE 6 (5), e19590.

Charlson, F.J., Baxter, A.J., Dua, T., et al., 2015. Excess mortality from mental, neurological and substance use disorders in the Global Burden of Disease Study 2010. Epidemiol. Psychiatr. Sci. 24, 121–140.

Cooper, J., Mancuso, S.G., Borland, R., et al., 2012. Tobacco smoking among people living with a psychotic illness: the second Australian Survey of Psychosis. Aust. N. Z. J. Psychiatry 46, 851–863.

Correll, C.U., Detraux, J., De Lepeleire, J., et al., 2015. Effects of antipsychotics, antidepressants and mood stabilizers on risk for physical diseases in people with schizophrenia, depression and bipolar disorder. World Psychiatry 14, 119–136.

Council of Australian Governments, 2017. The fifth National Mental Health and Suicide Prevention Plan. Australian Government Department of Health, Canberra.

De Hert, M., Correll, C.U., Bobes, J., et al., 2013. Physical illness in patients with severe mental disorders I: prevalence, impact of medications and disparities in health care. World Psychiatry 10, 52–77.

De Hert, M., Cohen, D., Bobes, J., et al., 2013. Physical illness in patients with severe mental disorders II: barriers to care, monitoring and treatment guidelines, plus recommendations at the system and individual level. World Psychiatry 10, 138–151.

Dipasquale, S., Pariante, C.M., Dazzan, P., et al., 2013. The dietary pattern of patients with schizophrenia: a systematic review. J. Psychiatr. Res. 47, 197–207.

Eastwood, K., Morgans, A., Stelwinder, J., et al., 2018. Patient and case characteristics associated with 'no paramedic treatment' for low-acuity cases referred for emergency ambulance dispatch following a secondary telephone triage: a retrospective cohort study. Scand. J. Trauma Resusc. Emerg. Med. 26, 8.

Erlangsen, A., Andersen, P.K., Toender, A., et al., 2017. Cause-specific life-years lost in people with mental disorders: a nationwide, register-based cohort study. Lancet Psychiatry 4, 937–945.

Farr, W., 1841. Report upon the mortality of lunatics. J. Stat. Soc. London 4, 17–33.

Ford-Jones, P.C., Chaufan, C., 2017. A critical analysis of debates around mental health calls in the prehospital setting. Inquiry 54, doi:10.1177/0046958017704608.

Happell, B., Platania-Phung, C., Scott, D., et al., 2015. Access to dental care and dental ill health of people with serious mental illness: views of nurses working in mental health settings in Australia. Aust. J. Prim. Health 21, 32–37.

Hiscock, H., Neely, R.J., Lei, S., et al., 2018. Paediatric mental and physical health presentations to emergency departments, Victoria, 2008–2015. Med. J. Aust. 208, 343–348.

Ho, C.S.H., Zhang, M.W.B., Mak, A., et al., 2014. Metabolic syndrome in psychiatry: advances in understanding and management. Adv. Psychiatr. Treat. 20, 101–112.

Holt, R.I.G., Mitchell, A.J., 2015. Diabetes mellitus and severe mental illness: mechanisms and clinical implications. Nat. Rev. Endocrinol. 11, 79–89.

Kisely, S., Lake-Hui, Q., Pais, J., et al., 2011. Advanced dental disease in people with severe mental illness: systematic review and meta-analysis. Br. J. Psychiatry 199, 187–193.

Kisely, S., Baghaie, H., Lalloo, R., et al., 2015a. A systematic review and meta-analysis of the association between poor oral health and severe mental illness. Psychosom. Med. 77, 83–92.

Kisely, S., Baghaie, H., Lalloo, R., et al., 2015b. Association between poor oral health and eating disorders: systematic review and meta-analysis. Br. J. Psychiatry 207, 299–305.

Knapen, J., Vancampfort, D., Moriën, Y., et al., 2014. Exercise therapy improves both mental and physical health in patients with major depression. Disabil. Rehabil. 37, 1490–1495.

Kritharides, L., Chow, V., Lambert, T.J.R., 2017. Cardiovascular disease in patients with schizophrenia. Med. J. Aust. 206, 91–95.

Krystal, A., 2012. Psychiatric disorders and sleep. Neurol. Clin. 30, 1389–1413.

Lambert, T.J.R., Reavley, N.J., Jorm, A.F., et al., 2017. Royal Australian and New Zealand College of Psychiatrists expert consensus statement for the treatment, management and monitoring of the physical health of people with an enduring psychotic illness. Aust. N. Z. J. Psychiatry 51, 322–337.

Lawrence, D., Kisely, S., 2010. Inequalities in health care provision for people with severe mental illness. J. Psychopharmacol. (Oxf.) 24 (11 Suppl. 4), 61–68.

Lawrence, D., Mitrou, F., Zubrick, S., 2009. Smoking and mental illness: results from population surveys in Australia and the United States. BMC Public Health 9, 285.

Lawrence, D., Considine, J., Mitrou, F., et al., 2010. Anxiety disorders and cigarette smoking: results from the Australian Survey of Mental Health and Wellbeing. Aust. N. Z. J. Psychiatry 44, 521–528.

Lawrence, D., Hancock, K., Kisely, S., 2013. The gap in life expectancy from preventable physical illness in psychiatric patients: a retrospective analysis of population based registers in Western Australia. BMJ 346, f2539.

Mangurian, C., Newcomer, J.W., Modlin, C., et al., 2016. Diabetes and cardiovascular care among people with severe mental illness: a literature review. J. Gen. Intern. Med. 31, 1083–1091.

Mascolo, M., Trent, S., Colwell, C., et al., 2012. What the emergency department needs to know when caring for your patients with eating disorders. Int. J. Eat. Disord. 45, 977–981.

McCall, W., V, Blocker, J.N., D'Agostino, R., Jr., et al., 2010. Insomnia severity is an indicator of suicidal ideation during a depression clinical trial. Sleep Med. 11, 822–827.

McKetin, R., Degenhardt, L., Shanahan, M., et al., 2018. Health service utilisation attributable to methamphetamine use in Australia: patterns, predictors and national impact. Drug Alcohol Rev. 37, 196–204.

McKibbin, C.L., Kitchen-Andren, K.A., Lee, A.A., et al., 2015. Oral health in adults with serious mental illness: needs for and perspectives on care. Community Ment. Health J. 51, 222–228.

Mental Health Commission of New South Wales, 2016. Physical health and mental wellbeing: evidence guide. Mental Health Commission of New South Wales, Sydney.

Mitchell, A.J., Hardy, S.A., 2013. Screening for metabolic risk among patients with severe mental illness and diabetes: a national comparison. Psychiatr. Serv. 64, 1060–1063.

Mitchell, A.J., Delaffon, V., Vancampfort, D., et al., 2012. Guideline concordant monitoring of metabolic risk in people treated with antipsychotic medication: systematic review and meta-analysis of screening practices. Psychol. Med. 42, 125–147.

Mitchell, J.E., Crow, S., 2006. Medical complications of anorexia nervosa and bulimia nervosa. Curr. Opin. Psychiatry 19, 438–443.

Morgan, V.A., McGrath, J.J., Jablensky, A., et al., 2014. Psychosis prevalence and physical, metabolic and cognitive co-morbidity: data from the second Australian national survey of psychosis. Psychol. Med. 44, 2163–2176.

National Mental Health Commission, 2016. Equally well consensus statement: improving the physical health and wellbeing of people living with mental illness in Australia. National Mental Health Commission, Sydney.

Naylor, C., Parsonage, M., McDaid, D., et al., 2012. Long-term conditions and mental health: the cost of co-morbidities. The King's Fund, London.

Naylor, C., Das, P., Ross, S., et al., 2016. Bringing together physical and mental health: a new frontier for integrated care. The King's Fund, London.

Nursing, Midwifery and Allied Health Professions Policy Unit, 2016. Improving the physical health of people with mental health problems: actions for mental health nurses. Department of Health, Public Health England, London.

Perera, J., Wand, T., Bein, K.J., et al., 2018. Presentations to NSW emergency departments with self-harm, suicidal ideation, or intentional poisoning, 2010–2014. Med. J. Aust. 208, 348–353.

Prochaska, J.J., 2011. Smoking and mental illness—breaking the link. N. Engl. J. Med. 365, 196–198.

Prochaska, J.J., Das, S., Young-Wolf, K.C., 2017. Smoking, mental illness, and public health. Annu. Rev. Public Health 38, 165–185.

Rethink Mental Illness, 2013. Lethal discrimination: why people with mental illness are dying needlessly and what needs to change. Rethink Mental Illness, London.

Royal Australian and New Zealand College of Psychiatrists (RANZCP), 2015. Keeping body and mind together: improving the physical health and life expectancy of people with a serious mental illness. RANZCP, Melbourne.

Rutters, F., Nieuwenhuizen, A.G., Lemmens, S.G., et al., 2009. Acute stress-related changes in eating in the absence of hunger. Obesity (Silver Spring) 17, 72, e7.

Saha, S., Chant, D., McGrath, J., 2007. A systematic review of mortality in schizophrenia: is the differential mortality gap worsening over time? Arch. Gen. Psychiatry 64, 1123–1131.

Sartorius, N., 2002. Iatrogenic stigma of mental illness begins with behaviour and attitudes of medical professionals, especially psychiatrists. BMJ 324, 1470–1471.

Scott, K., Lim, C., Al-Hamzawi, A., et al., 2016. Association of mental disorders with subsequent chronic physical conditions: World Mental Health Surveys from 17 countries. JAMA Psychiatry 73, 150–158.

Shaban, R., 2006. Paramedics' clinical judgment and mental health assessments in emergency contexts: research, practice, and tools of the trade. J. Emerg. Prim. Health Care 4, 369.

Sheals, K., Tombor, I., McNeill, A., et al., 2016. A mixed-method systematic review and meta-analysis of mental health professionals' attitudes toward smoking and smoking cessation amongst people with mental illnesses. Addiction 111, 1536–1553.

Stanley, S., Laugharne, J., 2010. Clinical guidelines for the physical care of mental health consumers. Community, Culture and Mental Health Unit, School of Psychiatry and Clinical Neurosciences, The University of Western Australia, Perth.

Stuart, H., 2008. Fighting the stigma caused by mental disorders: past perspectives, present activities, and future directions. World Psychiatry 7, 185–188.

Thompson, C.J., Grootemaat, P.E., Morris, D., et al., 2011. Ambulance service of NSW: responding to mental health frequent callers: final report. Centre for Health Service Development, University of Wollongong, Wollongong.

Thornicroft, G., 2013. Premature death among people with mental illness. BMJ 346, f2969.

Trent, S.A., Moreira, M.E., Colwell, C.B., et al., 2013. ED management of patients with eating disorders. Am. J. Emerg. Med. 31, 859–865.

Vancampfort, D., Knapen, J., Probst, M., et al., 2012. A systematic review of correlates of physical activity in patients with schizophrenia. Acta Psychiatr. Scand. 125, 352–362.

Vancampfort, D., Stubbs, B., Ward, P.B., et al., 2015. Why moving more should be promoted for severe mental illness. Lancet Psychiatry 2, 295.

Vancampfort, D., Correll, C.U., Galling, B., et al., 2016. Diabetes mellitus in people with schizophrenia, bipolar disorder and major depressive disorder: a systematic review and large scale meta-analysis. World Psychiatry 15, 166–174.

Vancampfort, D., Firth, J., Schuch, F.B., et al., 2017. Sedentary behavior and physical activity levels in people with schizophrenia, bipolar disorder and major depressive disorder: a global systematic review and meta-analysis. World Psychiatry 16, 308–315.

Van Hasselt, F.M., Oud, M.J., Loonen, A.J., 2015. Practical recommendations for improvement of the physical health care of patients with severe mental illness. Acta Psychiatr. Scand. 131, 387–396.

Whiteford, H.A., Degenhardt, L., Rehm, J., et al., 2013. Global burden of disease attributable to mental and substance use disorders: findings from the Global Burden of Disease Study 2010. Lancet 382, 1575–1586.

Ziedonis, D., Hitsman, B., Beckham, J.C., et al., 2008. Tobacco use and cessation in psychiatric disorders: National Institute of Mental Health report. Nicotine Tob. Res. 10, 1691–1715.

Mental health across the life span: Caring for the mental health of children and young people

8.1

Tim J. Crowley and Prue McEvoy

LEARNING OUTCOMES

By the end of this chapter, you should be able to:

* understand the nature of acute mental health disturbances in children and young people
* identify factors (genetic, developmental, environment, medical and cultural) that may have caused, or contributed to, the initiation and persistence of these problems
* evaluate a child or young person's normal level of functioning, and the extent this has been impaired by the mental health disturbance
* determine if transportation to the emergency department is required.

INTRODUCTION

Mental health problems in children and young people are common in the community. A national Australian survey established that 13.9% of children and young people aged 4–17 experience significant mental disorders (Lawrence et al., 2015). This equates to 560,000 Australian children and adolescents experiencing mental health problems per annum (Lawrence et al., 2015). Of these numbers, 8.3% had mild severity of impact, 3.5% had moderate severity of impact, and 2.1% had a severe disorder (Lawrence et al., 2015).

Evidence also tells us that:

* mental-health-related emergency department presentations had a higher proportion of patients aged 15–24 (77.0%) compared with all emergency department presentations (48.4%) in 2016–17 (AIHW, 2018)
* patients under 15 had the lowest rate per 10,000 population of mental-health-related presentations (25.0), whereas those aged 15–24 years had the highest (192.6) (AIHW, 2018)

- of all young people aged between 12 and 17 years old, 7.5% had experienced suicidal ideation in the past 12 months, 7.2% had made a suicide plan, and 2.4% had attempted suicide (Zubrick et al., 2016).

Limited statistical or clinical information exists that delineate primary precipitants, the level of mental health involvement and other socio-economic concerns. The issues with which children and young people present in an emergency are varied, and there are no universally accepted practice parameters for assessment and decision making in this context. Although there are practice parameters for the assessment and emergency management of suicidal behaviour, many do not address the underlying mental health issues, and when they do an adult diagnostic framework is used. Presenting symptoms differ vastly, and in adult psychiatry there is a greater focus on abnormal psychopathology rather than the deviation from the developmental trajectory or social and environmental factors.

Assessment of a child or young person differs from that of an adult in several respects:

- Children/young people rarely seek help on their own behalf.
- Children/young people are sometimes unable to provide certain historical and clinically necessary information. Greater emphasis is therefore also placed on the importance of multiple informants, including parents/carers, teachers, friends, bystanders or other persons who know the child/young person.
- The developmental level of the child/young person must always be considered when assessing the appropriateness of behaviour and functioning. To make accurate judgments about the child/young person's behaviour, a solid understanding of what is developmentally appropriate is required.

WHAT CAUSES MENTAL HEALTH PROBLEMS IN YOUNG PEOPLE?

Clinical experience and evidence tells us that child and adolescent mental health problems are rarely attributable to one single factor or event. Most presentations are multifactorial in their origins, and are impacted on by the young person's developmental history and current circumstances. The impact of each factor varies from problem to problem and child to young person.

FACTORS IMPORTANT FOR MENTAL HEALTH
PSYCHOLOGICAL
Affect regulation

Developmental trauma experienced early in life impacts on relational security and neurobiological integrity, and can lead to severe problems with affect regulation

(Cook et al., 2005). Affect regulation begins with the accurate identification of internal emotional experiences, which requires the ability to differentiate states of arousal, interpret these states, and apply appropriate labels (e.g. happy, scared).

Chronically traumatised children show impairments in both expressing and modulating their internal emotional experiences. These can manifest as dissociation, chronic numbing of emotional experience, dysphoria and avoidance of affectively laden situations (including positive experiences), and maladaptive coping strategies (e.g. substance abuse) (Cook et al., 2005). Consequently, these young people present with extreme emotional responses to minor stressors or precipitants.

Attachment and attachment difficulties

While secure attachment between the child and another can pave the way for successful cognitive, social and emotional development, insecure attachment can produce detrimental results for the child in these areas (Ohtaras, 2015). These successful foundations are critical to a young person's competencies, including distress tolerance, curiosity, sense of agency, and communication.

Within sensitive caregiving relationships, infants learn to trust both what they feel and how they understand the world (Van der Kolk, 2005). This allows them to rely on both their emotions and their thoughts to make sense of any given situation.

A basic problem for children and young people with disorganised attachments frameworks is the sense of mistrust that has emerged from their lack of a predictable, loving caregiver in early childhood. As a consequence, there are difficulties forming and sustaining helpful relationships, resulting in survival-based behaviours. Extreme relational trauma leads to a lifelong risk of physical disease and psychosocial dysfunction, including increased susceptibility to stress (e.g. difficulty focusing attention and modulating arousal) and an inability to regulate emotions without external assistance (e.g. feeling and acting overwhelmed by intense or numbed emotions).

BIOLOGICAL FACTORS

Young people exposed to appropriate caregiving environments learn to respond to both internal and external cues flexibly and with a sense of agency. Developmentally, the brain shifts and evolves. Cooke and colleagues (2005, p. 391) noted 'a gradual shift from right hemisphere dominance (feeling and sensing) to primary reliance on the left hemisphere (language, abstract reasoning, and long range planning) with an integration of neural communication across the two brain hemispheres (corpus callosum)'. Children and young people from challenging and complex family environments struggle to cognitively organise their feelings when under stress, resulting in disorganisation and a propensity to become behaviourally disturbed, marked by extreme helplessness, confusion, withdrawal or rage.

Developmental understandings and communication

The immense changes in emotional and cognitive functioning that take place during adolescence, heralded by puberty, have implications for emergency responders that are unique to this age group. Paramedics should make every effort to shape the questions to the child/young person's level of functioning, and to interpret responses through a developmental lens. This will ensure that the young person experiences your questions as trying to make sense of their situation in a meaningful and helpful way.

Not only are young people particularly vulnerable to new trauma during this developmental phase, but past early traumatic events can be re-triggered for which they may or may not have clear memories. This means that their response to a new stressor/trauma may seem out of context to what you as a paramedic are seeing in the here and now. Paramedic practice needs to be aware, then, that early childhood traumas can be reactivated in adolescence, leading to the re-emergence of problems that were thought to have been resolved in a very different context (Wilson & Thomas, 2004).

Children and young people's protective factors

From time to time, children and young people will show behaviour that suggests the presence of internal risk factors, which may be a part of their temperament or personality. Protective factors such as strong parent management skills and a functional peer group do not block the influence of risk. They do, however, act as a buffer against risk escalating into problem behaviour.

While risk exploration behaviour is a normal part of adaptive child/young person development, problems begin when the behaviour becomes entrenched. Building on a child/young person's internal protective factors (e.g. engagement at school, supportive peers, self-understanding, positive peer connection, etc.) will contribute to achieving developmental milestones, having a positive sense of self, and fostering resilience (the ability to adjust to changes and secure positive outcomes).

As paramedics, it is helpful to balance these considerations when undertaking an assessment.

CULTURAL AND LANGUAGE CONSIDERATIONS

Paramedics are increasingly required to interact with families whose race, culture, nation of origin, living circumstances and family composition are different from their own. Respect for different diverse cultural values is an integral consideration for all assessments and treatment.

For paramedics, being aware of the effects of the young person's experiences in their country of origin prior to migration and settlement will be critical in making sense of their presentation and that of their family.

OTHER SPECIFIC POPULATIONS

Young people presenting with self-harm and suicidal behaviour

The risk of both suicide attempts and suicide is significantly higher in those who have engaged in non-suicidal self-injury (Grandclerc et al., 2016). Suicide remains uncommon among young people aged 0–14, however it is the leading cause of death for young Australians aged 15–24 (ABS, 2016). Rates of suicide have been relatively stable over the past 15 years, but deliberate self-harm among young people has become an important focus of social policy and professional practice (Madge et al., 2008). Greater responsibility for personal decision making creates more opportunities for young people to engage in risky behaviours. For those aged 15 to 17 years, this independence occurs simultaneously at a time when peer acceptance is critical.

Young people are more likely to experiment with illicit substances and alcohol, rendering them susceptible to certain injuries, including falls, transport accidents, accidental poisoning and assaults. Of particular concern is the over-representation of young adults, especially young males, in road traffic accidents associated with risky driving behaviours such as speeding, driving when fatigued, and driving under the influence of substances (Vassallo et al., 2008).

Gender-diverse young people

Gender identity forms concurrently with physical and psychological growth. Although gender has traditionally been divided into 'male' and 'female', it is now recognised that there are a diverse range of gender identities. It is important to recognise that gender-diverse young people have high rates of mental illness and are particularly likely to experience bullying (Jones & Hillier, 2013). As a result, they may experience stressful situations that increase risk for conditions such as depression and anxiety, and have an increased propensity for self-harm and suicide.

Service transition from paediatric to adulthood services

Transition from child and adolescent to adult health services can create uncertainty. Changes in supports and services may exacerbate distress and interfere with appropriate help seeking, provoking increased contact with paramedic and emergency services. Young people who have experienced significant trauma and disruptions in their life will be most at risk during this transition period.

PREVALENCE OF COMMON MENTAL HEALTHCARE NEEDS IN CHILDREN AND YOUNG PEOPLE

The 2015 National Report on the Second Australian Child and Adolescent Survey of Mental Health and Wellbeing revealed that around one in seven (13.9%) children and adolescents aged 4–17 years experienced a mental disorder (Lawrence et al., 2015). This is equivalent to an estimated 560,000 Australian children and adolescents per annum.

The following is a focus on the common diagnoses seen in children and young people.

TRAUMA AND STRESS-RELATED DISORDERS

Acute trauma in children and young people occurs when they experience an event that causes actual harm or poses a serious threat to the child's emotional and physical wellbeing (Bartlett et al., 2017). Trauma is different from regular life stressors because it causes a sense of intense fear, terror and helplessness that is beyond the normal range for typical experiences (Perry, 2002).

Exposure to traumatic experiences can lead to the development of enduring mental and physical health problems (Ruzek et al., 2007). Compared with adults, children/young people may be more vulnerable to disasters or trauma, warranting special attention (Kousky, 2016).

Most psychological responses to trauma are relatively immediate, mild and transient (Norris et al., 2002), but some children and young people experience more intense stress reactions such as post-traumatic stress disorder and other mental health problems (Ruzek et al., 2007).

CASE STUDY

Carly

Carly is seven years old. Her school teacher called paramedics following an acute escalation in disruptive and aggressive behaviour. Her teacher tried to de-escalate Carly's behavior; however, the intervention seemed to make her more aggressive and agitated. Just prior to this, Carly was playing with a friend on the monkey bars and fell.

Five months ago, Carly was involved in a bushfire and was trapped inside the house with her parents and her younger sister. Her father and sister were able to escape, expecting her mother to follow with Carly. Unfortunately, Carly and her mother were unable to get out. Her father left her younger sibling outside and returned to the house for Mum and Carly. While he did this, her sister followed her father, and at this time some timber fell and she sustained a head injury requiring hospitalisation.

PRACTICE POINTS: TRAUMA AND STRESS-RELATED DISORDERS

- **Engage calmly and with confidence:** Take time to focus with the young person in the 'here and now'. Ground the young person in the present moment and reassure them that they are 'safe'.
- **Foster trust:** Encourage the relationship, ensure they are aware of you and your role, and of your goal to maintain and support them safely.
- **Self-reflect:** Do not panic. Make sense of what has happened using other people present. Maintain your self-confidence; do not replicate the internal worry of the child or young person in your own behaviour or responses.

COMPLEX DEVELOPMENTAL TRAUMA

The immediate and long-term consequence of children's exposure to maltreatment and other traumatic experiences are multifaceted. Emotional abuse and neglect, sexual abuse and physical abuse, as well as witnessing family violence, ethnic cleansing or war can interfere with the development of a secure attachment within the caregiving system (Cook et al., 2005). Complex trauma affects many key components of young people's development, including self-regulation and interpersonal relatedness, often leading to lifelong adjustment issues and, more commonly, a re-enactment of this abuse exposure in domains such as health, education, social, family and interpersonal (Van der Kolk, 2005).

Children and young people who have high and complex unmet mental health needs may present with:

- escalating behaviours that constitute a risk to themselves or others
- needs that are so complex (ongoing, persistent and unmet) that they cannot be effectively addressed by the usual services
- extremely challenging behaviours, including suicidal and risk-taking behaviours, antisocial behaviours, including aggression and substance abuse
- not living with families (e.g. homelessness) but in alternative care placements
- other mental health diagnoses, including autism spectrum disorder, intellectual disability, attention deficit disorder, conduct disorder and emerging borderline personality disorder
- experiences of abuse and neglect, family violence and parental mental illness
- behaviours that precipitate repeated trauma.

Intensive interventions are required to make an improvement for this group. Their circumstances place their family or alternative caregivers under extreme stress, often severely compromising their ability to provide adequate care. The very nature of this condition results in escalations in behaviours, often resulting in emergency services contact.

CASE STUDY

Jessica

Jessica is a 14-year-old girl with a complex developmental history. She has three half siblings and one full biological sibling. All children were removed and placed in the care of the Child Protection Service. Jessica's father has schizophrenia and her mother has a substance addiction.

Jessica was removed from her biological parents' care when she was aged 14 months because of neglect and physical abuse. The Child Protection Service placed her with foster carers (Peter and Sandra). She referred to them as 'Mum and Dad'. Child Protection Services had long-standing concerns about the placement, particularly relating to the appropriate level of emotional support.

Jessica felt closest to Peter, whom she described as supportive; however, she experienced Sandra as 'always blaming her'. Poor communication was a long-standing issue between the carers and her Child Protection social workers. Additional concerns were raised when Jessica was denied access to appropriate medical reviews under the basis that 'she was fine and never got sick'. There were reports of Jessica having dental appointments cancelled, along with optician and orthodontic appointments.

The foster placement broke down following a significant argument, with the family accusing Jessica of stealing something, which she vehemently denied. She was subsequently placed in a shared care house. While in this placement, she was being transported to and from her school by a specialist taxi service. Unfortunately, she was sexually abused by the driver of the car. He was later charged and prosecuted.

In the weeks following the alleged sexual assault, Jessica refused to return to the shared care house, so she was placed in another emergency care house in an unfamiliar area. Her distress intensified and, as her support workers were unfamiliar with Jessica, they frequently called paramedic services to assist with escalations.

PRACTICE POINTS: COMPLEX DEVELOPMENTAL TRAUMA

- Think about what might have led to the escalation and calling of paramedic services.
- Formulate an understanding about what may be going on with the child or young person. Consideration should also be given to what supports are available to the child or young person and the connection to these relationships (e.g. new foster care family).
- Gather an understanding or degree of urgency in terms of risk to the young person and others.
- Consider any relevant current and past medical history.

NEURODEVELOPMENTAL DISORDERS

Neurodevelopmental disorders (including intellectual disability, communication disorders, autism spectrum disorders (ASD), attention deficit hyperactivity disorder, specific learning disorder and motor disorders) are characterised by developmental deficits that produce impairments in personal, social, academic or occupational functioning. Many are associated with comorbid mental health conditions, including anxiety disorder and mood disorders.

Children and young people with neurodevelopmental disorders may have challenges with communication, emotional regulation and complex sensory needs. They can present with behavioural challenges such as aggression, self-injury, hyperactivity and temper tantrums. Non-verbal children or young people with neurodevelopmental problems may not have developed capacity to identify or communicate their physical distress. The distress associated with gastrointestinal problems, including constipation, and other medical conditions, such as seizures and pain (dental, earache), may be expressed with self-injurious behaviour. Hence, establishing communication preferences, verbal skills along with sensory needs at the outset may help to identify and manage the problems beyond the behavioural manifestations. Remember, chronological age is a poor indicator of developmental capacities, and so identifying true function (physical/emotional/cognitive) may assist in understanding the current presentation. Key assessment information includes medical comorbidities, medication history, pre-morbid functioning and developmental age.

For children with ASD, emergency departments with their high sensory environments can be overwhelming. This might lead to further disruptive and distressed behaviours. Careful and considered decision making about the presenting problem within the home environment might help to reduce such risks.

CASE STUDY
Joseph

The ambulance arrived at the house of 15-year-old Joseph, following a call from the police, who were in attendance. Joseph has ASD, is non-verbal and lives with his family. Joseph has a history of behavioural challenges and is supported by Child and Adolescent Mental Health Services (CAMHS). Parents report that in the last four days Joseph has become very distressed, hitting himself in the head and refusing to go to school. He has been tearful on occasions. Tonight he got aggressive, hitting out at his parents and smashing the television. He presents as hyperactive, agitated, with his hands over ears and screaming at the police. Parents report that he likes his routine and doesn't like going to the hospital. The ambulance called the after-hours CAMHS services, and it is established that this presentation is unusual. Given the reluctance of Joseph to attend hospital and the likelihood of needing physical restraint, further traumatising Joseph, the parents were advised to use oral benzodiazepines to reduce the distress. Further history from the parents points to the possibility of Joseph having an ear infection and constipation. Pain relief was given and an appointment with his regular general practitioner was suggested, along with a review with his CAMHS team.

PRACTICE POINTS: NEURODEVELOPMENTAL DISORDERS

- Tread carefully when attempting to reduce these behaviours, as they may be helpful for self-regulation of anxiety, agitation and/or frustration.
- Gather as much detail from parent/family or other significant people to build an understanding of what triggered the acute deterioration.
- Children and young people with neurodevelopmental disorders experience significant sleep disturbances that can lead to sleep deprivation for both the child and their family. Underlying medical issues (sleep apnoea, night tremors, seizures, anxiety, etc.) need to be identified as contributing factors.

DEPRESSION

Depression is a relatively common and treatable condition in children and young people. Depression can be accompanied by a range of physical and emotional symptoms in children and young people that can affect their capacity to attend and engage in routine, age-appropriate tasks, including school and social activities. It is, however, important to note that young people with depression have a significantly higher risk of suicide (Black Dog Institute, 2017).

A young person with depression may not only experience problems with how they feel but also with how they behave. This may cause difficulties at home and at school, as well as in relationships with family and friends. Some young people start taking risks. These can include missing school, harming themselves (e.g. by cutting), misusing drugs or alcohol, and having inappropriate sexual relationships. A change in functioning requires understanding.

CASE STUDY

Rebecca

At 9 p.m. a 16-year-old girl, Rebecca, contacts paramedic triage reporting that she is 'depressed'. She is speaking in a soft voice and not providing much information.

Rebecca lives with her mother, stepfather and one-year-old half-brother. Tonight, she had an argument with her stepfather and she is currently with a friend. She experiences her stepfather as mean and constantly putting her down. Rebecca was planning to walk to a bridge and jump off. She has had no past history with mental health services and is taking the medication Roaccutane to help with her acne.

Rebecca has had difficulty sleeping for the past six months and has not slept much over the past three days. She finds school hard, struggles to concentrate and remember things, and says her teacher often gives her a hard time for not completing work. Her mother is busy studying and cares for her grandmother, who was diagnosed with cancer six months ago. Rebecca is close to her grandmother.

Rebecca says she feels overwhelmed, can't cope and now she doesn't know whether she wants to live. She has never had thoughts of harming herself before.

PRACTICE POINTS: DEPRESSION

- In the assessment of a child or young person with depression, paramedics should ask the child or young person and their parent(s) or carer(s) directly about the child or young person's current alcohol and drug use, any experiences of being bullied or abused, self–harm and ideas about suicide.
- If a child or young person with depression presents following self-harm, the immediate management should focus on safe medical and physical health management, and safe transporting to the nearest metropolitan hospital.
- Assessment of depression requires an understanding of the young person's circumstances, including their family, social and cultural networks.

ANXIETY DISORDERS

Anxiety disorders are the most common mental health problem experienced by young Australians. Anxiety disorders are frequently comorbid with other mental illnesses, particularly with depression. Anxiety disorders during adolescence strongly predict subsequent onset and persistence of other mental and substance use disorders, and are associated with considerable burden of disease, including suboptimal social and occupational functioning.

CASE STUDY

Madeline

Madeline is a 10-year-old girl whose parents have called an ambulance due to Madeline describing worsening abdominal pain. The intensity of the pain has increased over a four-hour period. She reported that she was finding it difficult to breathe and was nauseated. Madeline's mother has recently been diagnosed with cancer. Madeline has no history of acute or chronic medical difficulties.

Her parents report that Madeline has missed about 17 days of school during the previous year because of this pain. They had taken Madeline to a GP, who did not offer an opinion but requested they keep 'an eye on it'.

On interview, paramedics discover that Madeline has avoided school out of concern that something may happen to her mother. She could not tolerate having her parents on a different floor of the house from herself. Her insecurity, need for constant reassurance, and school absenteeism were frustrating and upsetting for her parents.

PRACTICE POINTS: ANXIETY

- Work with the child or young person to understand the cause of their distress. Calmly provide support by example, showing the child or young person how they can remain calm when they are feeling anxious.
- Assist them to calm down by joining with them in taking long, deep breaths at slowed intervals.
- Provide consistent direction. Ground children and young people in the present moment. Give praise for every step they take in managing their distress and worry.

DISRUPTIVE, IMPULSE CONTROL AND CONDUCT DISORDERS

Externalising disorders such as oppositional defiance and conduct disorders refer to a group of children and young people who experience persistent difficulties with aggression towards people or property. Accompanying these difficulties are challenges with interpersonal relationships, emotional and mood management and difficulties complying with rules and law.

These difficulties can have functional impacts, such as the child or young person's engagement and attendance at school. The behaviour in the cluster of externalising disorders is more severe than general misbehaviour. Signs of these disorders often occur in the preschool years.

Conduct disorder is the more serious of the externalising disorders, and is marked by persistent breaking of social rules, acting aggressively towards people and animals, lying/stealing and clear violations of laws.

Treatment for this group is often best undertaken early in life through parental dyadic and family-based therapy, with a focus on challenging and managing overwhelming and dysregulated feelings.

CASE STUDY

Jacob

Jacob is 17 years old. He is one of 11 siblings, and his family environment is characterised by violence perpetrated by the father towards Jacob and other family members. Historically, Jacob has often changed schools, either due to his behavioural issues or the family moving. He has a short work history, commencing work in a bakery when he was 13 years old, before obtaining work as a mechanic from which he was dismissed after he became angry and smashed his employers' car.

Jacob became homeless at age 15. Information from accommodation services reported that Jacob has been banned from a number of services for stealing, lighting fires and assaulting staff.

Jacob has a long history of alcohol dependence, cannabis dependence and mood regulation issues. He was referred for paramedical support following arrest by the police for stabbing a male and later expressing suicidal ideation.

PRACTICE POINTS: IMPULSE CONTROL AND CONDUCT DISORDERS

- Paramedics may be involved at times of crisis.
- Gather and obtain as much history of the event as possible.
- Make your roles and responsibilities clear to the young person.
- Work with the police to ensure the safe transporting of the child or young person if they have been charged under the law.

PSYCHOTIC DISORDERS

Psychotic disorders can be severe and devastating illnesses that can seriously erode the quality of life of children and young people. The prevalence of children and young people under the age of 18 years with psychosis is low. Despite this, it is important to consider the intersection between developmental stage and acute presentation when requested to respond.

There are subtle differences in the clinical picture of psychosis in children and young people compared with that of adults. As an example, there tends to be higher levels of anxiety, poor concentration, florid and bizarre behavioural actions, and increased variability in emotional control and management.

Due to the noted intersection with developmental change, there tends to be some diagnostic confusion, particularly for those with severe developmental trauma. It is necessary to be clear about the nature of phenomenology in making the diagnosis of a psychosis.

It is essential to consider drug and alcohol misuse in the initial assessment when responding to a young person with a psychotic episode, as this may be an important differential factor or underlying cause.

CASE STUDY

Jane

Jane is a 16-year-old girl who lives with her mother and three siblings. Her mother has called an ambulance following a seven-day period of no sleep when she has been behaving in an increasingly bizarre manner. One week ago, Jane broke up with her boyfriend. Subsequently, Jane began contacting her now ex-boyfriend demanding an explanation for why he stopped their relationship. The intensity of this contact increased, and eventually resulted in his brother making threats towards Jane if she did not cease her contact. Coinciding with this were persistent conflicts between her separated parents over financial support of Jane. While Jane believed this was a parental issue, she felt challenged by the notion that her father was planning to withdraw his financial support. In addition, Jane's mother has commenced a new relationship and has been spending less time with Jane, resulting in Jane feeling isolated and disconnected in the family.

At the point of contact with emergency services, Jane was highly distressed, volatile and aggressive. She was affectively labile (emotions fluctuating from one extreme to another), her conversation was bizarre, but her behaviour was manageable and amenable to guidance and direction. Jane walked to the ambulance cradling a magazine with a baby on the front cover. Her eye contact was reasonable, but intermittently she would 'burst' into a fatuous smile with elaborate hand gesturing to indicate happiness, and other times she looked quite introverted, distressed and perplexed. Her conversation was of normal rate, themed with a persistent delusional, referential content about being a bunny or a butterfly (she over-identified with a bunny tattoo on her foot, and with the meaning of her name 'Jane' – 'butterfly').

Jane was transported to hospital, and after an assessment in the emergency department she was transferred to a mental health inpatient ward.

PRACTICE POINTS: ENGAGING WITH A YOUNG PERSON IN AN ACUTE PHASE OF PSYCHOSIS

- Use a calm, reassuring, professional and friendly manner.
- Negotiate flexibly for the best outcome.
- Understand the individual's circumstances.
- Provide simple, clear and coherent information/instructions to reduce arousal and provide relaxation.
- Provide a structured and predictable environment.
- Recognise that the patient may be nervous, wary or not want to see health professionals.
- Be aware that psychosis might distort patient's interactions and their ability to process information.
- Listen carefully to patients and take their views seriously.
- Identify common ground.
- Carefully explain any plans to the young person.

APPROACHES TO CARING FOR CHILDREN AND ADOLESCENTS

GOALS OF EMERGENCY ASSESSMENT

The goals of emergency assessment are to:

1. Determine whether the child or young person is at imminent risk of harm to self or others.
2. Establish the presence of significant mental health symptoms/disorders.
3. Identify the factors that may have caused or be contributing to the current problems and to their persistence (genetic, developmental, familial, social, medical).
4. Evaluate the child or young person's normal level of functioning and the extent this has been impaired by the symptoms.
5. Identify areas of strength (protective factors) as well as potential supports within the family and the wider social environment to ameliorate the current crisis.
6. Determine whether transportation to the emergency department is required.

DEVELOPMENTAL CONTEXT IN PERFORMING INTERVIEWS WITH CHILDREN AND YOUNG PEOPLE

Interviewing young people is different from interviewing adults. Young people are continuing to develop cognitive and language skills. They may not always present to appointments of their own volition, and may be concerned that contact with the mental health service implies that in some way they are 'crazy'. Stigma is a significant issue for young people.

Children and young people dislike repeating their story. Therefore, where and if possible, the child or young person should be interviewed by as few professionals as possible to assist cooperation and the formation of rapport.

Often clinicians prefer seeing a child or young person on their own first, and then together with a parent or significant other. For children, the opposite is often preferred: to see the child together with a parent first, and then interviewing the child alone. Children younger than 12 years of age are less likely to reliably answer questions about their mood, onset and duration of symptoms, and contributing factors, including family dynamics and psychosocial circumstances.

Once you have some understanding of the child or young person's developmental limits and capabilities you can apply appropriate, informed strategies for effective communication. A good grasp of a child or young person's developmental level will help facilitate a collaborative connection and minimise the propensity for the child or young person becoming further frustrated and invalidated.

Consider the following:

- **Language use:** Pitching language at a child or young person's developmental level will help obtain history that enhances your understanding. Think wisely about what language you use and the tone you deliver it in.
- **Use their language to describe their difficulty:** Use their phrasing, terms, names of people, places and feelings to validate the child or young person. This provides reassurance and validation that you are present with them.
- **Use language that conveys reassurance:** Calm, clear questioning that builds elaboration and enquiry is optimal. Take note of the young person's body language.
- **Non-verbal communication:** Position yourself in a safe, non-threatening way. Children and young people who have experienced adverse and cumulative trauma are adept at 'reading' adults. They are vigilant to adults withholding information, so consider what your non-verbal communication is conveying.
- If uncertain about a child or young person and their developmental stages, reflect on your own development and use this as a basis or guide for assessment.

ASSESSMENT OF YOUNG PEOPLE FROM CULTURALLY AND LINGUISTICALLY DIVERSE (CALD) BACKGROUNDS

Some children and young people from CALD backgrounds show increasing vulnerability to poor mental health due to the stress of migration and acculturation.

CALD children and young people also under-utilise mental health services (Bevan, 2000). Despite this, in practice CALD children and young people often present with issues arising from the loss of family and/or community supports, and trauma of the migration experience. Additionally, many struggle following an exposure to violence, community trauma and the effects of torture (experienced or witnessed).

To enhance communication, consider the following:

- Be aware that in some cultures there is stigma around mental health difficulties, which can lead to an uncomfortableness or unwillingness to discuss some topics.
- Utilise positive communication; for example, active listening and allowing the child or young person the time to express their needs.
- Reduce negative expectations by assuming capacity rather than incapacity.
- If required, utilise a phone interpreter service.

INTERVIEWING CHILDREN AND YOUNG PEOPLE ABOUT SUICIDE

Cognitive development and capacity appear variable among young people. While some young people may have suicidal intent, some may not fully appreciate the finality of death. It may be that they want the negative feelings to end, not their life.

Young children under the age of 12 years of age developmentally entertain the concepts that by hurting themselves it will improve their relationships with parents – the parents will realise how much they are loved. At other times, it is an expression of wanting things to stop, such as the aggression in domestic violence situations.

When focusing on assessment of suicidal ideation, areas of consideration include lethality, intent, plans, affect/mood and future plans. When assessing these concepts in children under the age of 12 years, consider specific examples and be mindful to deconstruct language: *'Do you think that every day?', 'How do you manage those uncomfortable feelings?'*

Assessment of the narrative around risk can also provide some further understanding of the young person's circumstances. Factors such as impulsivity, judgment and management of emotions in challenging situations require consideration. This may then provide useful information for intervention opportunities.

With children and adolescents, there is usually no clear relationship between medical lethality of attempt and intent (Spirito & Overholser, 2003). A strong focus on the young person's intentions needs to be maintained. Always remember to explore access to firearms (mandated notification), medication and knives.

Considering the difficulties in conducting assessments in emergency situations, a mnemonic can be helpful. A useful example of this would be a ***HEADSS*** assessment (Goldenring & Rosen, 2004). The key aspect to successfully using HEADSS is to provide open-ended questions.

> **H**ome: *Where do you live, and who lives there with you?*
> **E**ducation and Employment: *Are you in school? What are you good at in school? What is hard for you? What grades do you get?*

Activities: *What do you do for fun? What things do you do with friends? What do you do with your free time?*

Drugs: *Many young people experiment with drugs, alcohol or cigarettes. Have you or your friends ever tried them? What have you tried?*

Sexuality: *Are you involved in a relationship? Have you been involved in a relationship? How was that experience for you? How would you describe your feeling towards guys or girls? How do you see yourself in terms of sexual preference, i.e. gay, straight or bisexual?*

Suicide/Self-harm: *Have you tried this before? How long have you been thinking of this? What did you think/what did you hope would happen when you did this?*

EMERGENCY AND CRISIS CARE OF CHILDREN AND YOUNG PEOPLE

For children and young people there is often a very significant cross-over and interplay between 'psychosocial' crises and 'mental health' crises. Children and young people are inevitably affected by a range of circumstances. A crisis for young people is rarely due to a mental health problem alone: the breakdown in significant relationships, the impact of past or current trauma and abuse, or problems with money or housing are likely to present and be relevant to their presentation.

A crisis can present in the form of a deliberate ingestion, self-harm, or overwhelming feelings and emotions requiring containment and reassurance. This is made all the more complex by the developmental stage and supports surrounding children and young people. Outcomes in children and young people presenting in crisis are optimised when services are appropriately 'knitted' and connected together with good communication and clear plans. These plans, however, need to be driven by 'why has the young person presented now', and what may be situated in the shadows, contributing to or underlying the more obvious presenting concern.

FAMILY CONTEXT AND RELATIONSHIPS

Children and young people's problematic behaviour can often be a symptom of underlying family-based issues. At other times, it may be a sign of traumatic and unforeseen internal family incidents. These issues can overwhelm the general capacity of usual family-based problem-solving approaches, and the family can struggle to sustain its usual organisation.

In this circumstance the child or young person can be the symptom of the family distress. It is important to discuss and explore with family members what they believe may be underlying the child or young person's distress. These family enquiries can provide important perspectives.

As paramedics you will need to consider that while the child or young person is distressed, where does the origin of the problem exist? Is it internal to the child, or is the problem in the communication of the family or, in fact, is it a combination of both?

There has been increasing recognition of the caring role that many children and young people play in supporting a parent with a mental illness. It is estimated that between 21% and 24% of Australian children live in a household where at least one parent has a mental illness (Maybery et al., 2005). The caring role and the effects of mental illness in the parent may interrupt the development of attachment and a supporting and nurturing relationship, and potentially can affect the young person's emotional and social connectedness and development.

CONFIDENTIALITY AND LEGAL RESPONSIBILITIES

Consent to treatment and assessment is generally uncomplicated in situations of children and young people presenting in acute crisis. Presenting and participating in an assessment implies a level of consent by the young person or consenting adult(s). Generally, each state and territory has governing legislation for paramedics in acute mental health and medical crises. Within child and adolescent mental health, obtaining consent becomes increasingly complicated if biological parents are divorced, voluntary custody agreements exist, or the young person is 'in care'. Paramedics should, where possible, clarify who is the guardian and if there are currently any legal orders in relation to this. This may have little impact on the decision to commute the child or young person to hospital; however, it becomes integral once invasive forms of treatment occur in the referring hospital facility.

Regardless of legal obligations and opinions, where possible the paramedic should be clear with the young person about what can be done under current circumstances.

Confidentiality is of similar importance to this clinical assessment process. Paramedics should clearly explain the necessary legal aspects prior to commencing an assessment process. This should be revisited at the completion of the discussion. This approach will engender trust and connection between the child or young person and the paramedic.

Additionally, the following recommendations should always be considered when responding to children and young people:

- Assessment and treatment should be provided in the least restrictive manner and environment that is consistent with the child or young person's care and protection, treatment efficacy and public safety.
- The use of restrictive practices should be a last resort, and only occur where:
  - alternative strategies have failed to achieve or maintain safety for the child or young person who is experiencing distress, workers or others
  - behaviours and actions are assessed to be imminently or actually harmful to a child or young person, or to others, or
  - the health practitioner believes a failure to do so could put the child or young person, workers or public at a significant health or safety risk.

ASSESSMENT AND TREATMENT

Despite the inception of assertive outreach services and home treatments, the demand for inpatient treatment and care remains high. This contrasts with relatively low numbers of child and adolescent mental health inpatient beds. Despite this, admissions to inpatient treatment units can considerably disrupt the normal functional tasks of child and adolescent development, including engagement with education, family life and social relationships. As a result, the need for hospitalisation requires careful consideration.

The following considers the factors that surround hospital treatment and the required post-hospital supports.

WHEN TO TRANSPORT/ALTERNATIVE CARE PATHWAYS

Principles

The following key principles (adapted from Department of Health, 2014) should inform decisions about transporting children and young people with mental health concerns to hospital:

- The best interests of children and young people presenting with mental health issues should be listened to and strongly considered.
- The least restrictive means should be provided.
- The developmental aspects of the child or young person will be integrated into the formulation of the presentation.
- Privacy and the right to feel respected will be considered.
- The culture and identity of Aboriginal and Torres Strait Islanders children and young people will be recognised and responded to.
- Culture, religion, communication, gender and gender orientation, disability and sexuality should be considered at point of contact.
- Empowering appropriate lifestyle options should be encouraged to ensure children and young people build supports and skills.
- Service contact and assessment should aim to provide optimal therapeutic outcomes and re-engagement with school and community life.

INDICATIONS FOR CHILD AND ADOLESCENT MENTAL HEALTH INPATIENT STAYS

In children and young people, clear mental illness and disorders are rare; however, cumulative and adverse life traumas are common. As a result, the following are examples of conditions where an inpatient mental health admission may be of benefit:

- Clear evidence of psychotic phenomenology requiring further assessment and review.

- Where risk to self or others remains high and requires additional specialist assessment.
- Clear evidence of a mood disturbance with significant interruptions and disturbance to everyday functioning.
- Diagnostic uncertainty that requires further review by a specialist mental health service.

If hospital presentation is not indicated, the following recommendations are made for paramedics:

1. Most child and adolescent mental health services have a triage service. If possible, it will be beneficial to contact them and gather any history that may make your response efficient and safe.
2. If the child or young person does not require transporting to an emergency department, provide clear communication to the child/young person and parent/caregiver as to their responsibility and support/treatment options.
3. Ensure liaison and correspondence is provided to child or young person's paediatrician, general practitioner and mental health triage team.

MEDICATION IN CHILD AND ADOLESCENT MENTAL HEALTH EMERGENCIES

When considering administering medication, the primary position should be to 'do no harm'. Despite our very best intentions, utilising medications in crises with children and young people can potentially disrupt the anticipated assessment needed in hospital. As a result, it is suggested (where possible) to commute without medication. This is an imperative consideration to ensure optimal safety, but also to avoid unnecessary, time-consuming, restrictive, invasive or traumatic interventions.

FAMILY INVOLVEMENT

Generally, family support, parental attitude and involvement in treatment (including family-based treatment) are important predictors of treatment outcomes for children and adolescents with mental health concerns. In order to optimise care and treatment, contact and care is provided to the family to ensure progress and treatment is a shared responsibility. At other times, family therapy will be a core aspect of treatment. Family and family work are clear markers of difference with adult health services, as they are fundamental to ensuring appropriate progress.

COMMUNICATING CHILD PROTECTION CONCERNS WITH THE RELEVANT AGENCY

Child protection services must respond if someone reports that they think a child or young person 'in care' is at risk of serious harm. As a result, it will be important to consider your communication with child protection services and what information they require to support them in their decision making.

It is important to engage or a have a representative from your service engage and participate in interagency meetings to ensure safety of decisions in emergency situations.

TRAUMATIC DEATH (SUICIDE) AND POST-VENTION RESPONSES

Emergency personnel often have to respond to the needs of family members, witnesses and bystanders as well as the children and young people following traumatic death. As first responders, paramedics are at risk of stress-related conditions due to the nature of the situations they respond to. Strategies and approaches for debriefing and support embedded in organisational practice should be available to reduce the propensity for compassion fatigue and burnout.

SYSTEMIC SERVICE IMPROVEMENT

Local child and adolescent mental health services should have over-arching interface meetings with all key emergency services stakeholders. This should include representation from police, ambulance, child protection services, emergency departments and CAMHS. The goal of each committee should be to:

- identify high-risk and frequent hospital presenters, and systemically collaborate to develop interagency response plans
- explore ways and means to collaborate to improve interagency service cooperation and coordination
- identify and develop shared training that would be a benefit to either agency
- escalate systemic issues requiring attention (Department of Health, 2014).

ONGOING TRAINING AND EDUCATION

Paramedics engaged with children and young people should receive the necessary education and training to provide safe and effective clinical and emotional care. This focus should include training in approaches and updates on managing those with learning difficulties, as well as those children and young people placed in statutory care. This training should be interagency focused, and draw services and staff together to build mutual respect and appreciation for each service role.

CONCLUSION

The paramedic assessment and care for children and young people with emergency mental health issues is enhanced when the balance between the acute needs and long-term supports are considered from first contact. It is the skill of the paramedic responder to formulate an understanding using all of the key aspects and information and then provide a provisional plan that is centred on the child/young person and their family.

Child and adolescent mental health emergencies are varied and challenging for paramedics and emergency departments. There are a range of factors that need to be balanced and understood including: the nature of the presenting problem, family and developmental history, cultural considerations and medical history, while at the same time evaluating the quality of the information and the history of relationship supports. Despite this, it is essential that paramedics support the child/young person and/or family with dignity, respect and empathy to ensure care and treatment is optimal and in their best interest.

LINKS AND RESOURCES

- Hiscock, H., Neely, R., Lei, S., Freed, G. 2018. Paediatric mental and physical health presentations to emergency departments. Med. J. Aust. 7 May. 208 (8), 343–348
- Holmes, E., Ghaderi, A., Harmer, C. et al., 2018. The Lancet Psychiatry Commission on psychological treatments research in tomorrow's science. Lancet Psychiatr. Comm. 5 (3), 237–286. Online. Available: www.thelancet.com/psychiatry

REFERENCES

Australian Bureau of Statistics (ABS), 2016. Causes of death 2015. Online. Available: http://www.abs.gov.au/ausstats/abs@.nsf/mf/3303.0.

Australian Institute of Health and Welfare (AIHW), 2018. Mental health services in Australia. AIHW, Canberra. Online. Available: https://www.aihw.gov.au/reports/mental-health-services/mental-health-services-in-australia/report-contents/summary-of-mental-health-services-in-australia/prevalence-and-policies. October 2018.

Bartlett, J., Smith, S., Bringewatt, E., 2017. Helping young children who have experienced trauma: policies and strategies for early care and education. Child Trends April, 21.

Bevan, K., 2000. Young people, culture, migration and mental health: a review of the literature. In: Bashir, M., Bennett, D.L. (Eds.), Deeper Dimensions: Culture, youth and mental health. Transcultural Mental Health Centre, Sydney.

Black Dog Institute in association with Mission Australia, 2017. Youth Mental Health Report – Youth Survey 2012–2016. Online. Available: https://blackdoginstitute.org.au/docs/default-source/research/evidence-and-policy-section/2017-youth-mental-health-report_mission-australia-and-black-dog-institute.pdf?sfvrsn=6. November 2019.

Cook, A., Spinazzola, J., Ford, J., et al., 2005. Complex trauma in children and adolescents. Psychiatr. Ann. 35 (5), 390.

Department of Health, 2014. Protocol for the transport of people with mental illness. Victorian Government, Melbourne.

Grandclerc, S., De Labrouhe, D., Spodenkiewicz, M., et al., 2016. Relations between non-suicidal self-injury and suicidal behavior in adolescence: a systematic review. PLoS ONE 11 (4), doi:10.1371/journal.pone.0153760.

Goldenring, J.M., Rosen, D., 2004. Getting into adolescent heads: an essential update. Contemp. Paediatr. 21 (1), 64–90.

Jones, T., Hillier, L., 2013. Comparing trans-spectrum and same-sex attracted youth: increased risks, increased activisms. J. LGBT Youth 10 (4), 287–307.

Kousky, C., 2016. Impacts of natural disasters on children. Future Child. 26, 73–92.

Lawrence, D., Johnson, S., Hafekost, J., et al., 2015. Report on the second Australian Child and Adolescent Survey of Mental Health and Wellbeing. Department of Health, Canberra. Online. Available: https://www.health.gov.au/internet/main/publishing.nsf/Content/9DA8CA21306FE6EDCA257E2700016945/%24File/child2.pdf. June 2018.

Madge, N., Hewitt, A., Hawton, K., et al., 2008. Deliberate self-harm within an international community sample of young people: comparative findings from the Child & Adolescent Self-harm in Europe (CASE) Study. J. Child Psychol. Psychiatry 49 (6), 667–677.

Maybery, D., Reupert, A., Patrick, K., et al., 2005. VicHealth Research Report on Children at Risk in Families Affected by Parental Mental Illness. Victorian Health Promotion Foundation, Melbourne.

Norris, F., Friedman, M., Watson, P., et al., 2002. 60,000 disaster victims speak. Part I: an empirical review of the empirical literature, 1981–2001. Psychiatry 65, 207–239.

Ohtaras, A., 2015. Reactive attachment disorder in children: impacts on development, educational implications and the need for secure attachment. J. Stud. Engagement: Educ. Matters 5 (1), 28–38.

Perry, B., 2002. Stress, trauma and posttraumatic stress disorders in children: caregiver education series. ChildTrauma Academy, Houston, TX, p 9.

Ruzek, J., Brymer, M., Jacobs, A., et al., 2007. Psychological first aid. J. Ment. Health Couns. 29 (1), 17–49.

Spirito, A., Overholser, J., 2003. The suicidal child: assessment and management of adolescents after a suicide attempt. Child Adolesc. Psychiatr. Clin. N. Am. 12, 649–665.

Van der Kolk, B., 2005. Developmental trauma disorder. Psychiatric Annals May:35.

Vassallo, S., Smart, D., Sanson, A., et al., 2008. Risky driving among young Australian drivers II: co-occurrence with other problem behaviors. Accid. Anal. Prev. 40 (1), 376–386.

Wilson, J., Thomas, R., 2004. Empathy in the Treatment of Trauma and PTSD. Routledge, New York.

Zubrick, S., Hafekost, J., Johnson, S., et al., 2016. Suicidal behaviours: prevalence estimates from the second Australian Child and Adolescent Survey of Mental Health and Wellbeing. Aust. N. Z. J. Psychiatry 50, 899–910.

Mental health across the life span: Caring for the mental health of older people

Janine Stevenson

LEARNING OUTCOMES

By the end of this chapter, you should understand that:

- older adults are not just *older* adults
- mental illness may present differently in older people than in younger people
- it is often difficult to differentiate between medical/organic and psychiatric illness in the older person
- drug and alcohol abuse is sometimes 'hidden' in this population
- family/carers can provide both information and assistance in managing the older person.

INTRODUCTION

This chapter will explore the differences in presentation of mental illness in older adults: mood disorders, anxiety, suicide, drug and alcohol abuse and neurocognitive disorders. The chapter will explore how to connect with and communicate with the older person, challenges to assessment, how to manage aggression, the mental and emotional effects of ageing, and physical impediments to communication and their associated management.

Our population is ageing, the proportion of people over the age of 65 now in Australia is 15.3%, up from 12% in 1996 (Australian Bureau of Statistics, 2016), and this proportion continues to increase while younger age groups remain stable or decrease. Unfortunately, morbidity increases with age, including psychiatric morbidity, which will frequently be comorbid with physical illness. Both psychiatric and medical morbidity in older adults will more frequently need hospitalisation, and paramedics need skills in managing both.

PHYSIOLOGICAL CHANGES IN THE BODY WITH AGEING

There are normal changes in bones and joints due to loss of bone density. Muscle mass and strength decrease, beginning around the age of 30, but by no more than

10%–15%. Bed rest decreases muscle mass more dramatically. Body fat percentage increases with a person's age. Changes in vision occur, including loss of near vision, the need for brighter light, and changes in colour perception. Most 60-year-olds need three times more light to read than 20-year-olds. Hearing changes, making high-pitched sounds harder to hear, which can be challenging to communication. Skin becomes more fragile and heals more slowly. Thinking may slow, but dealing with complexity actually improves with age. Balance may not be as good. Endocrine function decreases with age, mainly estrogen, testosterone and growth hormone. This leads to menopause in women, and decreased muscle mass and strength in both sexes.

NEUROLOGICAL CHANGES WITH AGEING

The levels of chemicals involved in sending messages in the brain change, some down, some up. Blood flow to the brain decreases, and there is some nerve cell loss with ageing. However, the brain has ways of compensating by increasing connections between cells. Diseases such as Alzheimer's, Huntington's and Parkinson's disease all involve cell loss in various regions of the brain.

Actual disease processes, such as diabetes, metabolic syndrome, heart disease and hypertension, damage many bodily systems, affecting their function. This is in addition to naturally occurring changes with age.

EMOTIONAL CHANGES WITH AGEING

Negative emotionality (neuroticism) decreases with age. People become more content and outgoing as they age. Role reversal is common, with the wife becoming the dominant partner and making the family decisions after retirement. Depression is less common, but more severe when it does occur. Successful ageing has been found to be determined by non-smoking, a good marriage, good social connections and a feeling of wellbeing (not necessarily good health) (Dong et al., 2017). Older people are capable of more complexity of thought and emotions, being able to feel pride, anger, love and regret all at the same time. With their life experience they can have more insight into complex situations and relationships.

AGEISM

Ageism (also spelt 'agism') consists of prejudicial attitudes towards a group of people in a certain age group, especially the elderly but also towards youth. It also involves discrimination on the basis of age and institutional policies that stereotype all people in certain age groups.

Ageist beliefs are commonplace in today's society, even among the aged themselves, but elders who take control and independence in their lives are more likely to be active and healthy, both mentally and physically (Aw et al., 2017).

> **AGEISM – KEY CONCEPTS**
>
> - Implicit ageism refers to how we tend to think, feel and act towards older and younger people.
> - Stereotyping involves considering all people in a group (such as an age group) to have the same characteristics.

Prejudice against the elderly could lead the healthcare worker to be more pessimistic about the person's health outcome, and this attitude could be picked up by the patient resulting in 'giving up' or non-cooperation (Emlet, 2017). Health professionals tend to pursue less aggressive treatment options in older patients, even major surgery for a potentially curable condition, because of negative stereotyping and pessimistic thinking about older people (Emlet, 2017).

In other cultures (e.g. Eastern culture), the elderly are held in high regard, as having wisdom and experience to be passed on to the younger generation. In our multicultural society we find many different attitudes to ageing (Tam et al., 2016; Vauclair et al., 2017). Also, in Australian culture, the 'baby boomer' generation brings different expectations, lifestyle issues and attitudes compared with previous generations that experienced the Great Depression and World War II. The latter are now the 'old old', a group in their late eighties and nineties with even different attitudes and needs.

SPECIAL POPULATIONS – INDIGENOUS AUSTRALIANS

Aboriginal and Torres Strait Islander populations age at a greater rate than Caucasian Australians, developing age-related physical and mental changes in their forties and fifties. The high prevalence of diabetes, kidney disease and Alzheimer's disease shortens their life span by up to 20 years (Alzheimer's Australia, 2007; Emlet, 2017; Hart et al., 2009).

CASE STUDY
Fred

You have been dispatched at 2.30 p.m. to a car parked in a small reserve on the outskirts of town to attend to a 70-year-old male. It is summertime and the weather is a sunny 35 degrees. The local government council staff have been aware that the man has been living in his car in the park for up to a week. Council staff have been unable to move the man on and so they have called the police to assist.

The police attended and spoke to the man, Fred. Police were concerned for both his physical and mental health, and so have called an ambulance to assist.

On your arrival you are met by the police and council workers. Fred is still sitting in his car and has refused to unlock the door. He is willing to speak to the paramedics through a small opening in his window, but only if the police and council workers move away as he fears that they are imposters. He seems to believe that the council workers are from the taxation office and are here to seize his business assets, while the police are associated with a paedophile crime ring that were involved in his own son being kidnapped and taken overseas.

Fred tells you he has been living in his car for six months but can't remember where he previously lived. He parked in the reserve about a week ago because there was 'better reception' and it was easier to receive messages. The car battery has since gone flat and he has been unable to move the car. You enquire how he has managed to charge his phone, and he tells you that he doesn't have one, nor does he need one, because the government sends the messages through his car radio.

After a short time, Fred agrees to wind down his window far enough for you to take some observations:

Vital signs
- Glasgow Coma Score: 15
- Oxygen saturations: 97%
- Respiratory rate: 20
- Heart rate: 115
- Blood pressure: 165/95
- Electrocardiograph: unable to be obtained
- Pain score: 7/10 (mostly lower back pain)
- Blood sugar level: 17 mmol
- His mouth and lips appear dry, and his skin turgor is poor.

It is impossible not to notice Fred's dishevelled clothing as well as the strong fecal odour coming from the car. The car contains books, papers, clothes, personal belongings and rubbish.

Police tell you that they believe they have been there too long already and they want you to reach in and open the car door while you have the chance so they can get him in the ambulance and then go back to their other work. Fred becomes suspicious about you talking to the police and winds his window back up.

CRITICAL REFLECTION
- What are your main priorities at this time?
- Under what circumstances could you forcefully enter the car and remove Fred?
- What are the main risk factors to consider?
- How would you manage the communication with the police, the council workers and your patient, Fred?
- How would you maintain a therapeutic rapport with Fred while managing the scene?

Further information
Police provide you the phone number of his daughter Mary. Mary tells you that Fred was living independently in a retirement village until about five days ago when he suddenly left. She has tried to phone him, but his mobile phone had been left at home. Fred's medical background includes heart disease, type 2 diabetes, osteo-arthritis and anxiety. His regular medications are metformin, gliclazide, atenolol, sertraline, Panadol osteo, aspirin, frusemide. Mary reports that there had been a gradual decline in her father's general functioning over the past four years since her mother had died, but he had been able to maintain his independence with the support of the care workers from the retirement village. Fred had previously run his own small accountancy firm and still likes to tell people that he is an accountant.

CRITICAL REFLECTION
- Your partner tells you that Fred is 'schizophrenic' and probably needs to be locked up in the psych ward. What is it about Fred's history that suggests this is or is not schizophrenia?
- Discuss your differential diagnosis.

- What other information would you need to know to help you to make a diagnosis and plan treatment (assuming that you can get Fred out of the car)?
- Outline and document your mental state examination of Fred.

Fred eventually gets out of the car but refuses to go to hospital. Physical restraint is decided as necessary to get Fred into the ambulance. Fred believes that police are going to kidnap him and so he resists, which leads to the use of mechanical restraint of Fred while he is transported in the ambulance. Fred is concerned that his car and business documents are all being left behind, and that he is still waiting for the government to tell him the whereabouts of his son. He becomes increasingly distressed.

Vital signs en route to hospital

- Glasgow Coma Score: 15
- Oxygen saturations: 95%
- Respiratory rate: 32
- Heart rate: 155
- Blood pressure: 183/105
- Electrocardiograph: Sinus tachycardia
- Pain score: 10/10
- Blood sugar level: 16 mmol

CRITICAL REFLECTION

- What are your priorities for the care of Fred while you drive him to hospital?
- What would you do to try to calm Fred down?
- If in your scope of practice you were to administer sedatives in an older person, what would you need to consider and what would you administer? If not in your scope of practice but you believe sedation is required what steps would you take?
- Assuming that Fred is settled and participating in conversation, what other information would you like to ask him for?

MENTAL ILLNESS IN THE OLDER POPULATION

Generally, mental wellbeing increases with age, but the same mental illnesses that afflict younger adults also occur in older adults, namely depression (new onset or recurrence), anxiety, psychoses (new onset or recurrence), bipolar disorder and substance abuse.

SCHIZOPHRENIA

Psychoses such as schizophrenia usually have their onset in young adults, but can occur de novo in older adults, in which situation an organic cause needs to be excluded.

Schizophrenia and psychotic disorders in general speed up ageing in comparison with that of the general population, and the average life span is about 20 years shorter. Symptoms of schizophrenia include delusions (false beliefs), hallucinations (primarily auditory), disorganisation and poor functioning (as outlined in Chapter

13). Treatment is with antipsychotic drugs, but care needs to be taken as these drugs have more side effects in older people; for example, drowsiness, hypotension, falls, muscle stiffness, gait abnormalities, weight gain, constipation, vision impairment and abnormal movements (see Chapter 18).

People with schizophrenia tend not to take good care of themselves, often have poor diet, lack of exercise and comorbid substance abuse, and medical comorbidity is common (Chou et al., 2013). They may also lack insight into their illness, making effective management more difficult. Paranoid ideation is the most common symptom, such as fears the neighbour is spying on them. Cognitive impairment often accompanies schizophrenia in older adults. One result of these symptoms can be aggression and resistance to attempts at treatment. At these times it is important not to argue with the patient but empathise with their distress and reassure them that you are here to help.

Mood symptoms, especially depressive symptoms, complicate management, and the addition of antidepressant medication increases the rate and severity of side effects, especially hypotension, gastrointestinal upsets, constipation, hyponatremia and confusion. Depressive symptoms can also emanate from drug or alcohol abuse, some prescription medications and drug interactions. Post-psychotic depression occurs in a large number of people following a psychotic episode, and a dysthymia or chronic demoralisation can persist. These individuals have a decreased quality of life, decreased functional capacity and increased use of health services, as well as increased suicidality (Chou et al., 2013).

Treatment

Second-generation antipsychotics (such as risperidone) alone may treat psychotic as well as depressive symptoms, but the addition of a selective serotonin reuptake inhibitor (SSRI) such as citalopram is often used as well. Psychosocial interventions are also important in the management of the older person with schizophrenia.

ANXIETY DISORDERS

Anxiety in older people can be missed, as they tend to complain of somatic (bodily) symptoms and indeed do tend to have multiple psychiatric, medical and medication issues (Barton et al., 2014). Yet anxiety is more common in the elderly than depression, causing significant morbidity, and is often treated by GPs with benzodiazepines which have considerable problems in themselves. Ninety per cent of anxiety disorders in older people are either generalised anxiety or specific phobia. The rest include obsessive-compulsive disorders (OCD), post-traumatic stress disorder (PTSD) and panic disorder (Andreescu & Varon, 2015; Benshoff & Harrawood, 2003; Bryant et al., 2008; Jones et al., 2014; Markota et al., 2016).

Associated problems include hypervigilance, feeling vulnerable and feeling helpless. A recent stress or medical illness can re-activate or cause anxiety. Some medications can cause anxiety in older persons; for example, steroids, antihistamines and street drugs (more common now with the ageing of the baby boomers). Psychiatric causes of anxiety include PTSD, depression, OCD and psychosis.

Late-life anxiety impacts healthcare costs by being comorbid with physical problems, leading to multiple investigations (Weiss et al., 2016). Symptoms include excessive worry, restlessness, fatigue, muscle tension, fidgeting, agitation, wringing hands and insomnia, and often an associated depressive disorder. Agoraphobia is the most common phobia, and can follow an illness, assault or trauma. Panic may present with shortness of breath. Anxiety can be an early sign of developing dementia.

Treatment

Approaching the patient in a calm, empathic manner, taking things slowly, and distraction are important methods in reducing acute distress. Acute treatment of overwhelming anxiety can be the administration of a benzodiazepine, but chronic use has several deleterious effects, including cognitive impairment, dependence, incontinence and falls (Hallford et al., 2017). Selective serotonin reuptake inhibitors such as citalopram are first-line treatments. Cholinesterase inhibitors are of use to control anxiety in Alzheimer's disease. Other options include mirtazapine, and quetiapine. Cognitive behavioural therapy (CBT) is one type of long-term therapy for anxiety (Kishita & Laidlaw, 2017).

MOOD DISORDERS

Older adults can suffer from the same mood disorders as younger adults: depression, dysthymia, and bipolar disorders. Mood disorders tend to be more persistent in older people and are often associated with pain (Nicholl et al., 2014) or other medical comorbidity, worsening the outcome of the latter.

Depression affects sleep as well as appetite, concentration, memory and sociability (Han et al., 2016). People with depression can be irritable, withdrawn and feel hopeless. They may be uncooperative with treatment for any medical issues and pessimistic about the outcome. Suicidality is common, and attempts are more often fatal. Older persons complain less about mood and more about physical symptoms – fatigue, weight loss, insomnia, memory problems and constipation.

Recent loss such as the loss of a spouse, role (retirement), accommodation (moving into a nursing home), pet, friend or finances is often a precipitant (Shear et al., 2005). Some medications, such as beta-blockers used for hypertension, some pain medications and anti-glaucoma medications can cause depression. In older people women are more prone to depression.

Depression has an impact on medical mortality, increasing the death rate by four times following myocardial infarct and other medical disorders (Andreescu & Varon, 2015; Bryant et al., 2008). In severe depression people can have delusions; for example, *'I have no money'*, *'My brain has died'*. They can feel guilty and a burden on others.

Table 8.2.1 How to Distinguish Between Delirium and Dementia and Depression

	Delirium	**Dementia**	**Depression**
Course	Acute/subacute often twilight	Chronic, generally insidious	Coincides with life changes, abrupt
Duration	Shorter, diurnal fluctuations, worse at night and on awakening	Long, no diurnal effects, symptoms stable	Diurnal effects, worse in morning, situational fluctuations
Progression	Abrupt	Slow but even	At least two weeks but can be several months
Awareness	Reduced	Clear	Clear
Alertness	Fluctuates	Normal	Normal
Attention	Fluctuates	Normal	Minimal impairment
Orientation	Fluctuates, impaired	May be impaired	Selective disorienting

Manic symptoms in the older person

The older person with mania tends to be more irritable than euphoric, and resistive of medical intervention. Speech may be rapid and disorganised, and cognition impaired – resembling at times a delirium. Emergency transport to hospital can prevent retirement savings being depleted by reckless spending and reputations being destroyed by bizarre behaviour.

Treatment

Older people often need hospital admission, depending on risks and protective factors. Treatment with antipsychotic medications and mood stabilisers for mania and antidepressant drugs for depression may be required. Electroconvulsive therapy (ECT) is only used if the person is not eating/drinking, is psychotic, intensely suicidal or has not responded to several trials of medication. Support, education and counselling are vital. Psychological interventions such as CBT, social adjustments and management of medical comorbidities can lead to total recovery and improvement in physical health. Relapse is more likely if the person is over 80, lives alone, is socially isolated, has no family, has recently moved or is cognitively impaired (Mackenzie et al., 2014).

DEMENTIA

Dementia is a broad term that covers a variety of disorders that lead to deterioration in brain function. Three in 10 people over the age of 85 suffer from some form of dementia.

There are many causes of dementia, such as brain injury, tumour, stroke or metabolic, but there are four main types:

Alzheimer's disease

This is the most common form of dementia, but is not synonymous *with* dementia. It increases in prevalence with age, and results in memory disturbance, starting with short-term memory and progressing to medium- and long-term memory as well as affecting executive functioning and physical capabilities. Eventually, the sufferer needs full nursing care.

Vascular dementia

The second most common form of dementia, it is caused by tiny strokes in the brain and affects behaviour, speech and functioning. It can co-occur with Alzheimer's disease, but tends to follow a step-wise progression, becoming worse with each vascular event. It can also result from a series of major strokes. People with vascular dementia have greater disability and cognitive impairment.

Dementia with Lewy bodies

Lewy bodies are tiny protein deposits in the brain that disrupt function. They are also present in Parkinsonian dementia and, as well as cognitive symptoms, there are movement disorders, sleep disorder and emotional symptoms.

Frontal dementia

This usually presents not with memory problems, but with behavioural problems, such as disinhibition, hypersexuality, apathy, eating disorders, hoarding and psychosis.

Symptoms in common with all dementias include:

- memory loss, particularly short-term memory at first
- putting things away then forgetting where, and sometimes accusing others of having stolen them
- difficulty remembering words, names and people
- difficulty performing everyday tasks such as making a cup of tea
- becoming disorientated easily; for example, losing their way on a car trip
- change in mood or behaviour
- becoming withdrawn and depressed or apathetic.

Other symptoms depend on the type of dementia and can include:

- difficulty finding their way around, especially in new or unfamiliar surroundings
- difficulties with speech, substituting nonsense words for names of objects that they have forgotten
- disorientation to time
- inability to learn new tasks
- difficulty following a conversation, a book or a movie

- difficulty with balance, walking and getting out of a chair
- problems with coordination
- psychological changes, such as becoming irritable, saying or doing inappropriate things, or becoming suspicious or aggressive (Kales et al., 2017; Mavandadi et al., 2017)
- delusions and/or hallucinations
- incontinence, immobility.

When talking with someone with dementia the paramedic should do the following:

1. Approach from the front and position yourself so that you are face to face with the person you are speaking to. Refer to them by their name to ensure you have their full attention.
2. Speak one-on-one and remove distractions.
3. Speak slowly and simply.
4. Find a quiet environment.
5. Be brief and keep sentences short, direct and empathetic.
6. Ask closed questions with a 'yes' or 'no' answer.
7. Give them time to respond. Try to manage frustration and do not hurry them unless the situation requires it.
8. Do not interrupt.
9. Don't say you disagree with them. Accept it is their reality.
10. When they repeat themselves, realise that it is the 'first time' for them

Management of the disturbed patient with dementia needs patience and care. Providing a quiet, uncluttered environment will help (Soril et al., 2014). A strange environment, inability to meet another's expectations, a medical issue or an unexpected occurrence can trigger behavioural issues such as aggression or a catastrophic reaction (screaming, crying, shouting, making accusations, agitation). It is best not to attempt physical contact at that time. Leave them alone or enlist those on the scene to support if it is appropriate to do so. As a general rule, work with carers to best manage the situation.

Pre-hospital assessment of the dementia patient

Include an assessment of the environment and the social and family dynamic. Consider the strain on the carer(s) and whether they can cope with the care needs – paramedics might be dealing with two or more individuals with needs. Collateral information is important.

Be aware of the increased psychomotor movement/wandering or restless behaviour and how you position yourself so the person does not feel enclosed or threatened. Be aware that changes may be present in the visual and hearing ability of the person.

During a physical examination, look for issues with skin breakdown and pressure sores. A lack of support and elder abuse also need to be considered. Taking vital-sign observations may be challenging, but might be essential to help determine if there is an organic cause, such as urinary tract infection. Assess food and fluid intake (dehydration is a major concern), falls risk, risk to self if there is wandering behaviour or a decline in cognition has affected the ability to stay safe in their current environment. Check for any bruises or evidence of trauma, especially head trauma. Often initial signs of subdural bleeds are missed because of the challenges in behaviour and lack of ability to gain history.

Check for medications and the potential for overdose. Bring medications with you if you are going to hospital.

Search for common ground in terms of what you can engage the person in; for example, a common interest. Ask the carer what the person is normally engaged with.

Issues in the transporting of a confused older person from a familiar to an unfamiliar environment are discussed elsewhere, but are alleviated by the presence of a familiar relative or friend.

Further diagnostic assessment and testing

Neuropsychological testing by a neuropsychologist will delineate the extent of the cognitive changes. Blood testing for metabolic or hormone imbalance such as hypothyroidism, vitamin deficiency, such as in pernicious anaemia (vitamin B_{12}), or haematological disorders, such as anaemia, help to rule out reversible causes of cognitive decline. A CAT scan or MRI of the brain can show structural changes, and a PET scan can show functional changes.

Treatment

Treatment with cholinesterase inhibitors such as Aricept can slow progression of the disease but not stop it entirely. Other treatments are basically for the complications and behavioural effects of dementia; for example, sedatives for sleep disturbance, anticonvulsants for aggression, and psychotropics for treatment of depression or psychosis.

Other considerations for the long-term care of someone with dementia depend on the support available in the home by either a spouse or other relative. Home support involving housework, shopping, showering and dressing, administration of medications and general companionship is available depending on the requirements. Meals on wheels are available for those who cannot cook or prepare food. An occupational therapist assessment of the layout of the home is useful in determining if there is a need for structural changes such as railings in the shower, and removal of tripping hazards.

Access to GP, physiotherapist, occupational therapist for medical and physical care, possible attendance at a day centre for socialisation, advice on diet and exercise/lifestyle are all important to have in place.

DELIRIUM

Delirium is a transient organic psychiatric syndrome characterised by acute onset, fluctuating course, altered level of consciousness, global impairment in cognition, perception and memory, and widespread derangement of cerebral metabolism and behaviour. Terms used synonymously include metabolic encephalopathy, acute confusion state, and toxic psychosis.

The most common serious mental disorder in old age, delirium is reported to herald death in up to about 25% of the elderly. It is estimated that between one-third and half of hospitalised geriatric patients are likely to become delirious (Hendry et al., 2016; Malik et al., 2016). Despite this, it is usually transient resulting in full recovery. Prompt assessment, differential diagnosis and treatment are essential to reverse the medical disorder and control behaviour that might be life threatening. Despite this, delirium is frequently unrecognised, and the symptoms are often confused with other psychiatric illnesses (Andreescu & Varon, 2015; Bryant et al., 2008).

COMMON CHARACTERISTICS OF DELIRIUM

- Impaired attention
- Distractibility and diminished concentration
- Disorientation
- Mood changes
- Impaired memory
- Perceptual disturbances; in particular, visual and tactile hallucinations
- Reversal of the sleep/wake cycle
- Disorganised thinking
- Loss of judgment and insight
- Psychomotor disturbance – hyperactive, hypoactive or mixed
- Sudden onset (usually)

COMMON CAUSES OF DELIRIUM IN THE ELDERLY

- Infection (urinary tract infection)
- Polypharmacy, psychotropic medications, narcotic analgesics and some cardiovascular medications
- Alcohol and drug withdrawal
- Metabolic disturbances
- Vitamin deficiencies
- Neurological disorders
- Prolonged anaesthesia (especially if they have an underlying dementing illness)

Diagnosis and treatment by the paramedic must be rapid and thorough. A neurological examination should be performed, including looking for signs of stroke (unilateral muscle weakness, facial asymmetry), attention and concentration. A formal mental status examination repeated at frequent intervals is essential. The Mini Mental State examination is usually used to assess cognition and orientation. A full medical history must be taken, including the use of all prescribed and over-the-counter medications, and a complete review of biological systems (temperature, blood pressure, heart sounds, pain). In hospital, laboratory tests include full organic screens (bloods, urine, chest X-ray), serum drug levels, and CT scan. An EEG may be useful in both diagnosing and following the course of delirium (abnormal slow waves are seen in delirium, and persistence of cognitive impairment after resolution of brain activity may suggest an underlying dementia).

Delirium can be related to a medical emergency and would almost always require transportation to hospital. It may be necessary to use medication to treat anxiety, agitation or psychotic symptoms. A small dose of a benzodiazepine or antipsychotic can be used, enough to relieve distress, but care should be given not to over-sedate. An accompanying relative or carer can reassure the patient and help keep them calm.

Delirium leads to longer hospital stays, less chance of returning to independent living, exacerbates dementia, and has higher mortality rates, and increased rates of admission to long-term care units (Andreescu & Varon, 2015; Bryant et al., 2008). However, if recognised early and treated aggressively, full recovery is possible.

MEDICAL COMORBIDITIES – THE CHICKEN OR THE EGG?

In the older person it is often difficult to differentiate between medical/organic illness and psychiatric illness. Furthermore, in the older person it is common to have medical illnesses that contribute to or cause a psychiatric illness, and psychiatric illnesses that contribute to or cause medical illness.

Medical illnesses in the elderly that may lead to psychiatric illnesses or symptoms include:

- thyroid disorder – hyper or hypothyroidism
- Parkinson's disease
- autoimmune disorders
- pernicious anaemia
- brain tumours.

Psychiatric illness in the elderly that may lead or contribute to medical illnesses include:

- depression worsens the prognosis for myocardial infarction
- chronic anxiety worsens hypertension
- psychiatric medications affect blood pressure, weight, metabolic syndrome, diabetes, and movement disorders, and can impair functioning and mobility.

SUBSTANCE ABUSE

Substance abuse problems are common in the elderly but are largely ignored (Arndt et al., 2005; Benshoff & Harrawood, 2003). These people tend to be a 'hidden' population, but with the ageing of the baby boomers, a group with a greater use of substances, addiction of all types – alcohol, opioids, cannabis, nicotine, stimulants and benzodiazepines – is increasing (Andreescu & Varon, 2015; Bryant et al., 2008).

Chronic pain is common in older people, and so is opioid and prescription medication abuse. Benzodiazepine and other sedative hypnotic abuse increases linearly with age (Andreescu & Varon, 2015; Bryant et al., 2008). Being common, these substances also carry more risks for older addicts, such as falls, confusion, amnesia and sleepiness. They also tend to accumulate within the human body due to the older person's slower metabolism (Ozdemir et al., 1996).

Substance abuse remains largely undetected in older people and must be specifically looked for. *Asking specific questions is not the only means of obtaining the information.* An environment assessment may provide vital clues: it is important for the paramedic to check the house (kitchen, fridge, drug cabinet, etc.) and obtain as much collateral information as possible.

The symptoms of alcohol and drug abuse are often mistaken for the symptoms of ageing problems such as dementia, depression or other medical problems. Older adults consume more over-the-counter medication than any other age group, and benzodiazepines make up 17% to 23% of drugs prescribed for older adults (Markota et al., 2016; Reynolds et al., 2013). Drug use negatively affects the health of older people at a higher rate than other populations. Adverse drug reactions result in about 10% of hospital admissions in this age group (Kargar et al., 2018). Polypharmacy is common, leading to adverse drug interactions. Perhaps the largest contributing factor to drug abuse is family, caregiver and clinician complicity in the problem (Holzbach et al., 2010). Just being aware of this possibility and taking note of the home environment and the older person's access or otherwise to the drug helps subsequent medical personnel in their management. Other medical problems such as hepatitis, pancreatitis, hypertension, arrhythmia and pulmonary problems may be indicative of substance abuse.

Several screening tools exist to screen for alcohol and substance abuse, the CAGE being a four-question screen for alcohol abuse which is appropriate for use by paramedics. Unfortunately, few elderly-specific treatment resources have been developed, and most drug and alcohol treatment centres only accept clients who accept they have a problem and are motivated to change.

CAGE QUESTIONNAIRE

- Have you ever felt you ought to **C**ut down on your drinking?
- Have people **A**nnoyed you by criticising your drinking?
- Have you ever felt bad or **G**uilty about your drinking?
- Have you ever had a drink first thing in the morning to steady your nerves or get rid of a hangover (**E**yeopener)?

(Ewing, 1984)

SUICIDE IN OLDER ADULTS

CASE STUDY

Lew

You are dispatched at 9.15 a.m. to an 87-year-old man in an aged-care residential facility who has a deep laceration to his left wrist. Nursing staff attended his room after he failed to attend the dining room for breakfast. The nurses found him on the floor of the bathroom with a self-inflicted cut to his wrist from a sharp pocket knife. They estimate approximately 200 millilitres of blood loss. Lew states he has been on the floor since 5 a.m.

On arrival, the nursing staff provide the background history. Lew has been a resident at the home for just three weeks. He had been transferred from the psychogeriatric ward after an admission for depression. His discharge summary stated that he had been depressed for one month, with anhedonia (no enjoyment of life), sleep disturbance, poor appetite and numerous physical complaints. He has been very concerned about an upcoming driving test. He gave up care for his disabled son only recently – his son now lives across town in a supported care facility. He was the sole survivor of a helicopter crash while on a military training exercise, and migrated to Australia after medical discharge from the marines. He has enormous survivor guilt. Lew's wife died 25 years ago.

Lew had one prior episode of depression after the death of his wife. Medically, he has a history of atrial fibrillation, coronary bypass, hypertension, prostate problems and a bowel polyp. He was taking warfarin, digoxin, atenolol and allopurinol. He had grown increasingly isolated since his wife's death and now lives alone. Lew drank little alcohol and did not smoke. He was started on an antidepressant, mirtazapine, and was referred to the community mental health team for follow-up three days ago. Lew failed his driving test.

On the way to hospital, Lew disclosed that this was a planned attempt on his life. He spoke about a lifetime of losses: his parents at a young age, his navy mates, his wife, his son, and now his driver's licence and independence. He feels that he has nothing to live for. Last night Lew set his alarm for 4 a.m. He got up, had a cup of tea in his room, then had a shower. After his shower he sat on the bathroom floor and cut his wrist with his old navy knife that he had sharpened the night before.

Vital signs

- Glasgow Coma Score: 14
- Oxygen saturations: 96%
- Respiratory rate: 20
- Heart rate: 98
- Blood pressure: 102/65
- Electrocardiograph: Sinus tachycardia
- Pain score: 3/10
- Blood sugar level: 11 mmol

CRITICAL REFLECTION

- List the potential risk factors in Lew's history that the nursing staff and community mental health team should have been aware of.
- Discuss ways in which staff/care providers could try to mitigate against these risks.
- What would be important to include in your clinical handover to emergency medical staff as the paramedic caring for Lew?
- How would you communicate with Lew?
- What emotions might you have as the paramedic caring for Lew, and how would you manage your own responses when caring for Lew?

Most older adults who complete suicide have a mental illness, most often depression. There is a higher rate of suicide in our Indigenous population (Black et al., 2017). Risk factors include past suicide attempts, severe depression, chronic illness, pain, hopelessness, insomnia, psychosis and drug/alcohol abuse, but older people often do not disclose their feelings, so threats of self-harm should be taken seriously. Loss, social isolation and recent discharge from hospital may be triggers.

There is often less warning than in younger people and high lethality due to frailty or serious intent, as well as less likelihood of contacting mental health services due to shame, stigma and hopelessness. In young people, the number of attempts (100–200) far outweigh one completed suicide, but in older people there are only four attempts for every completed suicide (Vanyukov et al., 2017).

The elderly have a higher rate of completed suicide because they use more lethal methods such as firearms, hanging and drowning. Double suicides involving partners occur most frequently among the aged. There are also the 'silent suicides', such as overdoses, self-starvation and 'accidents'. Older adults often do not seek treatment for mental health problems. High-risk characteristics include increasing age, being male, and being divorced or losing one's life partner. Having a psychiatric illness such as depression is a further risk factor, as are alcohol use, medical illness, family conflict, financial problems, pain, perceived burdensomeness, loss and grief.

On attendance to what may appear as an accident or not a clear suicide attempt, paramedics need to be aware that further history taking and assessment are important, and to consider it potentially as self-harm or a suicide attempt in this age group. *Do not be afraid to ask the person directly about suicidal ideation.* Empathy, caring, concern and open communication with the person at this stage will help to understand the history and circumstances, and possibly assist the elderly person to obtain support at an early stage. Depression is not an inevitable consequence of old age, and intervention can change life for the better.

PSYCHOTROPIC MEDICATIONS IN THE ELDERLY

A psychotropic medication is a type of medication that affects mental functioning. These medications fall into four different categories: antipsychotics (also called major tranquillisers), antidepressants, mood stabilisers and minor tranquillisers (see Chapter 18).

Antipsychotics

Psychosis in the elderly is harder to treat and takes longer. The doses used are lower than in young people because side effects, hypotension and falls, movement disorders, sedation and confusion are all more severe. Drugs used include aripiprazole, quetiapine, risperidone and clozapine for resistant psychosis. Haloperidol in tiny doses (0.5 mg) is the treatment of choice in agitated delirium.

Antidepressants

The medications used for treatment of depression are described in Chapters 10 and 18. Tricyclic antidepressants such as amitriptyline, nortriptyline and dothiepin are effective antidepressants, but are lethal in overdose and cause hypotension, ECG changes and sedation, and therefore are rarely prescribed in the elderly. Many antidepressants can cause electrolyte imbalances in older adults, particularly hyponatremia, which could account for confusion and other symptoms.

Mood stabilisers

Lithium is used particularly for bipolar disorder. It needs a frequent check of blood serum levels as there is a narrow therapeutic range, and high levels cause kidney damage. Long-term use of lithium can result in renal failure in old age, so serum drug levels and renal function should be monitored. Sodium valproate is an anticonvulsant also used as a mood stabiliser. It is relatively safe and has a wide therapeutic range.

Benzodiazepines

These medications are minor tranquillisers used short term for anxiety, but are very addictive and should not be used long term. They are associated with drowsiness, falls, confusion and memory problems in the elderly (Markota et al., 2016; Reynolds et al., 2013; Verthein et al., 2013).

Safety issues with psychotropic medications

Great care must be taken with the use of psychotropic medication in the elderly. Patients should be monitored every three months for symptom recurrence, emerging side effects such as sedation and movement disorders, metabolic syndrome and diabetes.

All of these medications are associated with more side effects at lower doses in the older person, especially hypotension, somnolence, confusion, falls, constipation and effects on sodium levels (hyponatremia from inappropriate anti-diuretic hormone [ADH]). They can also interact with other medications the person may be prescribed, so it is important to gather all the information you can as to what medications and what doses the person is taking and communicate this information at handover. Do not rely on the patient themselves to provide the information as they frequently cannot tell you. The paramedic should look for scripts, Webster packs, and bottles or packets of medication in the person's home. Polypharmacy is common. It is also common for the elderly to retain medications they no longer use. If there is confusion or cognitive impairment, the elderly person may inadvertently take more or less than what is prescribed. Accidental overdoses are common.

PRE-HOSPITAL APPROACHES TO TREATMENT AND CARE
BE PRESENT, LISTEN, COMMUNICATE AND EDUCATE

'Just because you know what you're talking about does not mean that I do. Explain simply, give me options, and time to understand and ask questions. Don't just tell me what to do.'

– Ernestine, aged 73

Communication involves sending, receiving, understanding and utilising information. Talk WITH and not TO the older person.

1. LISTEN
2. Allow them to PARTICIPATE
3. ENGAGE them in the exchange of information
4. PROMOTE dignity and respect.

COMMON PROBLEMS TO CONSIDER WHEN COMMUNICATING WITH AN ELDERLY PERSON

- Hearing deficits
- Poor vision
- Poor memory
- Difficulty speaking (teeth problems, dry mouth due to medications)
- Stroke – aphasia, dysphasia (this may require other ways to communicate – writing, gesture, use of cards depicting an action or object, simple touch)
- Confusion (delirium, cognitive decline)
- The environment, including background noise
- Language/accent and culture

CREATING A SUPPORTIVE ENVIRONMENT

Many older people have a range of chronic illnesses, functional limitations and disabilities such as diabetes, Parkinson's disease, osteoporosis, hypertension and arthritis. They can be comfortable and functional in their familiar environment, but may have difficulty adjusting to a new environment such as a chaotic emergency department. They may feel anxious, helpless and confused in an ambulance or hospital. Taking a family member along with them may help to alleviate distress. Be aware that the decline of functional levels and loss of vitality associated with chronic illness, along with the experience of stressful life events, often leads to depression in older people.

The safety of the home environment can be enhanced by home modification – handrails, smoke detectors, and removal of tripping hazards. Accessible transportation and a supportive social environment with community-based medical and social services helps to avoid early institutionalisation.

MOBILITY

The changes that occur with ageing can lead to problems with mobility – unsteadiness, difficulty getting out of a chair, or falls (Bann et al., 2016). Many things contribute to mobility problems: muscle weakness, joint disease, pain, fear of falling, poor eyesight, certain medications (especially psychotropic and analgesia) and neurological problems such as Parkinson's disease and dementia. It is important to ask the person you are caring for or their carer about mobility problems and/or falls, because this may indicate other medical conditions and/or that the home environment is not safe (loose rugs, slippery flooring, lack of support railing) and will assist you in developing differential clinical formulations (diagnosis) which may be addressed on scene or crucial in clinical handover. Declining mobility can confine the older person to home and deprive them of meaningful and enjoyable activities, such as a walk to the shops or participating in social activities. A period of hospitalisation can result in an irreversible decline in mobility. 'Use it or lose it' is very true of mobility in old age.

MANAGING AGGRESSION

Aggression is a common behavioural symptom of dementia, especially frontotemporal dementia. It can also be due to delirium, acute pain or drug intoxication. It can include verbal abuse, threats, hitting out or physical violence towards another person.

Managing aggression involves being aware of warning signs such as agitation (increased psychomotor movement).

MANAGING AGGRESSION AND REDUCING RISKS TO THE PARAMEDIC AND THE PATIENT

- Eliminate possible causes of stress.
- Avoid confrontation.
- Ensure good communication.
- Maintain non-threatening body language. Approach the person from the front, and maintain a distance of two paces.
- Do not rush.
- Explain what you are going to do.

CONFIDENTIALITY AND LEGAL RESPONSIBILITIES

New privacy legislation requires all communication with your patient and all written medical information to be confidential, unless the person lacks capacity, in which case a guardian or carer can be involved. Of course, it is understood that medical information will be communicated to another health practitioner, but you cannot communicate with other friends or relatives without the person's or guardian's permission (preferably in writing). However, sharing information in an emergency is essential, and paramedics need to acquire as much information from as many sources as possible.

If the person has been placed under the Mental Health Act their information is still confidential apart from handover to the admitting medical team (see Chapter 6).

ASSESSMENT, DOCUMENTATION AND HANDOVER – KEY INFORMATION

Documentation of pre-hospital assessment by paramedics provides a vital baseline and insights to the further assessment and planning of care by the healthcare team.

Referral

Referrals can come from a variety of sources; for example, the person themselves, a relative, community mental health or aged-care team, general practitioner, police. The referrer can often supply you with extensive information, especially in regard to changes in behaviour, risk profile and functioning. These behaviours may be suggestive of a mental illness, but could also be due to a medical problem or developing dementia.

Family context and relationships

Any information regarding the relationships between the older person and their family will be vital for the healthcare team in planning ongoing care. Relationships in any family can vary from close and supportive, to openly hostile, to exploitative and abusive. While noting the family dynamics, it is important to listen to the older person's needs and preferences even when a son or daughter is trying to override them. This is so even if the older person has dementia – the person may still have the capacity and right to choose. If there is family conflict, a guardianship order may be necessary to be taken out so that the person's best interests are represented. The hospital or community social worker can arrange this. If paramedics have concerns for the welfare of the older person, then further help can be sought from team leaders, managers and state and territory reporting services.

Environmental assessment

Paramedics will often be the first of the healthcare team to see a person's living and social situation. This initial environmental assessment can provide vital information to the healthcare team regarding housing, social engagement and situation, and management of the activities of daily living. Where possible the paramedic should take note of the cleanliness and order of their environment, food, medications, disability aids, existing design, access and exits with the person's ability to manage their environment kept in mind.

Mental state examination (MSE)

The MSE can vary over the time taken to assess and transport a patient, so changes should be carefully documented. Furthermore, the MSE can often change from one environment to another, so documentation of a mental state of someone at home in their own environment can vary greatly from the MSE a few hours later in hospital. (Refer to Chapter 5 for detail on conducting an MSE.)

Cognitive testing

As per the MSE, an elderly person's cognition and orientation can fluctuate greatly over time and with changes of environment. Formal but brief cognitive testing by the paramedic in the pre-hospital setting is important to establish a baseline for further assessment in hospital.

Physical examination

This should be documented.

Risk assessment

A risk assessment for the elderly person should include a number of different criteria and not just the presence or absence of suicidal ideation – risk of falling, nutritional deficiency, activities of daily living (ADLs), and medication mismanagement, for example.

HOSPITAL AVOIDANCE/ALTERNATIVES TO TRANSPORT

For the paramedic, some call-outs (such as acute delirium) are likely to require transportation to hospital, while others (such as an acute but resolved aggressive incident in someone with an established diagnosis of dementia) may not. In fact, often the act of taking someone out of a familiar environment into an unfamiliar one will make the behaviour/situation worse. Paramedics must consider the risks and benefits of transporting or not transporting a patient. This decision will often rely on the presence of, and the information provided by, carers including family, support workers and community-based mental health and aged-care teams.

BIOPSYCHOSOCIAL APPROACHES TO LONGER-TERM CARE

It is not uncommon for hospitalisation to be the result of the older person no longer being able to cope in their own home, whether because of psychiatric morbidity or because physical morbidity precludes their being treated in their home. Subsequently, they may need to go into supported accommodation. This is usually organised by the hospital social worker, and may involve the selling of their primary residence. Both low-level care (supported and residential independent living) and high-level care (nursing home) are available. Before entering supported accommodation, an aged-care assessment team (ACAT) assessment is required. This can occur in the hospital or can be arranged in the home. Sometimes the older person lacks 'capacity', i.e. is not capable of making decisions about future care (usually because of cognitive impairment), in which case a guardianship order must be arranged with a relative as the guardian and decision maker, or a public guardian can be appointed. They then make decisions on behalf of the patient. This is different to a power of attorney, which only entitles the person to make financial decisions for the patient.

After discharge from hospital the older person's mental healthcare is provided by a Community Mental Health Care team (CMHT), which comprises psychiatrists, registrars, nurses, psychologists, social workers and occupational therapists. To be effective, the CMHT needs to establish and maintain good communication between themselves and inpatient teams to ensure comprehensive care for the patient. Families can also communicate with both inpatient and CMH teams in the interest of the patient, as they can advise on care pathways for family members with dementia. The importance of this for paramedics is to ensure handover is comprehensive (see above), because they are often the first on the scene and in the best position to assess not only the patient but the whole environment.

CONCLUSION

As an individual or a community, it is easy to underestimate the capabilities of older people. One of the key things contributing to an older person's wellbeing is how they feel they fit socially in the community and with their family. They, like all of us, need to feel valued. A caring, empathic response from a paramedic, communicating to them that they are valued could change the direction their life was heading. Paramedics are ideally placed to communicate a comprehensive assessment at handover, and have a good idea about any risks, but conversely can themselves be at risk in certain situations with an aggressive dementia patient or a person with a paranoid psychosis who could interpret attempts at care as attacks. Approach to a patient with a psychiatric problem should always be non-threatening, with a certain distance maintained until trust is achieved.

LINKS AND RESOURCES

- http://www.dementiatrainingaustralia.com.au
- http://www.dementia-australia.org
- https://www.alz.org/au/dementia-alzheimers-australia.asp
- http://www.carersaustralia.com.au
- https://agedcare.health.gov.au/
- Delirium Care Pathways, Department of Health and Aging, 2010. https://www.health.gov.au/internet/main/publishing.nsf/Content/FA0452A24AED6A91CA257BF0001C976C/$File/D0537(1009)%20Delirium_combined%20SCREEN.pdf
- Dementia – National Framework for Action 2015–2019, Department for Health and Aging. https://agedcare.health.gov.au/ageing-and-aged-care-older-people-their-families-and-carers-dementia/national-framework-for-action-on-dementia-2015-2019
- Living well at home: CHSP good practice guide. Commonwealth of Australia, Department of Social Services, 2015. https://agedcare.health.gov.au/programs-services/commonwealth-home-support-programme/living-well-at-home-chsp-good-practice-guide
- My aged care. Commonwealth of Australia. https://www.myagedcare.gov.au/
- De Bellis, A., Bradley, S.L., Wotherspoon, A., et al., 2009. Come into my world – how to interact with a person who has dementia: an educational resource for undergraduate healthcare students on person-centred care. Flinders University, Hyde Park Press, Adelaide. Online. Available: http://nursing.flinders.edu.au/comintomyworld (Includes video links within the document).

REFERENCES

Andreescu, C., Varon, D., 2015. New research on anxiety disorders in the elderly and an update on evidence-based treatments. Curr. Psychiatry Rep. 17 (7), 53. https://dx.doi.org/10.1007/s11920-015-0595-8.

Australian Bureau of Statistics, 2016. 3101.0 – Australian demographic statistics, June 2016. Online. Available: http://www.abs.gov.au/AUSSTATS/abs@.nsf/Previousproducts/3101.0Feature%20Article1Jun%202016.

Arndt, S., Gunter, T., Acion, L., 2005. Older admissions to substance abuse treatment in 2001. Am. J. Geriatr. Psychiatry 13 (5), 385–392.

Alzheimer's Australia, 2007. Beginning the conversation: addressing dementia in Aboriginal and Torres Strait Islander Communities. Online. Available: https://www.dementia.org.au/files/20061101-ATSI-Begining-Conversation-IndigenousForumReport.pdf

Aw, S., Koh, G., Oh, Y., et al., 2017. Explaining the continuum of social participation among older adults in Singapore: from 'closed doors' to active ageing in multi-ethnic community settings. J. Aging Stud. 42, 46–55. https://dx.doi.org/10.1016/j.jaging.2017.07.002.

Bann, D., Chen, H., Bonell, C., et al., 2016. Socioeconomic differences in the benefits of structured physical activity compared with health education on the prevention of major mobility disability in older adults: the LIFE study. J. Epidemiol. Community Health 70 (9), 930–933. https://dx.doi.org/10.1136/jech-2016-207321.

Barton, S., Karner, C., Salih, F., et al., 2014. Clinical effectiveness of interventions for treatment-resistant anxiety in older people: a systematic review. Health Technol. Assess. 18 (50), 1–59, v–vi.

Benshoff, J., Harrawood, L., 2003. Substance abuse and the elderly: unique issues and concerns. J. Rehabil. 69 (2), 43–48.

Black, E., Kisely, S., Alichniewicz, K., et al., 2017. Mood and anxiety disorders in Australia and New Zealand's indigenous populations: a systematic review and meta-analysis. Psychiatry Res. 255, 128–138. https://dx.doi.org/10.1016/j.psychres.2017.05.015.

Bryant, C., Jackson, H., Ames, D., 2008. The prevalence of anxiety in older adults: methodological issues and a review of the literature. J. Affect. Disord. 109 (3), 233–250.

Chou, S., Huang, B., Goldstein, R., et al., 2013. Temporal associations between physical illnesses and mental disorders: results from the Wave 2 National Epidemiologic Survey on Alcohol and Related Conditions (NESARC). Compr. Psychiatry 54 (6), 627–638. https://dx.doi.org/10.1016/j.comppsych.2012.12.020.

Dong, W., Wan, J., Xu, Y., et al., 2017. Determinants of self-rated health among Shanghai elders: a cross-sectional study. BMC Public Health 17 (1), 807. https://dx.doi.org/10.1186/s12889-017-4718-5.

Emlet, C., 2017. Stigma in an aging context. Interdiscip. Top. Gerontol. Geriatr. 42, 144–158.

Ewing, J., 1984. Detecting alcoholism: the CAGE questionnaire. JAMA 252, 1905–1907.

Hallford, D., Nicholson, G., Sanders, K., et al., 2017. The association between anxiety and falls: a meta-analysis. J. Gerontol. B Psychol. Sci. Soc. Sci. 72 (5), 729–741. https://dx.doi.org/10.1093/geronb/gbv160.

Han, K., Kim, W., Kim, S., et al., 2016. Sleep disorders and risk of hospitalization in patients with mood disorders: analysis of the National Sample Cohort over 10 years. Psychiatry Res. 245, 259–266. https://dx.doi.org/10.1016/j.psychres.2016.08.047.

Hart, L., Jorm, A., Kanowski, L., et al., 2009. Mental health first aid for Indigenous Australians: using Delphi consensus studies to develop guidelines for culturally appropriate responses to mental health problems. BMC Psychiatry 9, 47. https://dx.doi.org/10.1186/1471-244X-9-47.

Hendry, K., Quinn, T., Evans, J., et al., 2016. Evaluation of delirium screening tools in geriatric medical inpatients: a diagnostic test accuracy study. Age. Ageing 45 (6), 832–837.

Holzbach, R., Martens, M., Kalke, J., et al., 2010. Medication dependency and physician's role]. Bundesgesundheitsblatt Gesundheitsforschung Gesundheitsschutz 53 (4), 319–325. https://dx.doi.org/10.1007/s00103-010-1029-8.

Jones, C., Paulozzi, L., Mack, K., 2014. Alcohol involvement in opioid pain reliever and benzodiazepine drug abuse-related emergency department visits and drug-related deaths, United States, 2010. MMWR Morb. Mortal. Wkly Rep. 63 (40), 881–885.

Kales, H., Gitlin, L., Stanislawski, B., et al., 2017. WeCareAdvisorTM: the development of a caregiver-focused, Web-based program to assess and manage behavioral and psychological symptoms of dementia. Alzheimer Dis. Assoc. Disord. 31 (3), 263–270. https://dx.doi.org/10.1097/WAD.0000000000000177.

Kargar, M., Ahmadvand, A., Gholami, K., 2018. Comment on: 'Adverse drug reaction-related hospitalizations in elderly Australians: a prospective cross-sectional study in two Tasmanian hospitals'. Drug Saf. 41 (3), 321–322. https://dx.doi.org/10.1007/s40264-017-0612-4.

Kishita, N., Laidlaw, K., 2017. Cognitive behaviour therapy for generalized anxiety disorder: is CBT equally efficacious in adults of working age and older adults? Clin. Psychol. Rev. 52, 124–136. https://dx.doi.org/10.1016/j.cpr.2017.01.003.

Mackenzie, C., El-Gabalawy, R., Chou, K.L., et al., 2014. Prevalence and predictors of persistent versus remitting mood, anxiety, and substance disorders in a national sample of older adults. Am. J. Geriatr. Psychiatry 22 (9), 854–865. https://dx.doi.org/10.1016/j.jagp.2013.02.007.

Malik, A., Harlan, T., Cobb, J., 2016. Stop. Think. Delirium! A quality improvement initiative to explore utilising a validated cognitive assessment tool in the acute inpatient medical setting to detect delirium and prompt early intervention. J. Clin. Nurs. 25 (21–22), 3400–3408. https://dx.doi.org/10.1111/jocn.13166.

Markota, M., Rummans, T.A., Bostwick, J.M., et al., 2016. Benzodiazepine use in older adults: dangers, management, and alternative therapies. Mayo Clin. Proc. 91 (11), 1632–1639. https://dx.doi.org/10.1016/j.mayocp.2016.07.024.

Mavandadi, S., Wray, L.O., DiFilippo, S., et al., 2017. Evaluation of a telephone-delivered, community-based collaborative care management program for caregivers of older adults with dementia. Am. J. Geriatr. Psychiatry 25 (9), 1019–1028. https://dx.doi.org/10.1016/j.jagp.2017.03.015.

Nicholl, B., Mackay, D., Cullen, B., et al., 2014. Chronic multisite pain in major depression and bipolar disorder: cross-sectional study of 149,611 participants in UK Biobank. BMC Psychiatry 14, 350. https://dx.doi.org/10.1186/s12888-014-0350-4.

Ozdemir, V., Fourie, J., Busto, U., et al., 1996. Pharmacokinetic changes in the elderly. Do they contribute to drug abuse and dependence? Clin. Pharmacokinet. 31 (5), 372–385.

Reynolds, M., Fulde, G., Hendry, T., 2013. Trends in benzodiazepine abuse: 2007–2011. Emerg. Med. Australas. 25 (2), 199–200. https://dx.doi.org/10.1111/1742-6723.12035.

Shear, K., Frank, E., Houck, P., et al., 2005. Treatment of complicated grief: a randomized controlled trial. JAMA 293 (21), 2601–2608.

Soril, L., Leggett, L., Lorenzetti, D., et al., 2014. Effective use of the built environment to manage behavioural and psychological symptoms of dementia: a systematic review. PLoS ONE 9 (12), https://dx.doi.org/10.1371/journal.pone.0115425. e115425.

Tam, M., Aird, R., Boulton-Lewis, G., et al., 2016. Ageing and learning as conceptualized by senior adults in two cultures: Hong Kong and Australia. Curr. Aging Sci. 9 (3), 162–177.

Vanyukov, P., Szanto, K., Hallquist, M., et al., 2017. Perceived burdensomeness is associated with low-lethality suicide attempts, dysfunctional interpersonal style, and younger rather than older age. Int. J. Geriatr. Psychiatry 32 (7), 788–797. https://dx.doi.org/10.1002/gps.4526.

Vauclair, C., Hanke, K., Huang, L., et al., 2017. Are Asian cultures really less ageist than Western ones? It depends on the questions asked. Int. J. Psychol. 52 (2), 136–144. https://dx.doi.org/10.1002/ijop.12292.

Verthein, U., Martens, M., Raschke, P., et al., 2013. Long-term prescription of benzodiazepines and non-benzodiazepines]. Gesundheitswesen 75 (7), 430–437. https://dx.doi.org/10.1055/s-0032-1321756.

Weiss, S., Simeonova, D., Kimmel, M., et al., 2016. Anxiety and physical health problems increase the odds of women having more severe symptoms of depression. Arch. Women's Ment. Health 19 (3), 491–499. https://dx.doi.org/10.1007/s00737-015-0575-3.

Caring for a person with anxiety

Ellie Taylor

LEARNING OUTCOMES

This chapter's learning outcomes are to:

- demonstrate an understanding of anxiety disorders and their associated physical, autonomic and psychological signs and symptoms
- identify the causes of anxiety
- discuss the criteria for defining anxiety disorders
- discuss and identify strategies to assist someone who is suffering an anxiety disorder in the pre-hospital setting
- understand the non-pharmaceutical and pharmaceutical treatments commonly used in treating anxiety.

INTRODUCTION

Anxiety itself is a universal human experience; moreover, it is often a normal and beneficial reaction to stressful situations. Anxiety is manifest in physical, affective, cognitive and behavioural domains. It is important to consider when anxiety becomes pathological; that is, when it deviates from a normal or expected emotional response to an environmental event, as opposed to when it is considered to be a 'normal' response to the event.

For the diagnosis of an anxiety disorder to be made, the presence of a specific symptom profile associated with a significant level of distress or impairment is required.

The American Psychiatric Association's (APA's) *Diagnostic and Statistical Manual of Mental Disorders*, Fifth Edition (*DSM-5*) separates anxiety disorders into discrete categories based on purported similarities in phenomenology (lived experience of symptoms), aetiology and pathophysiology. In this chapter we will focus on three common anxiety disorders; namely, (1) panic disorder (PD), (2) social anxiety disorder (SAD) (or social phobia), and (3) generalised anxiety disorder (GAD). Separation anxiety, selective mutism and agoraphobia are other anxiety disorders which we will discuss briefly.

CASE STUDY

Andy

You have been dispatched to a residential address at 01.33 for a 25-year-old male medical student, Andy, who has woken with increasing shortness of breath, increased heart rate and chest pain. Andy has not been able to sleep for the last three to four days, and felt faint and nauseous when he attempted to get out of bed. The request for ambulance assistance was made by Andy's housemate and friend, Tim.

On your arrival, Tim meets you at the door and directs you to the bedroom. Tim mentions Andy seems to be getting worse and his breathing is becoming shallower and faster. Andy has a past history of asthma, but as far as Tim is aware it is well controlled and he has never seen Andy like this before.

Andy is sitting up in bed, leaning forward, using accessory muscles to breathe and appears pale and sweaty. Andy's facial expression is wide-eyed and he looks distressed. Andy expresses in short, coherent sentences a feeling of 'not being able to catch my breath'.

Vital signs

- Glasgow Coma Score: 15
- Oxygen saturations: 95%
- Respiratory rate: 30
- Heart rate: 110 strong / regular
- Blood pressure: 140/ 85
- Electrocardiograph: Sinus tachycardia
- Blood sugar level: 5.8 mmol
- Pain score: 7/10

CRITICAL REFLECTION

- What communication techniques would you use to reassure and build a therapeutic rapport with Andy?
- What would your priorities be?
- What assessments would you perform and why?

As part of your physical examination you listen to Andy's chest for changes in air entry. The examination reveals clear bilateral air entry with no obvious wheeze.

Andy speaks to you in short, hesitant sentences. He attempts to take deep breaths but finds it difficult to slow down his breathing. His body is shaking and he continually scans the room with his eyes. He states that he feels 'this is the end' and that he 'is going to lose consciousness and die'. He describes feeling as though the walls of his bedroom are going to collapse on him.

Tim informs you he believes Andy has recently broken up with his long-term partner of three years and knows Andy was upset by the breakdown of the relationship. Tim describes the past month as being very challenging for both of them with significant second-year medical exams in the near future, and that the study load has been exhausting. Andy has told Tim he feels as though he is 'falling behind and will not make it'.

Tim mentions he hears Andy moving around the house at all hours of the night and is concerned about the lack of sleep both he and Andy are experiencing. Andy states he is trying to sleep but feels he can achieve more at night in an attempt to catch up and complete his studies. The lack of sleep over the past three months has begun to affect Andy's ability to function at university and complete work.

CRITICAL REFLECTION

- Describe how you would manage Andy's breathing?
- Outline your mental state assessment of Andy at this point.
- Describe the key features in the case and link them to the key criteria for anxiety disorders.

PREVALENCE OF ANXIETY DISORDERS

Anxiety disorders have been shown to be some of the most prevalent mental health conditions in the community. Anxiety, when it becomes overwhelming and disrupts a person's ability to function, is debilitating and has negative effects on quality of life, work and social interaction as well as a person's ability to access and utilise healthcare. Anxiety often co-occurs with other mental health concerns such as depression, and has a similar economic burden on society (Bandelow & Michaelis, 2015).

According to the Australian Bureau of Statistics National Health Survey: First Results 2017–18 (ABS, 2018), it is estimated that 3.2 million Australians (13.1%) have experienced an anxiety-related condition. These numbers indicated an increase from 11.2% in 2014–15. The 2007 National Survey of Mental Health and Wellbeing (NSMHWB) of adults aged between 16 and 85 suggests that 14.4% of Australian adults self-reported experiencing an anxiety disorder in the previous 12 months (ABS, 2008).

The prevalence and experience of anxiety disorders can be significantly different depending on the social and cultural group and the perceived and real vulnerability experienced by those groups. For example, a cross-sectional study by Nasir and colleagues (2018) researching common mental disorders experienced by Indigenous peoples living in regional, remote and metropolitan Australia found that rates of anxiety are double that of the Australian general population.

Approximately 31.5% of individuals who identify as LGBTQI aged between 16 and 85 have experienced an anxiety disorder in the past 12 months. This is more than double the rate of heterosexual Australians (14.1%) aged 16 to 85 (Rosenstreich, 2013).

DEFINING ANXIETY DISORDERS

Anxiety disorders are characterised by strong feelings of being overwhelmed, worried and apprehensive with extended periods of negative emotions (Makovac et al., 2016). The negative emotions experienced in anxiety disorders often manifest with specific somatic (physiological), cognitive and behavioural signs and symptoms that as first-line clinicians are observable and form an essential part of your assessment. Anxiety disorders are often accompanied by avoidant behaviours, hyperarousal (always feeling 'on edge' and constantly checking and being very aware of what is happening around you), and fear that can disrupt everyday functioning and can be debilitating (Dattilo & Goddard, 2021; Kang & Harrison, 2013). Symptoms and the classification of anxiety disorders will be discussed later in this chapter.

Determining when anxiety becomes *pathological* – that is, when it deviates from a normal or expected emotional response to an environmental event – can be informed by considering the following criteria:

1. *excessiveness* – is the anxiety experienced disproportionate to the current circumstances or environmental stimuli?
2. *intensity* – how severe is the distress experienced by the person?
3. *duration* – does the anxiety response persist for longer than would be expected?
4. *impairment* – is there impairment in social, occupational, educational, health or daily function? (Calkins et al., 2016).

ANATOMY AND PHYSIOLOGY OF ANXIETY DISORDER

Specific regions of the brain and neural pathways associated with anxiety are being understood with the use of functional and structural imaging of the brain. Changes in the amygdala, anterior cingulate cortex and hippocampus are implicated across all anxiety disorders. Functional neuroimaging shows hyperactive amygdala response, hyperactive hippocampus and hypoactivation of the anterior cingulate cortex (Ahrens et al., 2018; Duval et al., 2015; Martinez et al., 2007).

Anxiety disorders are triggered by a combination of biological and environmental factors. Several neurotransmitters are thought to play important roles in the pathophysiology of stress, mood and anxiety disorders (Martin et al., 2009). In the central nervous system noradrenaline (norepinephrine), serotonin, dopamine and gamma-aminobutyric acid (GABA) appear to be major mediators of symptoms of anxiety. Decreased levels of GABA and serotonin receptor sensitivity are common, as well as overactivity of the central noradrenaline system and elevated sensitivity to lactate and carbon dioxide (Kang & Harrison, 2013; Krystal et al., 2001; Martin et al., 2009).

The autonomic nervous system, in particular the sympathetic nervous system, mediates many of the symptoms of anxiety. The autonomic nervous system functions to regulate unconscious actions known as the 'fight or flight' response or the sympatho-adrenal response of the body. Activation of the sympathetic nervous system results in a massive release of adrenaline and to a lesser extent noradrenaline. Stimulation of this system causes increased heart rate, increased cardiac contractility, increase in blood pressure, increased respiration rate, bronchial dilation, sweating, piloerection, increased glucose into the blood, inhibition of insulin secretion, reduction in blood-clotting time, mobilisation of blood cells by contraction of the spleen, and decrease in gastrointestinal activity (Hall & Hall, 2021; Richerson, 2017).

However, it is important to recognise that the responses involve a wide range of cognitive, motor, neuroendocrine and autonomic systems and thus are not limited to manifestations of sympathetic nervous system activity (Lyness, 2020).

CHARACTERISTICS OF ANXIETY DISORDERS

Anxiety many be accompanied by a variety of somatic, cognitive and physical signs and symptoms which will vary from person to person. Most individuals experience one or more somatic symptoms that may be referrable to virtually every body organ system (Table 9.1). The physical symptoms (Table 9.2) that a person may experience are similar to those of excitation; they may have a normal physical exam or may exhibit physical symptoms (Table 9.3) (Kang & Harrison, 2013; Lyness, 2020).

Many different types of anxiety disorders include panic attacks. Panic attacks are acute discrete periods of symptoms when a person experiences a sudden surge in anxiety, fear-related thoughts and somatic symptoms in the space of a few

Table 9.1 Somatic Manifestations of Anxiety

Cardiorespiratory	Genitourinary
Palpitations	Urinary frequency or urgency
Chest pain	**Neurological/Autonomic**
Dyspnea or sensation of being smothered	Diaphoresis
Gastrointestinal	Warm flushes or chills
Sensation of choking	Dizziness or presyncope
Dyspepsia	Paraesthesis
Nausea	Tremor
Diarrhoea	Headache
Abdominal pain/bloating	

(Lyness, 2020)

Table 9.2 Physical Manifestations of Anxiety

Repetitive behaviour	Atypical affect
Restlessness	Avoidance of stressor
Increased startle response	Diaphoresis
Stiffness	Hyperkinesis
Tachycardia	Hypervigilance
Tachypnoea	Pressured speech
Tremor	Hyperventilation

(Kang et al., 2013)

Table 9.3 Cognitive Manifestations of Anxiety

Amnesia	Apprehension
Depersonalisation	Derealisation
Distractibility	Emotional liability
Fear	Irritability
Racing thoughts	Intrusive thoughts
Flashbacks or recurrent images	

(Kang et al. 2013)

minutes. They are sudden and unprovoked and can be severe and debilitating. In these circumstances the symptoms resolve usually within one hour (Lyness, 2020).

The *DSM-5* defines a panic attack as an abrupt surge of intense fear or intense discomfort that reaches a peak within minutes, and during which time four or more of the following symptoms occur:

1. Palpitations, pounding heart or accelerated heart rate
2. Sweating
3. Trembling or shaking
4. Sensations of shortness of breath or smothering
5. Feelings of choking
6. Chest pain or discomfort
7. Nausea or abdominal distress
8. Feeling dizzy, unsteady, light-headed or faint
9. Chills or heat sensations
10. Paraesthesia
11. Derealisation (when things or people around seem unreal) or depersonalisation (specifically a sense of detachment from oneself *and* one's identity)
12. Fear of losing control of 'going crazy'
13. Fear of dying.

The combination of symptoms can vary, and subsequently the appearance of panic can vary significantly (APA, 2013).

CLASSIFICATIONS OF ANXIETY DISORDERS

The anxiety disorders are a group of conditions in which the hallmark is idiopathic anxiety (due to an unknown cause), typically accompanied by psychological and somatic symptoms. Anxiety is a common accompanying symptom in many other psychiatric disorders, but the primary anxiety disorders lack the neurocognitive deficits, depressive or manic symptoms or psychosis seen in the other disorders. There are many manifestations of anxiety, and each person will experience them differently. Anxiety disorders include panic disorder, social anxiety disorder, generalised anxiety disorder, separation anxiety, agoraphobia and selective mutism.

PANIC DISORDER

The characteristic feature of panic disorder is the presence of recurrent panic attacks, or paroxysms of extreme anxiety, which are sudden, intense bursts of anxiety or fear accompanied by an array of physical symptoms (APA, 2013).

These are unexpected attacks that are accompanied by cognitive and behavioural effects related to perceived consequences of the panic. It is a common disorder associated with negative outcomes in emotional and physical health.

The diagnosis of panic disorder requires the presence of recurrent unexpected panic attacks, along with at least one month of worry about the possibility of future attacks, worry about the implications or consequences of panic attacks, and/or the development of maladaptive behavioural changes related to the attacks. As well as this, the person must experience marked levels of distress and/or functional impairment that results from their panic symptoms (APA, 2013).

SOCIAL ANXIETY DISORDER

Social anxiety disorder (SAD) is recognised as prevalent in our society and is often incapacitating (Calkins et al., 2016). Diagnosis requires the presence of marked fear or anxiety about one or more social situations in which the individual is exposed to possible scrutiny by others. They fear they will act in a way or show symptoms of anxiety that will be negatively evaluated by others (APA, 2013).

It is a common psychiatric condition with lifetime prevalence rates in Western countries ranging between 7% and 13%, and being more common in women than in men, with a ratio of approximately 3:2 (Furmark, 2002). It is characterised by early onset, typically appearing by age 11 years in 50% of patients and age 20 years in 80% of patients (Stein et al., 2008).

According to data from the national epidemiological survey, quality of life improves with anxiety symptom improvement; however, in people with SAD there is a lower quality of life even after symptom reduction (Rubio et al., 2013).

GENERALISED ANXIETY DISORDER

Generalised anxiety disorder (GAD) is a common and chronic psychiatric condition associated with significant distress, functional impairment and poor health-related outcomes (Calkins et al., 2016).

It is characterised by persistent, excessive and difficult-to-control worry and tension about one's daily life. Common worries concern financial matters, work or school matters, relationships and health concerns. Worries can also include minor things such as punctuality, small household repairs or visiting friends (Calkins et al., 2016, Spitzer et al., 2006).

Worry is a universal human experience. It can be defined as 'a chain of thought and images, negatively affect-laden and relatively uncontrollable' (Borkovec et al., 1983).

In GAD the worry must be associated with at least three out of six of the following psychological and somatic symptoms:

1. Feeling keyed-up, restless or on edge
2. Being easily fatigued
3. Having impaired concentration
4. Irritability
5. Muscle tension
6. Sleep disturbance (APA, 2013).

For the diagnosis of GAD, the person's worry and feelings of anxiety and tension must be present for more days than not for at least six months, with significant distress or marked impairment in social, occupational or daily function (APA, 2013; Calkins et al., 2016).

OTHER ANXIETY AND ANXIETY-LIKE CONDITIONS

PD, SAD and GAD are three types of anxiety disorders that are commonly encountered by paramedics. There are other types of anxiety that can be equally common and equally debilitating but less likely to be encountered by paramedics. In addition, there are also anxiety-like conditions such as obsessive-compulsive disorder (OCD) and post-traumatic stress disorder (PTSD), which are no longer classified as anxiety disorders under the *DSM-5*, but which are summarised here in this chapter as they will generally present with anxiety-like symptoms.

Separation anxiety disorder

This is an excessive fear or anxiety of being separated from a person's home or their attachment figures (e.g. mother, father, etc.) and this anxiety must exceed what is expected at that person's developmental level. These people experience excessive distress when separated from their home or attachment figure; they worry about the wellbeing or death of these figures, and need to know where they are at all times.

Selective mutism

Seen in children, they don't initiate speech or reciprocally respond when spoken to by others in social interaction. They will speak with immediate family members in their home; however, they often won't speak in front of others, including cousins, grandparents, etc.

Agoraphobia

This is an intense fear or anxiety triggered by real or anticipated exposure to a wide range of situations. These people experience these symptoms when using public transport, being in open spaces (parking lots, marketplace), being in enclosed spaces (shops, cinemas), standing in line or being in a crowd, or being outside of the home. The amount of fear experienced can vary from person to person.

Obsessive-compulsive disorder

Obsessions are defined as recurrent and persistent thoughts, urges or images that are intrusive and unwanted, causing anxiety or distress. Compulsions are defined as repetitive behaviours or mental acts that the person feels driven to perform. These are aimed at preventing or reducing anxiety or distress, or even preventing some dreaded event or situation.

Obsessive-compulsive disorder (OCD) is where a person has repetitive thoughts (obsession), or they feel the need to perform certain actions or routines repeatedly (compulsion) to the point where it causes distress and/or impairs daily functioning. These thoughts, actions or activities are not able to be controlled by the person. These compulsions can include hand-washing, repeated checking to see if doors are locked or counting things, and often are in response to the negative obsessive thoughts as a way to manage those thoughts (e.g. fear of germs leading to compulsive hand-washing). The individual is aware that these behaviours don't make sense; however, they cannot control them, which causes them great distress.

The symptoms people experience are diverse; however, there are three main dimensions that occur: contamination obsessions with cleaning compulsions, symmetry obsession with ordering and repeating compulsions, and intrusive thoughts related to religious, sexual, aggressive and somatic themes with checking compulsions. Affected individuals can experience multiple symptoms at any given time, and these symptoms tend to change over the course of the person's illness.

The onset of OCD peaks in pre-adolescence and early adulthood, with females and males being affected equally. Males, however, have an earlier onset than females. OCD is often associated with tics, anxiety disorders and an increased risk of suicide. It is common for there to be a delay in a diagnosis of OCD. There are many reasons for this, including under-recognition by clinicians and the shame that these individuals feel about their OCD. This delay in diagnosis is associated with worse outcomes.

Treatment of OCD involves the combination of both medication and therapy. Medications include selective serotonin reuptake inhibitors (SSRIs) and tricyclic antidepressants (TCAs). Therapies that are effective in the treatment include cognitive behavioural therapy (CBT), and psychoeducation and support groups. CBT for OCD includes exposure and response prevention (ERP). ERP works by exposing the person to a feared OCD stimulus and working with them not to act out their compulsion.

As well as OCD there is a separate category of obsessive-compulsive-related disorders (OCRDs) which are also no longer classified as anxiety disorders. These disorders are differentiated from OCD by the lack of intrusive thoughts. OCRDs are categorised by repetitive behaviours which can be related to body appearance. The OCRDs include hoarding disorder, body dysmorphic disorder, trichotillomania and skin picking (excoriation) disorder.

Hoarding disorder: This is the persistent difficulty discarding or parting with possessions. The difficulty is due to a perceived need to save items and the significant distress associated with discarding them. This results in the accumulation of possessions that clutter the person's house and compromise its use.

Body dysmorphic disorder: This is the preoccupation with perceived defects or flaws in physical appearance. These flaws are not observed by others or only appear very slight. The person will perform repetitive behaviours such as mirror checking, or excessively comparing themselves to others.

Trichotillomania: This is the recurrent pulling of hair resulting in hair loss, which causes clinically significant distress or impairment.

Skin-picking (excoriation) disorders: This is the recurrent skin picking that results in skin lesions.

(Stewart et al., 2016)

POST-TRAUMATIC STRESS DISORDER

Post-traumatic stress disorder (PTSD) is a psychiatric disorder that involves a particular set of reactions and health complications that follow a traumatic event that threatened the life or safety of the person or those around them. These events can include a terrorist act, war or combat, rape, sexual violence, serious accident or natural disaster.

The diagnosis of PTSD requires a presumptive cause (i.e a traumatic event) as well as the typical symptom constellation. The presumptive cause can include directly experiencing the traumatic event, witnessing a traumatic event, learning that a traumatic event has occurred to a close friend or family member, or experiencing repeated or extreme exposure to aversive details of the traumatic event (e.g. emergency first-responders).

The symptoms of PTSD are categorised into intrusive symptoms, avoidance symptoms, negative alterations in mood and cognition, and a negative emotional state. For a diagnosis of PTSD, the duration of these symptoms must be present for more than one month and cause clinically significant distress or impairment in social, occupational or other areas of functioning.

Many people who have been diagnosed with PTSD often have other comorbid psychiatric disorders. The three most common comorbid psychiatric conditions are major depressive disorder, alcohol abuse and anxiety disorders (generalised anxiety disorder, panic disorder, specific phobias). PTSD also has a risk of suicide ideation (three- to five-fold increase) and suicide attempts (three- to six-fold increase).

There are a variety of psychological interventions that have been effective in the treatment of PTSD. These include prolonged exposure therapy, cognitive therapy, stress management, psychodynamic therapy, and eye-movement desensitisation and reprocessing (EMDR). Pharmacotherapy is another important aspect of patient care and has shown to be effective in treating the symptoms of PTSD. Commonly used drugs are selective serotonin reuptake inhibitors (SSRIs), monoamine oxidase inhibitors (MAOIs), serotonin-noradrenaline reuptake inhibitors (SNRIs), tricyclic antidepressants (TCAs) and mirtazapine.

SYMPTOMS OF POST-TRAUMATIC STRESS DISORDER

Intrusive symptoms

These symptoms must have begun after the event(s).

- Recurrent, involuntary and intrusive distressing memories of the event(s).
- Recurrent distressing dreams in which the content and/or effect of the dream are related to the event(s).
- Dissociative reactions (a feeling of being disconnected from yourself and the world around you) such as flashbacks in which the person feels or acts like the event(s) is/are recurring.
- Intense or prolonged psychological distress at exposure to internal or external cues that symbolise or resemble the event(s).
- Marked physiological reactions to internal or external cues that symbolise the event(s).

Avoidance symptoms

These symptoms must have begun after the event(s).

- Avoidance or efforts to avoid distressing memories, thoughts or feelings associated or closely associated with the traumatic event(s).
- Avoidance or efforts to avoid external reminders that bring about distressing memories, thoughts or feelings about the event(s).

Negative alterations in cognition or mood

These must be associated with the event(s) and begin or worsen after the event(s) occur(s).

- Inability to remember an important aspect of the traumatic event(s).
- Persistent and exaggerated negative beliefs or expectations about oneself, others or the world.
- Persistent distorted cognitions about the cause or consequences of the traumatic event(s) that lead to the person blaming themselves or others.
- Persistent negative emotional state – e.g. fear, anger, guilt.
- Markedly diminished interest or participation in significant activities.
- Feelings of detachment or estrangement from others.
- Persistent inability to experience positive emotions.

Alterations in arousal and reactivity

These must be associated with the event(s) and begin or worsen after the event(s) occur(s).

- Irritability and angry outbursts with little or no provocation, typically expressed as verbal or physical aggression towards people or objects.
- Reckless or self-destructive behaviour.
- Hypervigilance.
- Exaggerated startle response.
- Problems with concentration.
- Sleep disturbance.

(Dekel et al., 2016)

It should be noted that The American Psychiatric Association made many changes to the *DSM* when they published the *DSM-5*. Some of the changes they made were in relation to obsessive-compulsive disorder and post-traumatic stress disorder. Obsessive-compulsive disorder is no longer included in the anxiety chapter. Post-traumatic stress disorder has also been removed from the chapter on anxiety and has been included in a new chapter 'Trauma and Stressor-related Disorders'. This does not mean that these conditions do not present with significant anxiety and anxiety-like symptoms; however, it has been identified that these are disorders that are more than just anxiety and so are now in separate categories.

ANXIETY IN MEDICAL CONDITIONS

It is important to remember that anxiety can occur for many reasons, and that it isn't always a psychiatric disorder. It is important for the paramedic to always consider that anxiety may be due to a medical condition or as an effect of medication.

The symptoms of anxiety can include chest pain, shortness of breath, palpitations, tachycardia, headache, irritability and abdominal discomfort. These symptoms can also be indicative of a primary medical condition which could be life-threatening. People presenting with symptoms of anxiety must be evaluated for potential medical causes of the presenting symptoms.

Depression and cardiac disorders present a major comorbidity – abnormalities of mental function are common in individuals with heart failure. When the heart is severely compromised in advanced heart failure people can present with symptoms of anxiety. This can also occur due to the drugs used to treat heart failure, which can cause electrolyte disturbances and hypotension which may exacerbate or induce anxiety and anxiety-like symptoms (Kang & Harrison, 2013; Testa et al., 2013).

Myocardial infarction, angina and cardiac arrythmias can all present with similar clinical findings to that of a panic attack or anxiety. These clinical findings include chest pain, shortness of breath, palpitations, dizziness and apprehension (Kang & Harrison, 2013).

Acute and chronic respiratory disorders can also produce anxiety-like symptoms or anxiety itself. Hypoxemia, hypercarbia and acidosis can all produce psychiatric symptoms, more specifically pulmonary oedema, pulmonary embolism, asthma and chronic obstructive pulmonary disease can present with a sensation of choking or not being able to breathe, fear, chest tightness, hyperventilation, diaphoresis, agitation and a fear of impending death, all of which are associated with anxiety (Kang & Harrison, 2013; Patel & Hurst, 2011; Testa et al., 2013).

In diabetic patients, reactive hypoglycaemia is often considered a cause of anxiety, and in patients with hyperthyroidism 30–50% of female patients will suffer from panic and generalised anxiety disorders (Bunevicius et al., 2005; Testa et al., 2013).

Transient ischaemic attacks, temporal lobe seizures and brain tumours may promote anxiety, and many emergency department presentations for the above have anxiety as an accompanying symptom (Kang & Harrison, 2013; Testa et al., 2013).

Other medical conditions that can mimic, exacerbate or initiate anxiety or anxiety-like symptoms include nutritional deficiencies, anaemia, sickle cell disease, epilepsy and degenerative neurological disorders (Testa et al., 2013).

Those with chronic medical illness are also at an increased risk of developing anxiety, and studies have shown that there is a relationship between chronic disease and the emergence of depression and anxiety symptoms. Those with chronic medical illness and comorbid anxiety and depression reported a significantly higher number of medical symptoms. This could also make it difficult to control their medical condition and quality of life (Gerontoukou et al., 2015; Katon et al., 2007).

NON-PSYCHIATRIC CAUSES OF ANXIETY AND ANXIETY-LIKE SYMPTOMS

- **Cardiac**: Angina, arrythmias, hypertensive emergency, myocardial ischaemia
- **Endocrine:** Addison's disease, diabetes, Cushing's syndrome, thyroid disease
- **Exogenous:** Stimulant use (including caffeine), dietary supplements, acute intoxication (alcohol and illicit substances), withdrawal (alcohol, benzodiazepines, sedatives, heroin)
- **Gastrointestinal:** Dyspepsia, gastro-oesophageal reflux disease, irritable bowel syndrome
- **Immunological:** Allergic reaction, early anaphylaxis
- **Medications:** Amphetamines, salbutamol/Ventolin, SSRIs, anticholinergics, histamine 1 and 2 blockers
- **Metabolic:** Electrolyte abnormalities, nutritional deficiencies
- **Neurologic:** Brain tumours, cerebrovascular accidents, degenerative disorders, delirium, dementia, meningitis, some seizure disorders
- **Pulmonary:** Asthma, chronic obstructive pulmonary disease, pulmonary embolism, upper respiratory tract infection

(Adapted from Kang & Harrison, 2013)

TREATMENT AND MANAGEMENT OF ANXIETY

The treatment of anxiety can involve psychotherapy or medication as first-line treatment, or a combination of both approaches. Therapies include (but are not limited to) cognitive behavioural therapy (CBT), acceptance and commitment therapy (ACT) and solution-focused brief therapy (SFBT). There are a variety of medications available for the treatment of anxiety, from short-term relief to long-term management.

In the pre-hospital environment, paramedics will have to develop and use a wide variety of knowledge and skills to assist people presenting with symptoms of anxiety.

PSYCHOLOGICAL THERAPIES

Cognitive behavioural therapy (CBT)

This is a proven effective psychotherapeutic treatment for anxiety spectrum disorders as well as other psychiatric conditions. CBT has been extensively researched and is considered by many to be the first-line therapy in the treatment of generalised anxiety disorder, panic disorder and social anxiety disorder.

CBT is an individualised collaborative approach to psychotherapy that emphasises the importance of thought, feeling and expectations. It is a structured and goal-orientated intervention that targets core components of a given disorder.

CBT combines two effective kinds of psychotherapy: *cognitive therapy* and *behavioural therapy*. Cognitive therapy teaches individuals how certain thinking patterns contribute to their symptoms, and behavioural therapy helps individuals weaken the learned connections between troublesome situations and their habitual behavioural reactions to them. It focuses on how certain thinking patterns and/or beliefs cause symptoms, and by recognising that emotions and behaviours are best addressed by considering the faulty thought processes that precede such feelings and acts.

CBT centres on the elimination of core features of each disorder; for example, treatment for panic disorder targets fears of anxiety and panic symptoms; treatment for social phobias targets fears of negative evaluations by others.

As with many psychological therapies, a key feature of CBT involves the establishment of a strong collaborative working alliance with the individual. This is often initiated in the context of educating the individual about the nature of his or her disorder, explaining how CBT came about, how it works and what is expected from each person involved (Dattilo & Goddard, 2021; Glass et al., 2018; Sprich et al., 2016; Vaughan et al., 2020)

Acceptance and commitment therapy (ACT)

ACT belongs to the family of behavioural and cognitive therapies. Its primary aim is to encourage individuals to adopt positive life values and to accept adverse experiences that are an inevitable consequence of life. It is a modern form of CBT that is based on a distinct philosophy and the basic science of cognition.

The foundational principle of ACT emphasises psychological flexibility to manage suffering that is an unavoidable part of the human experience. By being able to adopt psychological flexibility individuals may pursue goals in meaningful or valued domains.

It achieves psychological flexibility by strengthening six core skills:

1. *Acceptance* – experiencing both pleasant and unpleasant thoughts, feelings, memories and impulses instead of trying to control or avoid them.
2. *Contact with the present moment* – consciously engaging in any moment, being mindful of thoughts, feelings, bodily sensations and potential actions, even during distressing experiences.
3. *Diffusion* – stepping back and observing thoughts as a representation of thought processes.
4. *Self as context* – developing a broad perspective on thinking and feeling.
5. *Values* – clarifying and defining fundamental values and goals.
6. *Committed action* – taking effective action guided by values.

ACT has overlapping processes with other psychosocial interventions; however, it differs from these in that its emphasis is on appraising and changing the relationship with one's thoughts rather than changing those thoughts themselves. It doesn't attempt to eliminate or modify negative thoughts or feelings, rather it encourages the person to accept that these feelings exist and move towards more important values.

The ultimate goal of ACT for people with anxiety disorders is to help them function better with the anxiety they are experiencing, not necessarily lessen the experience. When a person with psychological flexibility experiences anxiety it has less of an impact on the behavioural choices that are made (Coto-Lesmes et al., 2020; Coyne et al., 2011; Kim et al., 2021; Twohig et al., 2017; Wynne et al., 2019).

PHARMACOLOGICAL THERAPIES

There are many different pharmacological treatment options available for the treatment of anxiety disorders. Some individuals who receive pharmacological interventions will still remain symptomatic and will require a combination of psychotherapy and medication.

Medications that are commonly used in the treatment of anxiety include selective serotonin reuptake inhibitors (SSRIs), serotonin-noradrenaline reuptake inhibitors (SNRIs), tricyclic antidepressants (TCAs) and benzodiazepines. Other classes of drugs do play a role in the treatment of anxiety; however, the focus here will be on the more commonly used drugs.

Selective serotonin reuptake inhibitors (SSRIs) and serotonin-noradrenaline reuptake inhibitors (SNRIs)

SSRIs along with SNRIs are first-line agents in the treatment of anxiety disorders as they have an excellent spectrum of efficacy with a low side-effect profile and a lack of cardiotoxicity.

Serotonin is a neurotransmitter that affects autonomic function, motor activity, and cognition, as well as complex processes associated with affection, emotion and reward.

SSRIs work by inhibiting the reuptake of serotonin in the synaptic cleft; in other words it increases the amount of serotonin that is available for use by neurotransmitters.

Like SSRIs, SNRIs work by inhibiting the uptake of serotonin as well as inhibiting the uptake of noradrenaline, thereby enhancing neurotransmission. They have also been shown to be effective in people who don't respond to SSRIs.

Common side effects experienced by people taking these drugs include sexual dysfunction, sleep disturbance, weight gain and gastrointestinal disturbance (Bui et al., 2016; Sangkuhl et al., 2009).

Tricyclic antidepressants (TCAs)

TCAs are efficacious in panic disorders, and were originally the first-line gold standard for the treatment of anxiety disorders. However, they have since been replaced as first-line treatment by SRRIs and SNRIs. TCAs are still very effective in the treatment of anxiety; however, they are used less frequently due to their side-effect burden, cardiotoxicity and potential lethality in overdose.

TCAs work by blocking the reuptake of serotonin and noradrenaline, increasing the synaptic concentrations of neurotransmitters, which leads to an enhancement of neurotransmission. As well as this, they also act as a potent antihistamine and anticholinergic agent, providing a sedative which in the setting of anxiety is very useful.

The other pharmacological effects of TCAs are sodium channel blockade, potassium channel blockade, and peripheral alpha-1 receptor blockade. These lead to widening of the QRS complex and prolonged QTc interval that can result in the development of torsade de pointes, vasodilation, decreased perfusion and hypotension. It is these effects that make TCAs potentially lethal in an overdose (Bui et al., 2016; Christian & Bryant, 2013).

Monoamine oxidase inhibitors (MAOIs)

MAOIs are not commonly used in anxiety disorders, especially as a first-line therapy, due to dietary restrictions and the risk of a hypertensive crisis associated with these interactions. There is some suggestion that MAOIs may be effective in the treatment of those with refractory anxiety disorders. MAOIs work by inhibiting monoamine oxidase isoenzymes. These isoenzymes remove neurotransmitters including adrenaline, noradrenaline, serotonin and tyramine. By inhibiting the enzyme there will be an increase in these neurotransmitters available to the brain.

The use of MAOIs must be accompanied by a very strict diet and careful monitoring of the individual's diet to ensure they don't consume food containing tyramine. The ingestion of tyramine-containing foods while taking MAOIs can lead to a hypertensive crisis and/or serotonin syndrome (Bui et al., 2016; Christian & Bryant, 2013).

Benzodiazepines

Benzodiazepines are widely used for panic and anxiety disorder due to their effectiveness, tolerability and rapid onset of action. They are commonly prescribed as an 'as-needed' medication, meaning that they can be taken when a person is experiencing an increase in anxiety symptoms due to an event or if a person develops an acute panic or anxiety attack.

Benzodiazepines enhance the effect of gamma-aminobutyric acid (GABA). GABA is a chief inhibitory neurotransmitter, with its principal role being the reduction of neuronal excitability throughout the nervous system. By enhancing the effect of GABA, benzodiazepines have a sedative effect, a hypnotic (sleep-inducing) effect, anxiolytic (anti-anxiety) effect, anticonvulsant effect, and muscle-relaxant properties.

Long-term use of benzodiazepines can lead to dependence, a decrease in the effectiveness of the medication, and withdrawal syndrome if discontinued. These medications should not be used as monotherapy, but rather be part of a treatment regimen which includes appropriate medications, therapy and supervision by a medical practitioner (Bui et al., 2016; Griffin et al., 2013).

COMMONLY PRESCRIBED DRUGS FOR ANXIETY

SSRIs

* Citalopram (Celexa)
* Escitalopram (Lexapro)

- Fluoxetine (Prozac)
- Fluvoxamine (Luvox)
- Paroxetine (Paxil)
- Sertraline (Zoloft)

SNRIs
- Venlafaxine (Effexor)
- Desvenlafaxine (Pristiq)
- Duloxetine (Cymbalta)

TCAs
- Amitriptyline (Endep)
- Nortriptyline (Allegron)
- Clomipramine (Anafranil, Placil)
- Dothiepin (Dothep)
- Doxepin (Deptran, Sinequan)
- Imipramine (Tofranil, Tolerade)

MAOIs
- Phenelzine (Nardil)
- Tranylcypromine (Parnate)

Benzodiazepines
- Temazepam
- Nitrazepam
- Diazepam
- Oxazepam
- Lorazepam

PARAMEDIC MANAGEMENT IN THE PRE-HOSPITAL ENVIRONMENT

Treating a person who is anxious or having a panic attack should always begin with creating a calm, quiet and soothing environment, and then creating a trusting rapport. In the pre-hospital environment this can sometimes be difficult to achieve. As you enter the room you need to observe your surroundings (who is in the room, what is in the room) and get that first impression of not only the mood of the person but the tone of the room (is everybody stressed/upset/heightened, are people frustrated/angry/aggressive). This skill, which you will develop over time, will help you to identify what is going to help the situation and what isn't. Always remember to ask the individual what they need to feel safe, and, where possible, accommodate those needs.

There are many different treatment options that paramedics can use to help people who are feeling anxious or having a panic attack. These include but are not limited to: creating a safe environment, breathing techniques, grounding techniques, muscle relaxation, and communication/brief psychotherapy.

There is no one technique that will work for every person; it will be different for every person every time. What may have worked the last time on one person may not work the second time. It will also depend on what symptoms the person is experiencing as to what the most appropriate and effective approach would be.

CREATING A SAFE, CALM ENVIRONMENT

Creating a safe and calm environment can help people who are having acute anxiety or a panic attack. For paramedics, achieving a calm environment where the individual can feel safe and secure is incredibly beneficial.

There are many ways to create this type of environment, and it will all depend on the location and the needs of the individual involved. Some basic, easy-to-implement suggestions include:

- moving the person to a quiet place
- creating a private environment where they are not in view of the public
- dim lighting
- removing any stressors or triggers, e.g. TV, people, noises, animals, etc. (be aware that some people have therapy dogs and these should not be removed)
- including supportive people who will help de-escalate the situation.

The goal is to ensure the individual feels safe, supported and understood, so they will be receptive to other techniques to help them with their anxiety and panic.

BREATHING TECHNIQUES

Coaching an individual through breathing exercises is of great help, especially if they are hyperventilating due to anxiety.

It is important that the paramedic speak in a calm yet firm voice when talking through breathing exercises. It may also be beneficial to do the breathing exercises with them, not only so that they can see what to do, but so that they can also be drawn in by using more than one of their senses.

The simplest breathing exercise that a paramedic can coach someone through is breathing in for a set amount of time, then breathing out for a set amount of time. The length of time can be modified as required, either to gradually slow down the breathing, or to encourage a deeper breath.

Many people will struggle initially, so gentle encouragement and perseverance will help. It is always beneficial for the paramedic to sit in front of the person and breathe with them; for example, slowly counting to four each time. For some people, talking through the exercise may be enough, but for others a visual representation of a square may assist. By slowly running your finger around the perimeter of the square, the person can visualise the timing of each section.

BREATHING TECHNIQUE

To perform this, you need to ensure that you have the person's attention so that you can clearly explain what you need them to do. To achieve this, there needs to be no other noise in the room, such as TVs or conversations.

They should be in a comfortable position, either sitting, lying or standing – whichever position they want.

In a slow, calm voice, instruct them to breathe in slowly for 4 seconds, pause, then breathe out slowly for 4 seconds and pause again. Counting out loud so they can hear is very important, i.e. 'we are breathing in for four seconds, one … two … three … four, and out for four, one … two … three … four and back in for four …'.

This is repeated until they feel like their breathing and/or anxiety is under control.

GROUNDING TECHNIQUES

Grounding is an excellent way to bring the person back to the moment and recentre their focus on the here and now. It works by allowing the person to notice things around them using their five senses.

There are many different types of grounding techniques. The 54321 method is simple to use pre-hospital and can be effective with both adults and children. This method allows them to stop and think about each of their five senses and identify what they can see, hear, feel, smell and taste in that moment.

This is a simple yet effective technique that paramedics can implement, and it can be repeated more than once.

54321 GROUNDING TECHNIQUE

To implement this technique the individual should be in a calm and safe environment. They should be in a comfortable position for them, which can be sitting, lying or standing.

Position yourself where they can see you but not in their direct line of sight.

Start by getting them to take a few deep breaths, and then ask them the following questions:
1. First, tell me 5 things you can hear in your immediate surroundings.
2. Now tell me 4 things you can see.
3. Now tell me 3 things you can touch/feel.
4. Now tell me 2 things you can smell.
5. Finally, tell me 1 thing you can taste (if they can't taste anything identify what their favourite taste is).

This process can be repeated as many times as required, and can be particularly useful for children.

Progressive muscle relaxation

This method helps relieve any tension they may have in their body, and it is particularly helpful for those who feel like their muscles are tense and they can't relax.

This is best done in a quiet, private environment with no distractions. While it is preferable for the individual to lie down, this can also be done sitting in a comfortable position.

For this to work, the person needs to be comfortable and to be able to freely move and feel each part of their body. Encourage them to remove their shoes and loosen tight clothing, if this will help.

As with all of these techniques, this needs to be clearly explained and done slowly, and you can repeat the process if needed. The goal is that by relaxing the body, reducing the tension in the muscles, and controlling the breathing, it should help to relax the mind.

PROGRESSIVE MUSCLE RELAXATION SEQUENCE

As you are talking the individual through these steps, the environment should be quiet, calm and free of distractions or stressors. The person should be in a comfortable position of their choosing – either sitting, lying or standing.

In a calm, soft, even-toned voice you will guide them through the steps of muscle relaxation.

This process can be repeated as much or as little as required. The goal of this is to help the individual to relax and release some tension, worry or anxiety.

The following is an example of a script for progressive muscle relaxation.

1. As you take a breath in, squeeze your toes and feet tight, and, as you breathe out, relax your toes and feet releasing the tension.
2. As you take a breath in, squeeze your calves tight, and, as you breathe out, relax your calves releasing the tension.
3. As you take a breath in, squeeze your thighs tight, and, as you breathe out, relax your thighs releasing the tension.
4. As you take a breath in, squeeze your bottom tight, and, as you breathe out, relax your bottom releasing the tension.
5. As you take a breath in, squeeze your stomach tight, and, as you breathe out, relax your stomach releasing the tension.
6. As you take a breath in, squeeze your hands into a fist, and, as you breathe out, relax your hands releasing the tension.
7. As you take a breath in, squeeze your biceps tight, and, as you breathe out, relax your biceps releasing the tension.
8. As you take a breath in, squeeze your shoulder blades together tight, and, as you breathe out, relax your shoulder blades releasing the tension.
9. As you take a breath in, squeeze your shoulders up to your ears, and, as you breathe out, relax your shoulders down releasing the tension.
10. As you take a breath in, clench your jaw tight, and, as you breathe out, relax your jaw releasing the tension.
11. As you take a breath in, squeeze your eyes shut tight, and, as you breathe out, relax your eyes releasing the tension.

COMMUNICATION

All of the above techniques are effective in relieving anxiety and panic. However, it is important that these are used in combination with an appropriate communication style. While it may be appropriate to allow someone to talk about why they are feeling anxious, a focus on the stress, trigger or symptoms during a time of acute panic may actually intensify the feelings of anxiety. In most situations, it would be more appropriate to focus on the relief of symptoms before completing an assessment of possible psychosocial causes. However, in some situations concurrent assessment and intervention is required; for example, if it was thought that the anxiety symptoms were related to a cardiac event then an assessment of stressors and triggers can occur later.

A brief therapy approach such as solution-focused brief therapy (SFBT) may be used as a stand-alone approach or an adjunct to other interventions. While most other therapies start with an examination of what's wrong, SFBT moves straight to talking about the solution; for example, what life would look like when they get through the current problem, and what things they would both notice and be doing differently as they move towards a healthier state. A discussion would include an examination of the person's strengths, including past achievements and how they have gotten through previous events. An approach such as this can assist a person to build hope and to see their way through the problem (Henden, 2017). It is an approach that is not limited to anxiety disorders, but can be used in virtually any scenario where there is distress and high levels of emotions (Smith, 2021).

CONCLUSION

Anxiety is a normal human experience, and for most people it will not impair their daily functioning. However, for some people, an anxiety disorder can develop where the symptoms are so severe that it impacts on functioning, behaviour and decision making. There are many types of anxiety and many causes, which could be psychiatric, medical or related to social stressors. It is imperative that the paramedic can understand the signs of anxiety and be able to differentiate between anxiety due to a mental health condition and anxiety due to an underlying medical event.

Pre-hospital, paramedics have a wide variety of skills and techniques they can use to help someone suffering with anxiety or a panic attack. The skills and knowledge to talk to people having an episode of acute distress are essential for paramedics, and these same skills can be transferable to working with consumers in a wide variety of scenarios and disorders.

REFERENCES

Ahrens, S., Wu, M., Furlan, A., et al., 2018. A central extended amygdala circuit that modulates anxiety. J. Neurosci. 38 (24), 5567–5583. doi:10.1523/JNEUROSCI.0705-18.2018.

American Psychiatric Association (APA), 2013. Diagnostic and Statistical Manual of Mental Disorders, fifth ed. DSM-5. APA, Washington, DC.

Australian Bureau of Statistics (ABS), 2008. 2007 National Survey of Mental Health and Wellbeing: summary of results. ABS cat. no. 4326.0. ABS, Canberra.

Australian Bureau of Statistics (ABS), 2018. National Health Survey: first results. Online. Available: https://www.abs.gov.au/ausstats/abs@.nsf/mf/4364.0.55.001. 17 May 2021.

Bandelow, B., Michaelis, S., 2015. Epidemiology of anxiety disorders in the 21st century. Dialogues Clin. Neurosci. 17 (3), 327–335. doi:10.31887/DCNS.2015.17.3/bbandelow.

Borkovec, T., Robinson, E., Pruzinsky, T., et al., 1983. Preliminary exploration of worry: some characteristics and processes. Behav. Res. Ther. 21 (1), 9–16. doi:10.1016/0005-7967(83)90121-3.

Bui, E., Pollack, M., Kinrys, G., 2016. The pharmacotherapy of anxiety disorders. In: Stern, T., Fava, M., Wilens, T., et al. (Eds.), Massachusetts General Hospital Comprehensive Clinical Psychiatry, second ed. Elsevier, Philadelphia.

Bunevicius, R., Velickiene, D., Prange, A., 2005. Mood and anxiety disorders in women with treated hyperthyroidism and opthalmopathy caused by Graves' disease. Gen. Hosp. Psychiatry 27 (2), 133–139.

Calkins, A., Bui, E., Taylor, C., et al., 2016. Anxiety disorders. In: Stern, T., Fava, M., Wilens, T., et al. (Eds.), Massachusetts General Hospital Comprehensive Clinical Psychiatry, second ed. Elsevier, Philadelphia, pp. 353–366.

Christian, M., Bryant, S., 2013. Antidepressants and antipsychotics. In: Adams, J.G., Barton, E.D., Collings, J.L. (Eds.), Emergency Medicine: Clinical Essentials, second ed. Elsevier, Philadelphia.

Coto-Lesmes, R., Fernandez-Rodriguez, C., Gonzalez-Fernandez, S., 2020. Acceptance and Commitment Therapy in group format for anxiety and depression, a systematic review. J. Affect. Disord. 263, 107–120.

Coyne, L., McHugh, L., Martinez, E., 2011. Acceptance and Commitment Therapy (ACT): advances and applications with children, adolescents and families. Child Adolesc. Psychiatr. Clin. N. Am. 20 (2), 379–399.

Dattilo, N., Goddard, A., 2021. Generalized anxiety disorder. In: Kellerman, R.D., Rakel, D.P. (Eds.), Conn's Current Therapy 2021. Elsevier, Philadelphia.

Dekel, S., Gilbertson, M., Orr, S., et al., 2016. Trauma and posttraumatic stress disorder. In: Stern, T., Fava, M., Wilens, T., et al. (Eds.), Massachusetts General Hospital Comprehensive Clinical Psychiatry, second ed. Elsevier, Philadelphia.

Duval, E., Javanbakht, A., Liberzon, I., 2015. Neural circuits in anxiety and stress disorders: a focused review. Ther. Clin. Risk Manag. 11, 115–126. doi:10.2147/TCRM. S48528.

Furmark, T., 2002. Social phobia: overview of community surveys. Acta Psychiatr. Scand. 105, 84–93.

Gerontoukou, E., Michaelidoy, S., Rekleiti, M., et al., 2015. Investigation of anxiety and depression in patients with chronic disease. Health Psychol. Res. 30 (2), 2123. doi:10.4081/hpr.2015.2123.

Glass, S., Pollack, M., Otto, M., et al., 2018. Anxious patients. In: Stern, T.A., Freudenreich, O., Smith, F.A., et al. (Eds.), Massachusetts General Hospital Handbook of General Hospital Psychiatry, seventh ed. Elsevier, Philadelphia.

Griffin, C., Kaye, A., Bueno, F., et al., 2013. Benzodiazepine pharmacology and central nervous system mediated effects. Ochsner J. 13 (2), 214–223.

Hall, J., Hall, M., 2021. Nervous regulation of the circulation and rapid control of arterial pressure. In: Hall, J., Hall, M. (Eds.), Guyton and Hall Textbook of Medical Physiology, fourteenth ed. Elsevier, Philadelphia, pp. 217–228.

Henden, J., 2017. Preventing Suicide: The Solution Focused Approach, second ed. Wiley Blackwell, Chichester, UK.

Kang, C., Harrison, B., 2013. Anxiety and panic disorders. In: Adams, J.G., Barton, E.D., Collings, J.L., et al. (Eds.), Emergency Medicine: Clinical Essentials, second ed. Saunders Elsevier, Philadelphia, pp. 1644–1647.

Katon, W., Lin, E., Kroenke, K., 2007. The association of depression and anxiety with medical symptom burden in patients with chronic medical illness. Gen. Hosp. Psychiatry 29 (2), 147–155.

Kim, L., Khanna, V., Yanez, V., et al., 2021. A comprehensive approach to psychosocial distress and anxiety in breast and gynecological cancers. In: Cristian, A. (Ed.), Breast Cancer and Gynecologic Cancer Rehabilitation. Elsevier, Amsterdam.

Krystal, J., D'Souza, D., Sanacora, G., et al., 2001. Advances in the pathophysiology and treatment of psychiatric disorders: implications for internal medicine. Med. Clin. N. Am. 85, 559–577.

Lyness, J., 2020. Psychiatric disorders in medical practice. In: Goldman, L., Schafer, A.I. (Eds.), Goldman-Cecil Medicine, twenty-sixth ed. Elsevier, Philadelphia, pp. 2305–2315.

Makovac, E., Meeten, F., Watson, D.R., et al., 2016. Alterations in amygdala-prefrontal functional connectivity account for excessive worry and autonomic dysregulation in generalized anxiety disorder. Biol. Psychiatry 80 (10), 786–795.

Martin, E., Ressler, K., Binder, E., et al., 2009. The neurobiology of anxiety disorders: brain, imaging, genetics, and psychoneuroendocrinology. Psychiatr. Clin. North Am. 32, 549–575.

Martinez, R.C., Ribeiro de Oliveira, A., Brandão, M.L., 2007. Serotonergic mechanisms in the basolateral amygdala differentially regulate the conditioned and unconditioned fear organized in the periaqueductal gray. Eur. Neuropsychopharmacol. 17 (11), 717–724.

Nasir, B.F., Toombs, M.R., Kondalsamy-Chennakesavan, S., et al., 2018. Common mental disorders among Indigenous people living in regional, remote and metropolitan Australia: a cross-sectional study. BMJ Open 8 (6), e020196.

Patel, A., Hurst, J., 2011. Extrapulmonary comorbidities in chronic obstructive pulmonary disease: state of the art. Expert Rev. Respir. Med. 5, 647–662.

Richerson, G., 2017. The autonomic nervous system. In: Boron, W.F., Boulpaep, E.L. (Eds.), Medical Physiology, third ed. Elsevier, Philadelphia, pp. 334–352.

Rosenstreich, G., (2013) LGBTI People: Mental Health and Suicide (revised second ed.). National LGBTI Health Alliance, Sydney.

Rubio, J., Olfson, M., Villegas, L., et al., 2013. Quality of life following remission of mental disorders: findings from the National Epidemiologic Survey on Alcohol and Related Conditions. J. Clin. Psychiatry 74, 445–450.

Sangkuhl, K., Klein, T., Altman, R., 2009. Selective serotonin reuptake inhibitors (SSRI) pathway. Pharmacogenet. Genomics 19 (11), 907–909. doi:10.1097/FPC. 0b013e32833132cb.

Smith, S.W., 2021. Solution Focused Interactions in Nursing: Growth and Change. Cambridge Scholars Publishing, Cambridge.

Spitzer, R., Kroenke, K., Williams, J., et al., 2006. A brief measure for assessing generalized anxiety disorder: the GAD-7. Arch. Intern. Med. 166, 1092–1097. doi:10.1001/archinte.166.10.1092.

Sprich, S., Olatunji, B., Reese, H., et al., 2016. Cognitive-behavioural therapy, behavioural therapy and cognitive therapy. In: Stern, T., Fava, M., Wilens, T., et al. (Eds.), Massachusetts General Hospital Comprehensive Clinical Psychiatry, second ed. Elsevier, Philadelphia.

Stein, M., Stein, D., 2008. Social anxiety disorder. Lancet 29 (371), 1115–1125. doi:10.1016/S0140-6736(08)60488-2.

Stewart, S., Lafleur, D., Doughterty, D., et al., 2016. Obsessive-compulsive disorder and obsessive-compulsive and related disorders. In: Stern, T., Fava, M., Wilens, T., et al. (Eds.), Massachusetts General Hospital Comprehensive Clinical Psychiatry, second ed. Elsevier, Philadelphia.

Testa, A., Giannuzzi, R., Daini, S., et al., 2013. Psychiatric emergencies (part III): psychiatric symptoms resulting from organic disease. Eur. Rev. Med. Pharmacol. Sci. 17, 86–89.

Twohig, M., Levin, M., 2017. Acceptance and commitment therapy as a treatment for anxiety and depression. Psychiatr. Clin. North Am. 40 (4), 751–770.

Vaughan, M., Khanna, S., Buelt, E., et al., 2020. Cognitive behavioral therapy for addiction. In: Johnson, B.A. (Ed.), Addiction Medicine: Science and Practice, second ed. Elsevier, Philadelphia.

Wynne, B., McHugh, L., Gao, W., et al., 2019. Acceptance and commitment therapy reduces psychological stress in patients with inflammatory bowel diseases. Gastroenterology 156 (4), 935–945.

Caring for a person with changes in mood ('affective' disorders)

Michael Keem and Cate Houen

LEARNING OUTCOMES

On completion of this chapter, you should be able to:

- understand the significance of mood and affect in health and functioning
- identify the signs and symptoms of an affective disorder
- complete and understand a biopsychosocial assessment of someone with a possible mood disorder, and consider causes of behavioural disturbance and dysregulated affect
- understand short- and long-term treatments for mood disorders.

INTRODUCTION

Every day, we experience and communicate anywhere from a cacophony to a harmony of feeling states, or emotions. They are both primitive and elegant, being able to be modified by any number of qualifiers or experiences to communicate entirely different canvases of feeling. Little separates an experience of fear from excitement, for example, in the absence of expectations that modify our perception of the experience. Emotions can enrich or command our lives. Occasionally they can overtake us, give us purpose – or overcome us completely.

But at what point does the natural ebb and flow of emotions become a disorder prompting treatment? The distinction between normal sadness and clinical depression, or bombastic confidence and mania, can be imprecise. Mood changes are considered abnormal when they are severe, pervasive and persistent, leading to suffering in life; be that functioning at work, school, within relationships, or in spirits, leading to distress and psychic pain.

MOOD VERSUS AFFECT

Mood reflects a person's subjective, longitudinal experience of feeling states that is elicited on history; and if abnormal, distressing or impairing, it may represent a symptom. **Affect** represents a transient manifestation of emotion influenced by this mood, and is a key component elicited on a mental state examination; namely, an objective assessment of expressed emotion that, if persistent, prolonged and not congruent with circumstance, may constitute a sign of illness. A person who glances at the ground, looks miserable in their facial expression, and is low in vocal volume and tone may appear downcast to the assessing clinician, demonstrating a low, depressed affect. How they state they feel overall within themselves, or their 'spirits', represents their mood.

The oft-cited adage that 'mood is to affect as climate is to the weather' captures this distinction. A tumultuous, depressing climate of mood can be manifested in more frequent overcast days, hailstorms of emotion and dampened spirits, but can be punctuated by sunny days. The observed, objective presence of sunny days of expressed affect does not invalidate a person's subjective self-assessment of a colder climate of mood; the distinction between the two is useful diagnostic data. Furthermore, several affects can be apparent at once, and over the course of an assessment.

Affect and mood are both described by their **quality**, **range** and **appropriateness**. Affect is also described by the degree of its **communication**.

Quality refers to how the elicited affect or mood would be described: for example, 'euthymic' (normal), upset, angry, cheerful, bright, euphoric, warm, curious, guilty, anxious, ashamed, suspicious, irritable, frustrated, perplexed, depressed or elevated.

Range can vary from normal, labile (rapidly shifting extremes of emotion, a common feature of mania or disinhibited states), restricted (reduced emotional response), flattened (heavy restriction; an awareness but lack of capacity to respond emotionally, as seen in depression), and blunted (emotional detachment; an inability to emotionally respond appropriately, due to diminished comprehension of the emotional significance of events, as seen in psychotic states with pronounced negative symptoms).

Appropriateness refers to whether the expressed affect or mood matches what is occurring or being said during an assessment. Affective disorders are associated with appropriate affects.

Mood should be explored and assessed on history taking. Its congruence with affect, determined by observing the mental state, should then be assessed as part of an evaluation of appropriateness. For example, a person who states they are depressed (subjectively; their mood), and have felt so for months, may smile warmly and laugh appropriately in response to comments; this incongruence between depressed mood and bright affect makes melancholic depression (see below) less likely, for example, and raises the index of suspicion for a stress reaction, chronic dysthymia, or another form of dysphoric state, such as an anxiety disorder.

Communication of affect is an imprecise but diagnostically useful observation of the degree to which feeling states are empathically experienced by the assessor. An elevated, euphoric person experiencing mania may induce similar feelings of energetic cheerfulness in the assessor during their assessment. In the presence of a depressed person, it is common to feel sad, despondent or even to experience their feelings of guilt, hopelessness and helplessness. Communication of affect is not only diagnostically valuable, but also essential to recognise when providing interventions and debriefing. For example, acknowledging a sense of hopelessness after talking to someone who is depressed can help prevent the development of therapeutic nihilism or burnout in the helping professional.

PERCEPTIONS

Assessment and treatment of mood disorders can be complicated by prevailing perceptions of mental illness, distress and wider societal acceptance of these. People with mental illness, or who are being assessed by medical professionals for distress or socially unacceptable behaviours, will often feel overwhelmed, frightened and judged. They are often subject to systematic discrimination or stigmatisation (Royal Australian and New Zealand College of Psychiatrists [RANZCP], 2016). The experience of stigma, including self-stigmatisation, may accompany embarrassing or acute disturbances in behaviour, hospitalisation, treatment or 'labelling' with a psychiatric diagnosis. Embarrassment about seeking or receiving treatment is a significant barrier to accessing care. Healthcare professionals are prone to a negative 'physician bias' about prognosis for recovery, and 'diagnostic overshadowing' (misinterpreting physical signs and symptoms for psychopathology), exacerbating wider social stigma towards mental illnesses and leading to disengagement of those with mental illness from their care, or from seeking care at all (Thornicroft et al., 2017).

People with mental illness may internalise this stigma, diminishing their self-determination, restricting their support network, limiting opportunities to participate in their community, and damaging their self-esteem. Misconceptions of illness signs and symptoms, such as amotivation as 'laziness' and 'self-pity', or lability as 'hysteria', fuel social isolation, leading to disconnection from support networks and services. Social withdrawal, self-stigmatisation, exclusion from community and social processes, and healthcare professionals' therapeutic nihilism can exacerbate distress, increase the burden on carers, and impede prompt diagnosis, the establishment of a therapeutic alliance, and recovery.

People affected by mental illness are among the most vulnerable and marginalised within our society. Affective disorders are notable for both stigmatisation of sufferers and, at times, counter-productive awareness campaigns. Depression is frequently categorised as a 'chemical imbalance'. However, only a minority of those presenting with depression – albeit a significant one – have a 'chemical imbalance' (a term that greatly oversimplifies the changes that occur in the brain) necessitating pharmacological, electroconvulsive or transcranial magnetic therapies. Feelings of sadness and normal grieving may be pathologised, leading to sufferers being diagnosed as 'sick' and receiving unnecessary biological treatments with the risk of developing side effects. 'Mood swings' are commonly equated to 'being bipolar'. Conversely, those with severe depressive symptomatology can feel stigmatised as lazy, reclusive, intentionally apathetic and 'not trying' to get better; and those with manic symptoms as erratic, 'silly', scatter-brained, aggressive, unpredictably violent, or humorous in the extent of their 'crazy antics'. Sensitivity and empathic curiosity can facilitate the establishment of rapport and an accurate history.

CASE STUDY

Charmaine

Charmaine is a 27-year-old graphic designer, who has been in a stable relationship for two years. Her partner called emergency services after she expressed a wish to 'throw myself from the stairs and end it all'. He reported to 000 that Charmaine has been depressed since her employer had lambasted her work a month ago after failing to obtain a key contract, and had threatened to terminate her employment. She recovered from a 'cough from a chest infection' the week after this, but otherwise has no past medical history of note, including no previous psychiatric diagnoses that he is aware of, and has no forensic history nor history of violence. Her only regular medication is the oral contraceptive pill, and her substance use history is notable only for an occasional glass of wine in social settings. On attendance at her home, paramedics find Charmaine sitting on the couch with her partner. She is overtly anxious, tearful, softly spoken and fidgety. At interview, after a lengthy introductory silence, she begins to exhaustively detail her frustration with her employer, and feelings of inadequacy and meaninglessness that had plagued her on several occasions in the past decade, but not in recent years since meeting her partner. She explains that her statement about throwing herself from the stairs was made in exasperation, not with intent, however tempting the thought of dying is. Charmaine has not slept for more than a few hours each night for the past fortnight. Her appetite is poor; she has lost 3 kg of weight in recent weeks. She reports poor concentration and has found it difficult to get through the working day, and thus has taken the past week off, feeling increasingly guilty for doing so. Her family history is notable for her mother's Graves' disease (a hypothyroid condition) and grandmother's diagnosis of bipolar affective disorder. She has always got on well with her family and has held the same job for the past five years. She reports no concerns about her health or safety beyond feeling overwhelmed, and has never been treated for depression or mania. Her mood is 'depressed' and 'horrible'; her symptoms do not fluctuate over the day.

Vital signs

- Glasgow Coma Scale: 15
- Respiratory rate: 22
- Heart rate: 72
- Blood pressure: 105/75
- Temperature: 36.3
- Blood sugar level: 4.8

On examination, Charmaine's vital signs are stable, she has no physical signs of hypothyroidism, and has no injuries. Mental state examination is notable for psychomotor agitation, soft volume of speech but normal rate and no latency, a dysphoric and miserable affect that is well-communicated, linear thought form with preserved thought stream, guilty and self-critical ideation with hopeless themes, no paranoid or mood-congruent delusional content, passive suicidal ideation with expression of a vague wish to die, orientation to time, place and person, and reasonable insight into her depressive symptoms. On further clarifying, Charmaine and her partner report that she has always been 'a bit of a worrier', prone to perfectionism and ruminating on 'little mistakes' at work. She appears distressed when discussing crisis numbers to call if suicidal thoughts were to resurface. Charmaine agrees to go to hospital for further assessment, but prefers for her partner to transport her. After discussion with your team leader, you agree to this.

Charmaine is admitted to the mental health inpatient unit. While her feeling of being overwhelmed abates a day into her inpatient admission, she confides that she has planned to drive her car off a bend on a nearby cliffside, and continues to present as restless, has a poor appetite, is vaguely angry at her employer, and distressed. Admission bloods, including thyroid function tests, were normal. While several neurovegetative symptoms remain present, her perfectionistic personality tendencies, clear precipitant stressor with her job, prominent symptoms of anxiety, and ability to extensively detail an accurate account of her recent stressors (signifying intact concentration) are more in keeping with a non-melancholic depression, with emergent melancholic signs, and no evidence of bipolarity. An antidepressant is prescribed and positive coping strategies imparted via the inpatient team. Eight days later, she feels 'much better' and, while somewhat apprehensive about facing the challenges off the ward, is prepared to do so and engage with a weekly community mental health team follow-up, including a course of cognitive behavioural therapy.

THE PREVALENCE OF DEPRESSION AND OTHER MOOD (AFFECTIVE) DISORDERS

Affective disorders are common. While variable between studies, depression is frequently cited as having a prevalence in Western populations of up to 10%, with a lifetime risk of up to 20% (Bromet et al., 2011). Bipolar affective disorder has a lifetime prevalence of 1% for type 1, and up to 5% including type 2, in which manic symptoms are less severe and do not necessitate hospitalisation.

Neuropsychiatric disorders have overall been estimated to comprise 10% of the total global burden to disability-adjusted life years, with unipolar affective disorders (i.e. depressive symptoms only) and bipolar affective disorder representing 29% and 5% of this, respectively (Whiteford et al., 2015). Unipolar affective disorders thus represent the fourth leading cause of disability worldwide.

Other estimates have calculated that mental illnesses account for 37% of the worldwide burden to disability-adjusted life years specifically due to non-communicable diseases (World Health Organization [WHO], 2011), representing a $2.5 trillion impact in 2010 and projected to reach $6 trillion in 2030 (Bloom et al., 2011). This represents the largest categorical contributor to the total costs of non-communicable diseases worldwide, outstripping cardiovascular disease, diabetes and cancer. Nearly two-thirds of the economic burden can be accounted for with indirect costs, such as psychosocial supports and unemployment.

RECOGNISING DEPRESSION AND BIPOLAR DISORDERS: DEFINITIONS, SIGNS AND SYMPTOMS
DEPRESSION

Broadly, depression is a severe, pervasive and persistent lowering of mood lasting at least two weeks, and is commonly described as unipolar or bipolar.

Unipolar depression can be further categorised under several different models. The most prevalent but reductionistic is the unitary model, found in the *Diagnostic and Statistical Manual of Mental Disorders (DSM-5)* of the American Psychiatric Association (2013), which posits that depression is a homogeneous syndrome that can be subclassified by severity (mild, moderate or severe) and specifiers (with melancholia or with psychotic features). This model is simple to apply, but is limited by its equally unitary approach to prognosis and treatment; a 'one size fits all' model of care, with scant regard to the factors that have led to the depression. Other models favour subcategorisation by the course of the illness, such as a seasonal affective disorder and postpartum depression, or the state of the illness, such as atypical and catatonic depressions. A clinically useful approach is to consider a unipolar depressive episode under one of two broad categories: **melancholic depression**, and **non-melancholic depression**, ascribing further descriptors to better characterise the illness and direct treatment. A careful assessment allows for the most effective treatment to be chosen first, minimising the patient's suffering and helping prevent recurrence. Prolonged illness or failure to achieve remission can lead to more frequent relapses and future treatment difficulties.

As depression overall represents a clinical syndrome, there are common **emotional features** that all subtypes share, and may or may not be present during a given depressive episode:

- anhedonia, the loss of interest in activities that usually provide pleasure, which includes:
  - anticipatory anhedonia, the expectation of finding no pleasure in ordinarily pleasurable activities, and
  - consummatory anhedonia, the inability to take pleasure from activities in the present
- a sensation of misery, despondency, pessimism, despair or an empty emotional vacuum
- hopelessness
- helplessness
- guilt, a feeling characterised by self-blame and remorse for the perceived wrongdoing (this differs from shame, frustration or self-criticism).

Suicidal and parasuicidal behaviours may also be present; their assessment and management are discussed separately.

Melancholic depression

Also referred to as 'biological' or 'endogenous' depression, melancholic depression is characterised by the presence of **neurovegetative features**:

- psychomotor disturbance, such as difficulty moving or a sensation of agitation and restlessness
- insomnia, including poor sleep quality and duration, and typically featuring early-morning waking
- anorexia (loss of appetite – not to be confused with 'anorexia nervosa') with resultant weight loss
- sensitivity to cold temperatures
- loss of libido
- constipation
- anergia (no energy) and fatigue
- impaired concentration, which should be qualified and distinguished from usual fluctuations in concentration – for example, an emergent inability to read books or pay attention to TV
- restricted and flattened affect, giving so-called 'mask-like faces'
- repetitive diurnal variation of these symptoms, which are classically worse in the morning.

More prevalent in melancholic depressions than non-melancholic are **psychic symptoms of depression**:

- pervasive social withdrawal, with attempts to help the patient socialise often proving counter-productive and potentially worsening their symptoms
- self-neglect, including with their appearance or their attention to activities of daily living
- self-devaluation, including demeaning, ashamed or accusatory thoughts about oneself

- depression and non-reactivity of mood; at its most extreme, this can constitute a total freezing of emotional experience
- psychomotor changes:
  - the more common sign is psychomotor retardation, in which the patient's movements are slowed and less prevalent; this is accompanied by speech changes, chiefly their response to questions being delayed and limited; decreased thought stream (slowing and poverty of thought); and restriction and flattening of affect
  - less common is psychomotor agitation, which may be present during brief periods in an otherwise psychomotor-retarded patient: this is characterised by excessive, agitated motor activity; other associated findings on mental state examination include speech or motor perseveration (seamlessly repetitive statements or goal-directed motor activities), stereotypies (spontaneous, purposeless motor activities), importuning (repeated questions that continue despite reassurance), repetition of preoccupations or themes, and an agitated affect.

Unlike non-melancholic depressive episodes, melancholic depression can be defined by genetic susceptibility, poor response to placebos and psychotherapy, greater response to ECT and antidepressants, and the presence of a gamut of neurovegetative and psychic symptoms. Those with high genetic susceptibility to developing depression may exhibit more neurovegetative features with a relatively less severe depressive episode.

Psychotic depression

Psychotic depression is considered to be a particularly severe form of melancholic depression, or a similar depressive subtype. It is most frequently characterised by the aforementioned psychic and neurovegetative symptoms of depression, together in the presence of mood-congruent psychotic symptoms: delusions of guilt, poverty, persecution, worthlessness, punishment, inadequacy and nihilism (belief that something does not exist, including oneself), which include 'Cotard' delusions (belief that one is already dead), and hallucinations, most commonly auditory. Pseudo-dementia, or cognitive impairment that has emerged in the context of a depressive episode, is common; obtaining collateral history of premorbid intellectual and cognitive functioning is crucial in assessment. While less common, mood-incongruent psychotic symptoms may also be apparent. In the absence of treatment, this condition is often complicated by catatonia (stupor, mutism). Unlike non-psychotic, melancholic depressions, psychotic depression frequently does not have diurnal variation in symptoms, including mood.

There are significant risks associated with psychotic depression due to the level of distress the patient experiences, together with the likely presence of mood-congruent beliefs that they act upon, and cognitive impairment. For example, a patient may believe that their bills have not been paid for years, they will have nowhere to live, they have let their loved ones down and have 'heard' them say this, they are consequently being prosecuted by authorities, that life is not worth living, and that their food is poisoned. Social withdrawal, self-neglect, starvation, dehydration and misadventure may arise. Psychotic symptoms present during a depressive episode are accordingly dangerous and always warrant transport to hospital for inpatient treatment.

Non-melancholic depression

Non-melancholic, or characterological, depressive episodes are the most common form of depression, yet are frequently confused with the far less common melancholic depressive illnesses. While some consider them a category of residual cases that do not meet criteria for a melancholic or bipolar depression, several features raise the clinical index of suspicion for a non-melancholic depression:

- The patient identifies that their depressive episode was triggered by an environmental or psychosocial factor that appears, to the examiner, relatively minor; patients will often attach a great deal of symbolic value to these triggering factors.
- Chronic helplessness or hopelessness that is marked by anger, rather than depression of mood – for example, a patient expressing (via speech content or affect) anger at having been let down by their loved ones after a stressful incident several years prior, citing this as a factor for why they feel depressed.
- A high degree of symptom fluctuance.
- Variation of symptoms with social context – for example, a patient being depressed in mood during the week and reporting significant difficulties finding energy to address the day, but fulfilling social commitments they find relaxing or enjoyable on the weekend; or a patient reporting depressed mood in context of being in a particular environment only, like the family home.
- A history of a personality disorder or traits thereof.
- Premorbid personality is notable for features consistent with dysfunctional personality traits – important to corroborate on collateral history.
- There has been a long period of reportedly stable illness – for example, a patient who states they have experienced the same, depressed mood for years. Caution should be exercised, however, given the possibility of a 'double depression' (melancholic superimposed on non-melancholic presentation) or of treatment-resistant melancholic depression.

Non-melancholic depressions are typically subcategorised based on the most significant identifiable precipitant.

Melancholic and non-melancholic depressions not only have different features, but also significantly different treatment priorities. Careful observation of these features at the scene can lead to more targeted and efficient history taking, collection of collateral information and provision of pre-hospital supports. Non-melancholic presentations may benefit from simple problem solving, brief counselling and lifestyle advice at the scene, for example, whereas melancholic presentations will often warrant transport to hospital. The key differences between melancholic and

Table 10.1 Comparison Between Melancholic and Non-melancholic Depression

Melancholic Depression	Non-melancholic Depression
Pervasive symptoms	Symptoms vary, particularly with social context
Consistent pattern of symptom intensity over the day, usually worse in the mornings	Symptoms significantly fluctuate with social and environmental stressors
Insomnia with early-morning waking	Insomnia from ruminating, and feeling overwhelmed and anxious
Many neurovegetative symptoms	Limited number of neurovegetative symptoms
Pervasive psychomotor changes on MSE	No consistent or pervasive psychomotor changes
Pervasive social withdrawal	Fluctuant or intact social engagement
Restricted, low affect on MSE	Miserable affect, often with anger at others
'Frozen', depressed mood more likely; minimal reactivity	Dysphoric, despondent mood more likely; some reactivity common
Can have delusions	No delusions
Can have hallucinations	No hallucinations; can have pseudo-hallucinations
Can develop catatonia	No pervasive catatonic symptoms
Objective difficulty concentrating – poor attention, cognitive slowing, 'pseudo-dementia'	Subjective difficulty concentrating; ruminating on negative thoughts; cognition intact on MSE
'Biological' causes	'Psychological' or 'social' causes
Prior (or family history of) episodes that responded well to antidepressants or ECT	History of personality vulnerabilities, crisis presentations, or 'always' feeling depressed over several months or years
Responds well to antidepressants or ECT	Responds well to social interventions and psychotherapy

non-melancholic depression to ascertain in the pre-hospital setting are outlined in Table 10.1.

Dysthymia

Under *DSM-5* criteria, dysthymia represents a mild depressive illness lasting longer than two years in duration. It typically emerges due to underlying personality or temperamental vulnerabilities and can be exacerbated by psychosocial stressors.

Reactive depression (adjustment disorder with depressed mood)

A reactive depression represents a depressive episode emerging in response to a notable stressor lasting for longer than two weeks. While primarily emerging reactively to a stressor, pervasive low mood rarely persists beyond two weeks without an underlying personality vulnerability. It is rarely necessary to hospitalise a person with this kind of depressive reaction, but helping to identify and deal with the underlying stressor is useful.

In summary

The distinction between a melancholic (endogenous) and non-melancholic (characterological) depression can be distilled to careful evaluation of four key factors.

Favouring melancholic depression are the presence of:

- more psychic symptoms
- constant or increasing neurovegetative symptoms.

Favouring non-melancholic or characterological depression are the presence of:

- a personality disposition
- environmental triggers which may appear relatively insignificant to the assessor.

Favouring 'double depression' is the presence of:

- all of the above.

Aim to treat the melancholic depression first.

BIPOLAR AFFECTIVE DISORDER

Bipolar affective disorder (BPAD) is an illness marked by recurrent, debilitating episodes of affective extremes – at 'both poles' of mania and depression. Under DSM and International Classification of Diseases (ICD) diagnostic criteria, a diagnosis of BPAD requires the presence of at least one major depressive episode and one manic (type 1) or hypomanic (type 2) episode. In practice, BPAD is typically diagnosed after assessment of a manic or hypomanic state. Identifying manic and depressive symptoms (detailed below) is an essential component of assessment. However, the use of symptom checklists or leading questions can often lead to manic symptoms being erroneously elicited on history. For example, impulsive purchasing of unnecessary items, insomnia, agitation and racing thoughts may be present in someone presenting in crisis who is distressed and overwhelmed, rather than manic.

The 'affect storms' and chronic emotional instability of a diffused, borderline personality structure (typically from cluster B – see Chapter 16) are commonly confused with hypomanic and manic states. A person with a severe personality disorder presenting in crisis with labile affect and expansive mood, and a person presenting with mania (bipolar type 1), can often be differentiated by the breakdown of reality testing present in the latter. The presence of psychotic symptoms such as paranoid (including persecutory, referential and grandiose) delusions and hallucinations, the extent of disorganised and socially inappropriate behaviour that proves difficult or impossible to control by others, lack of insight into their symptoms, or hallmark features on mental state examination, such as flight of ideas, indicate deteriorated capacity to reality test, suggesting that these symptoms and signs are due to mania. This distinction is less apparent in a hypomanic state, where reality testing may be intact, or psychotic symptoms less pronounced or absent. Bipolar type 2 is thus commonly confused with severe personality disorders or acute situational crises, particularly borderline personality disorder. Careful evaluation of the patient's long-term relationships with others can prove invaluable in making this differentiation:

- Those with BPAD only, regardless of type, will likely have a healthy degree of social and occupational functioning between manic, hypomanic or depressive episodes. Their mood, affect and behaviour will noticeably change during an episode of illness compared with their baseline as identified via collateral history.
- Those with BPAD type 1 will likely experience delusions, perceptual disturbances and a loss of reality testing while manic, but not pervasively or between episodes.
- Those with a severe personality disorder only, will likely have an absence of affective stability – that is, they will likely have no consistent periods of non-labile or stable affect – together with an absence of mature relations with others, and instability in work record, romantic relationships and self-assessed identity. Collateral history will likely indicate a past pattern of similar behaviour and pervasively unstable affect.
- Note, however, that people may have both a personality disorder and a bipolar affective disorder.

Thus, the easiest means of differentiating a manic or hypomanic state from other causes of affective instability is to establish whether the patient has exhibited out-of-character behaviour over the course of several days compared with their usual, or premorbid, behaviour.

This differentiation is important diagnostically, therapeutically and prognostically. An episode of BPAD – depressive, manic or mixed – that is left untreated, is prolonged, or does not reach full remission, which may increase the chance of recurrence and treatment resistance: the so-called 'kindling hypothesis'. Mood stabilisers will constitute the hallmark intervention in someone with bipolar affective disorder, whereas psychosocial and psychotherapeutic interventions are the key treatments for a personality disorder or crisis. Pre-hospital interventions also substantially differ, as detailed later in this chapter.

Bipolar affective disorder, type 1 (bipolar 1 disorder)

This subtype of BPAD is defined in practice by the presence of a manic syndrome on clinical assessment. Manic features typically arise over the course of a few days, often in response to common triggers such as substance use (alcohol being common), jet lag, increased psychosocial stress and poor sleep. Manic signs on mental state examination include the following:

- hyperactivity
- pressured speech: speech seemingly marked by a sense of urgency, with few natural pauses, that is difficult to interrupt
- speech that can become loud, incomprehensible, rapid and expansive in tone
- flight of ideas: increased volume and rate of thought stream with marked tangentiality; that is, an accelerated production of thoughts that rapidly jump and continuously flow into each other with potentially little coherent connection (this is analogous to a surging river, with an accelerating current while the river breaks from the banks constantly to form newer and newer rivers); patients with insight into this will often describe 'racing thoughts' that they cannot stop
- irritability, commonly observed when the manic patient feels challenged
- euphoric affect and mood: highly energetic, cheerful and exuberant affect and mood that is often well-communicated, thus proving somewhat infectious
- elevated, expansive affect and mood: unrestrained and increased intensity of affect and mood
- attentional difficulties evident on cognitive examination
- dysexecutive features on cognitive examination, particularly disinhibition and impulsivity
- impaired judgement.

Psychotic features can also feature on mental state examination in manic presentations:

- grandiosity: a belief of having special significance, abilities, talents, powers or importance
- other forms of delusional thinking, typically mood-congruent
- hallucinations
- a loss of reality testing of their impairments, and thus reduced insight.

Other symptoms of mania include:

- decreased need for sleep, often quite markedly
- functional impairment: difficulties with social, educational, community or occupational obligations
- odd, driven behaviours that result from the constellation of disinhibition, impulsivity, loss of reality testing, flight of ideas, grandiosity and hyperactivity, commonly including:
  - reckless driving (check for a recent history of speeding and dangerous driving)
  - sexual disinhibition
  - excessive spending, including on unneeded items or services and excessive gambling
  - poor, impulsive social and business decisions, often in pursuit of a grandiose goal.

Bipolar affective disorder, type 2 (bipolar 2 disorder)

This BPAD subtype is defined by the presence of both hypomanic and depressive episodes across the life span. 'Hypomania', literally 'under mania', can be conceptualised as mania with two key distinctions: the absence of psychotic symptoms during the episode; and minimal functional impairment despite the presence of affective symptoms, with fulfilment of activities of daily living, occupational duties and social obligations being possible.

Therefore, elevation of mood being severe enough to warrant hospitalisation would, by definition, constitute a manic symptom of BPAD type 1.

Note that hypomanic episodes can also occur in BPAD type 1. Therefore, a diagnosis of BPAD type 2 can only be made in the historical absence of functional impairment or psychotic symptoms during episodes of elevated mood.

Bipolar affective disorder, mixed states

The definition of a 'mixed state' – namely an experience in which both manic and depressive symptoms are simultaneously present – was changed between the fourth and fifth versions of the *DSM*. Previously, a mixed state required diagnostic criteria for both a manic and depressive episode to be consistently met for over a week, limiting the diagnosis to a subgroup of patients with BPAD type 1 who presented with depressed mood yet manic symptoms on mental state examination. Patients with this presentation are at increased risk of suicide and distress.

A mixed state can now be diagnosed with only three symptoms of the 'opposite pole' present on mental state, including those with 'agitated depression' and people with mania with some depressive thought content. People with agitated depression may need treatment with a mood stabiliser and an antipsychotic, and require close follow-up.

CYCLOTHYMIA

This syndrome is defined by mild, episodic mood swings, occurring independently of experiences that may increase or decrease mood, and that do not meet the diagnostic criteria for major depression or hypomania.

ORGANIC MANIA

Manic symptoms may be evident due to an underlying comorbidity or treatment, described below during the discussion on physical comorbidities. This includes neurological and cerebrovascular diseases, several common medications (e.g. prednisolone), substance intoxication, and hyperactive or mixed delirium. Treatment of the precipitating cause or revision of the causative medication are the staples of management.

CAUSES OF MOOD (AFFECTIVE) DISORDERS

The aetiology of an affective disorder is often multifactorial across the biopsychosocial spectrum. However, some generalisations can be made:

- melancholic depression, including psychotic depression, and bipolar affective disorder typically have greater biological contributing factors, and may or may not involve key psychosocial precipitants, whereas
- non-melancholic depression typically has greater psychosocial contributing factors.

BIOLOGICAL

There is no unifying neurobiological cause for melancholic depression or BPAD, given both diagnoses represent clinical syndromes and likely reflect a variety of heterogeneous yet similar pathological conditions. However, several underlying neurobiological factors have been implicated in affective disorders, particularly those that disrupt neural connectivity and communication between brain regions.

Underlying polymorphic genetic vulnerabilities can predispose people to melancholic depression and BPAD. They are thus more common in those with a family history of these conditions. Some genes have been implicated in certain temperaments and thus potential personality vulnerabilities (including for non-melancholic depression).

The monoamine hypothesis of depression underpins the oft-cited 'chemical imbalance' view of depression: that a deficiency in monoamines active in the limbic regions of the brain responsible for mood and cognition, such as dopamine or the catecholamines serotonin and norepinephrine, induces a depressive state; and treatments that regulate their expression or activity in the brain thus reverse the neurotransmitter imbalance and consequent depression. This hypothesis has been recognised as a gross oversimplification in recent years. It has been demonstrated that complex and interrelated changes in a variety of hormones, neurotransmitters and immunological factors, determined by both genetic and environmental influences, are involved in the pathology of mood disorders. Medications and other physical and psychological treatments for mood disorders can influence these factors, helping to restore normality if treatment is successful.

Acute episodes of melancholic depression and mania can be precipitated by factors influencing neuronal activity, including poor sleep, substance use, illnesses triggering an inflammatory response and medications.

PSYCHOSOCIAL

Depressive and manic episodes are often preceded by a key stressor, although this is not always the case with melancholic depression or BPAD. The nature, severity and personal significance of a given stressor heavily determines its impact.

PSYCHOLOGICAL

The personal significance of a given stressor varies with personality – our individual pattern of feeling, thinking and consequently behaving, determined by the interplay of temperament (genetic) and experience (upbringing). Some personality types predispose to developing depression, particularly histrionic, borderline, narcissistic, obsessive, perfectionistic, dependent and anxious-avoidant.

Depression has been conceptualised as an overreaction to loss in those sensitised by a vulnerability stemming from early childhood (Klein, 1935). Adverse childhood events and disruptions to healthy parental bonds can result in an enduring sense of loss that may be unconsciously relived, or exacerbated, by additional perceived losses later in life. Ambivalent feelings towards an object of this loss, such as a neglectful parent, can lead to resentment; this anger can lead to guilt, particularly if unacknowledged, reducing self-esteem or ultimately manifesting as suicidality. Parental abuse and/or neglect also lead to feelings of unworthiness, shame and self-loathing, which can be manifest in adulthood as a chronic vulnerability to depression. People with this kind of vulnerability may seek relief in recreational drugs, sexual promiscuity or other 'exciting' activities aimed at compensating for their negative feelings. Sometimes these can imitate the recklessness and compulsive overactivity of mania, but, unlike in mania, are not sustained for prolonged periods of time.

SOCIAL

Stressful experiences can be disruptive, painful, confusing, strip people of their sense of agency and meaning, cause emotional turbulence, and overwhelm their capacity to cope. These experiences can range from significant trauma to otherwise positive events, such as marriage, the birth of a child, relocating home or another major life decision that involves uncertainty and change. A paucity of social supports erodes resilience and removes a key protective factor, increasing the risk of developing depression, mania, parasuicidal behaviours and suicidal gestures.

Given that the impact of most social circumstances is determined by a person's psychological makeup and circumstances, it is difficult to detail a comprehensive list of social precipitants of mood disturbance. However, some common examples include:

- close, intimate or romantic relationship difficulties
- bereavement
- occupational difficulties – job loss, being bullied or overwhelmed at work
- trauma – sexual, physical, emotional, financial, social or incurred in perceived life-threatening situations
- other forms of abuse and threatened danger within close relationships
- experiences involving a loss of control, promoting 'learned helplessness'

- familial stressors
- isolation
- a chaotic living situation.

Social precipitants of mood disturbance are often volunteered by the patient with use of open questions, establishment of rapport and the assessor listening with the intent to understand.

SPECIFIC ASSESSMENT AND EXPLORING DIFFERENTIAL CLINICAL FORMULATIONS
ASSESSMENT

Assessment of mood disorders is complicated by their inherent nature; they impair the ability of patients to regulate their mood, therefore limiting their ability to relate or connect with others. Definitive diagnosis is further fraught in the pre-hospital setting as a multitude of differential diagnoses and stressors can precipitate mood disturbance. Thus, assessment of a person presenting with mood or affective disturbance follows that of general assessment principles – refer to Chapter 5 for further details – and comprises:

- history of presenting complaint
  - characterising the reason for the call-out and the major symptoms
- background history:
  - psychiatric, medical, medication, substance use, forensic, social, personal
  - assessment of neurovegetative features (sleep, appetite and weight, energy, motivation, or libido changes)
  - any previous or current treatments
  - support networks (social and professional)
- mental state examination
  - assessing for the features listed earlier in this chapter
- physical examination
  - particularly important in helping establish comorbidities and physical complications requiring treatment, or precipitants to the change in mood
  - vital signs should always be collected and may suggest underlying physical comorbidities triggering a mood disturbance, substance intoxication, or physical compromise secondary to a mood disorder – for example, tachycardia, hypotension and hypothermia in someone who has had poor oral intake secondary to mood-congruent delusions in psychotic depression (see below for common physical comorbidities and precipitants that may inform a targeted examination)
- collateral history (if available)
  - helpful in determining the longitudinal course of a person's illness, the integrity of their interpersonal functioning, the occupational and social

impacts of their illness, and their symptomatology, especially if there is a breakdown of their reality-testing (as occurs in psychotic depression and manic states)

- establishing the severity of the illness
  - how does the illness or symptoms impact on the person's functioning?
  - how does the illness or symptoms impact on the person's risk factors?
- establishing the presence of comorbidities
  - which, as a rule, are present in those presenting with affective disorders (see below)
- evaluating safety and risk factors
  - including dynamic and static risks of harm to self and others, deterioration in mental state, and deterioration in physical health, as well as protective factors.

In the pre-hospital setting, gathering as much of these data as possible allows for more informed and accurate decision making.

Complicating assessment are the common comorbidities of anxiety and substance use disorders, personality vulnerabilities, and other precipitant medical conditions (RANZCP, 2015). Low mood and suicidal ideation are frequently present in those presenting with a psychotic illness, eating disorder, somatoform disorder or cognitive impairment, and may represent an overlying mood disorder. Substance abuse as a primary condition or means of self-medication is often missed on assessment, and should be carefully screened for to maximise the chances of recovery, help address maladaptive coping strategies and rule out common mimics of an affective syndrome: substance withdrawal, substance intoxication and medication side effects.

Physical comorbidities are common and complicate recovery from both the mood disorder and the comorbid physical illness. Affective disorders may arise secondary to physical illnesses – 'organic depression' and 'organic mania' – or their treatments. Organic mood disorders may arise in context of neuropsychiatric and cognitive disorders, including cerebrovascular disease, dementing processes, other neurodegenerative conditions such as Creutzfeldt-Jakob disease and Parkinson's disease, genetic diseases such as Huntington's disease or Niemann-Pick disease, epilepsy, acquired brain injury, space-occupying lesions (such as neoplasms), multiple sclerosis, cerebral lupus, encephalitis, HIV encephalopathy, or tertiary syphilis. Endocrine disorders often have an affective component – for example, emotional lability and irritability in hyperthyroidism, or depressive symptoms in hypothyroidism, Cushing's disease, Addison's disease, or steroid therapy prescribed to treat these. Medications may lead to the development of mood symptoms, with common culprits being antihypertensives such as beta-blockers, chemotherapeutic agents, antibiotics and steroid (hormonal) treatments, including the oral contraceptive pill.

Furthermore, comorbidities – whether psychiatric or physical – carry a poorer prognosis, particularly if unaddressed. They can exacerbate and prolong an episode of an affective illness, impede optimal treatment, limit recovery, worsen disability, increase risks and lead to higher relapse rates.

For the paramedic, all patients should be screened for contributing or underlying physical illness. All medications should be noted including a record of how the person engages with their medication regimen.

EVALUATION

Evaluating a patient to determine their primary diagnosis and comorbidity is difficult, particularly when several symptoms overlap within syndromes, or may represent symptoms of two or more concurrent illnesses – for example, a 'double depression' of a major depressive episode superimposed on chronic dysthymia. One suggested clinical approach involves careful evaluation of several key factors in a patient's presentation when exploring differential diagnoses for mood disturbances and affective disorders (Kernberg & Yeomans, 2013). A modified version for the pre-hospital setting is as follows.

On arrival at the scene, ascertain each of the following in sequence:

1. Is this an emergency?
   - See below, 'dealing with emergencies', for more details.
   - If this is an emergency: liaise with an emergency department, mental health services, or both, as described below, while initiating emergency interventions.
   - Some patients with frequent emergency presentations may have an enhanced treatment plan or equivalent, which local mental health clinicians can then use to outline a holistic approach to the patient's management.
   - If this is not an emergency: note why this is the case, as this will be helpful on subsequent assessments and reviews.
   - While commencing emergency interventions, continue as much of the below assessment as is feasible to help clarify the differential diagnosis and stratify the risks apparent in a patient's presentation, even if this is limited to simple and brief points for clarification at the emergency department later.
2. What depressive signs and symptoms does the patient demonstrate?
   - Reference to Table 10.1, which differentiates features of melancholic from non-melancholic depressions, may prove helpful.
3. The presence and nature of suicidality, and other self-destructive behaviours and thoughts.
   - Helps to understand risk, and may help distinguish between an affective disorder and a crisis. See Chapters 11 and 12 for further details.
4. The presence of manic or hypomanic episodes either presently or historically.
   - Helps distinguish a bipolar from a unipolar illness.
   - A breakdown of reality-testing – leading to a lack of insight into one's symptoms and impairments – in the presence of a mood disturbance warrants further assessment.

- Refer to the brief descriptions of mental state examination findings and symptoms of BPAD subtypes detailed above for key features to be aware of, and assess if there is clinical suspicion of manic symptoms.

5. What are the patient's cognitive functions?
   - Important in evaluating for neurovegetative symptoms of melancholic depression; elucidating a patient's testamentary capacity, or their ability to explain their story, thoughts, concerns, feelings and circumstances; and screening for comorbid cognitive impairment (e.g. dementia), delirium or drug-affected states.
   - Cognition can be broken into several domains. While a detailed assessment of these is not feasible in the pre-hospital setting, any impairment in these cognitive domains should be noted.
   - Attention: does the patient demonstrate a poor ability to concentrate on your assessment, or appear easily distracted? Attentional difficulties may indicate underlying formal thought disorder, such as flight of ideas in mania, objective concentration impairment and the so-called 'pseudodementia' of melancholic depression, or reflect that the patient is consumed by ruminations in non-melancholic depression.
   - Visuoconstruction refers to spatial abilities and planning and coordination of these with fine motor skills. This domain is not typically impaired in non-melancholic depression. Can the patient draw a clockface with a given time (a useful screen for delirium) or perform simple arithmetic? Do they write in a childlike, regressed manner with inconsistent spelling and grammar compared with their baseline (common in manic presentations)? Impairments signify likely difficulty with other visuoconstructional tasks such as driving, a key factor in stratifying risk.
   - Memory: do they recall recent events or autobiographical details? Memory impairment is not consistent with a non-melancholic depressive presentation unless the patient has comorbidities or otherwise presents in crisis. Do they confabulate (suggestive of Wernicke-Korsakoff syndrome in alcohol use disorder, or dementia)?
   - Executive function: do they appear disinhibited, impulsive and difficult to redirect, suggestive of mania, or are they acting in a manner uncharacteristic of their usual behaviour?
   - Language impairments are uncommon in mood disorders unless the patient presents with the 'pseudodementia' of a melancholic depression, demonstrates formal thought disorder (in manic or melancholic depressive episodes), or otherwise is suffering from a comorbidity – such as substance intoxication or delirium.

6. Is there any substance abuse, or any evidence of substance (including alcohol) intoxication or withdrawal?
   - This is important to assess given the high rates of comorbidity, poorer prognosis if left unaddressed, and possible presence of a drug-induced state, intoxication or withdrawal accounting for the patient's mood symptoms.

The following are difficult to comprehensively assess in the pre-hospital setting, but important details can be collected, particularly from collateral history, and are invaluable in formulating both an immediate and long-term recovery plan for a patient – refer to the below sections on pre-hospital and longer-term treatments:

7. The quality of a person's interpersonal relations.
    - This may be difficult to assess in a pre-hospital setting, but remains important in characterising underlying challenges in connecting with or understanding self-identity and personality vulnerabilities, in turn helping distinguish characterological depression from melancholic depressive states.
8. Their personality characteristics.
    - Evaluation of personality characteristics will be limited in a pre-hospital setting and (if undiagnosed or unavailable in a patient's history) requires longitudinal assessment. Nonetheless, it is an important component of a comprehensive psychiatric assessment and helps target therapy by addressing underlying, predisposing personality contributions to affective disturbances.
    - It may be helpful to enquire how they find their interactions with others, how they perceive their environment, what is significant to them in the way they act and react to life around them, and if and how this has changed over time. This may establish trends that will help inform further care.
9. The presence and degree of antisocial traits.
    - These carry poor long-term prognosis and increase the risk of deliberate self-harm, suicidal and homicidal gestures.

CRITICAL REFLECTION

In reference to the case study of Charmaine:
- Identify any possible factors for an organic cause of her low mood.
- Identify any possible personality factors as contributing to her low mood.
- What further information would you need to know in order to differentiate between organic and personality factors? Where (or who) would you get this information from?
- Complete a risk assessment, identifying both risk and safety factors as well as (potential) protective factors.

PRE-HOSPITAL APPROACHES TO TREATMENT AND CARE
BE PRESENT, LISTEN, COMMUNICATE AND EDUCATE

As a general guide to crisis intervention and pre-hospital care of someone presenting with features of a mood disorder:

- be present – avoid multitasking and distractions
- listen – with the intent to understand, not to reply
- check their safety – including an assessment of risk and suicidality as indicated (detailed above); those who have presented to healthcare professionals in crisis

previously may have a 'safety plan', which the patient should be encouraged to follow

- complete an assessment (detailed above) – starting with open-ended questions, and avoiding use of potentially patronising remarks (such as requests for the patient to 'calm down') and judgmental questions
- acknowledge their feelings/distress/emotions
- make a plan (with them, if possible) – identify if transport to an emergency department is indicated, find mutual goals, and otherwise negotiate to find common ground; solution-focused brief therapy (SFBT), detailed below, can be used at the scene to help a patient problem solve
- explain what is happening – provide psychoeducation, if feasible, and communicate the next steps with them
- offer further support services and alternative care pathways, if suitable, to them and their loved ones (detailed below).

Good interviewing technique involves adopting an empathic approach of authenticity, curiosity, warmth and consistency. These traits may be evident through simple measures such as gentle encouragement of the patient to talk, providing (true) hope, courtesy, sensitivity and being present with the patient. While it can be anxiety-inducing on the assessor's part, it may be necessary to pause and allow extra time for a depressed and psychomotor-retarded patient to reply. Silence can be therapeutic; it allows the patient space to express their thoughts and feelings without fear of foreclosure. Similarly, while it can feel impolite, it is often necessary to interrupt a manic patient to direct the assessment and help them stay on topic – and potentially diagnostic, should they prove difficult to interrupt due to pressure of speech. Interruptions should be made with tact and warmth. Many people experiencing mania will not take offence at interruptions due to their euphoria, while those with underlying irritability will likely be redirectable from expressions of anger due to their underlying thought disorder.

Note, however, that people who are particularly unwell with a melancholic depressive or manic state are likely to experience some distortion in reality-testing of their symptoms. They may not be able to recognise their symptoms as abnormal, their thoughts as non-reality-based, or even that they are unwell. Impaired insight into their condition is thus likely to lead to poorer judgment, increasing the rationale for inpatient assessment and treatment. Those with impaired insight and judgment may not agree to assessment or treatment, and instead may appear to lack capacity to understand the severity or significance of their signs and symptoms. There may also be reasonable suspicion that their or others' health would deteriorate without treatment, potentiating assessment under the relevant Mental Health Act. Psychotic symptoms may emerge in severe depressive states (psychotic depression) or manic states (BPAD type 1) and warrant urgent inpatient treatment. Patients who cannot guarantee their safety may also require transport to an emergency department for further assessment.

HOLISTIC LIFESTYLE ADVICE AND POSITIVE COPING STRATEGIES

It may be prudent to provide simple interventions, such as: providing healthy life-style advice pertaining to diet, exercise, activity and social engagement; providing sleep hygiene advice; advising them to journal or keep a mood diary; encouraging them to reach out to their familial and wider social supports; brainstorming and providing the patient with a list of online, phone, crisis or NGO supports (see the resources section at the end of this chapter), stepping through when and how the patient will contact these supports, and what they may say; safety planning; and encouraging positive coping strategies, such as mindfulness, relaxation techniques, and deep breathing techniques. Risk of misadventure should be accounted for; for example, someone with manic symptoms should be encouraged not to drive and to keep credit cards and social media login details in the care of a loved one until further medical assessment.

DEALING WITH EMERGENCIES

An emergency is a life-threatening or imminently harmful situation requiring an immediate response to protect the health of a patient or others. It is not the same as a crisis, when a stressor overwhelms a person's capacity to cope; note that a crisis may, but not necessarily, result in an emergency. Likewise, suicidal and deliberate self-harming behaviours constitute a psychiatric emergency, but may not warrant transport to hospital if the assessed risks are low, a reasonable outpatient follow-up plan is in place, and the patient consents to this. Mental health emergency or out-patient crisis teams may be better equipped to implement these follow-up plans and should be contacted if doubt about the degree of risk remains. Suicidal, manic and psychotic patients may superficially agree to treatment, but if there are any doubts about their safety, caution should be exercised, and the patient transported to hospital. The use of the relevant Mental Health Act and rationale for its use should be provided, but the least restrictive approach to care and treatment should always be attempted first (see Chapter 2).

The priority during an emergency is guaranteeing the safety of the patient and others, including bystanders. A patient or environment should only be approached when and if it is safe to do so. This may involve collating collateral information to determine if there is any risk of aggression or history of violence. Impulsivity and agitation, as are typical of mania, may underscore immediate risks of harm to self or others; whereas a risk of harm to others is significantly less common in depressive episodes. Should risks of physical harm be posed to the patient, attending clinicians or others that cannot be readily mitigated, further supports should be made available, such as police presence. Support from community mental health clinicians may also be available. Multiple clinicians should be present, but be cautious about creating confusion or overstimulating the person. Assessment should be conducted in a calm, respectful manner, in as private a setting as is feasible, and as comprehensively as is practicable. In the event of a suicide attempt for example, initial history taking and examination will likely be brief. Significant comorbidities should be screened for, such as substance intoxication or delirium, by collecting vital signs, assessing gross neurological status, and performing a brief cognitive screen, including orientation to time, place and person.

Medication may be indicated in the acute pre-hospital setting in helping relieve a patient's distress or mitigate risks of harm sufficiently to facilitate transport. This is more likely to be indicated when the patient is agitated due to a psychotic state, such as psychotic depression or mania, or is otherwise demonstrating a marked degree of impulsivity or disorientation. Sedative and anxiolytic medication should be used sparingly or not at all if these risks are not present. Benzodiazepines, such as oral diazepam, intramuscular lorazepam and intravenous midazolam are common pre-hospital choices. Medications should be administered in the lowest possible dose to relieve distress but not to sedate, as further assessment will be required by subsequent clinicians. Physical restraint can be utilised if prominent risks due to patient agitation are present, but it is potentially traumatising and often risky, and therefore should be avoided where possible. Police transport of patients to hospital is another measure that can be utilised as a last resort to manage acute risks of physical harm.

CRITICAL REFLECTION

In relation to the case of Charmaine:
- If Charmaine did not want to go to hospital, what other information would you require in order to consider leaving her at home?
- What risk mitigation strategies could be put into place (by you or by others) to support leaving her at home?

BIOPSYCHOSOCIAL APPROACHES TO LONGER-TERM CARE

The Royal Australian and New Zealand College of Psychiatrists guidelines on the treatment of mood disorders are a useful reference; a link is provided at the end of the chapter.

PSYCHOLOGICAL

Various psychological therapies are available in the management of mood disorders and are first-line for treatment of non-melancholic depression. They are particularly efficacious in addressing underlying personality vulnerabilities and in relapse prophylaxis, but have limited benefit in acute episodes of BPAD or melancholic depression. They are covered in more extensive detail in Chapter 17. Some prominent examples are given below:

- Cognitive behavioural therapy (CBT) comes in many forms, although all strive to emphasise problem solving, the present reality rather than the past, personal responsibility, and unhelpful thoughts and behaviours to the patient. The 'cognitive' therapy involves identification of negative thoughts and challenging the patient to realistically reframe them. The 'behavioural' aspect involves provision of 'homework' tasks for the patient to gradually master related to their 'cognitive' therapy.

- Dialectical behavioural therapy (DBT) is a modified form of CBT, useful in those with cluster B personality traits and maladaptive behavioural responses to certain emotions. DBT aims to explore a maladaptive behaviour the patient has exhibited in the previous week, brainstorm alternative solutions and coping strategies to the scenario that triggered that behaviour, and analyse the barriers that prevented the patient from using these alternative solutions.
- Psychoeducation with the patient and their family can involve explanation of their illness, its prognosis, its aetiology, current treatments, treatment options, the risks and benefits of these, and methods of supporting the patient through their illness. It is particularly effective in relapse prevention.
- Family or couples therapy may be indicated if prominent familial or relationship stressors are thought to be precipitating episodes of a patient's mood disorder.
- Interpersonal therapy (IPT) was designed specifically for the management of depression. It emphasises present circumstances over the past, and involves a combination of psychodynamic, cognitive and behavioural approaches to exploring maladaptive patterns in the patient's relationships.
- Psychodynamic psychotherapy including manualised therapies such as transference-focused psychotherapy are long-term, highly effective treatments if the patient is both psychologically minded and motivated to recover.
- A useful psychotherapeutic option at the scene is solution-focused brief therapy (SFBT), which aims to explore a patient's own solutions to their problems, rather than focusing on the problems themselves, by goal-setting and subsequently asking the patient what would have changed in their life if a 'miracle' had occurred and steps had been taken to resolve these problems. Other therapeutic questions pertain to quantitative scaling of progress and mood, coping methods, and 'exception-seeking' (what was different when the problem was less severe). It can be used in tandem with the above psychotherapies.

PHARMACOLOGICAL

Several types of medications are used in management of mood disorders. They are described in more detail in Chapter 18 (Psychopharmacology).

All antidepressants increase the concentration of monoamines (serotonin, noradrenaline or dopamine) at the synaptic cleft. However, this does not necessarily reflect their antidepressant properties, or mechanism of action. They take approximately two weeks before clinical improvement is noted, and up to six weeks before their full benefit is felt. If no clinical improvement is noted at six weeks, the diagnosis should be reviewed. If melancholic features are present, then either the dose is increased, or the medication switched. Patients with ongoing melancholic depression after six weeks of assertive antidepressant treatment are referred to as treatment-resistant.

Choice of antidepressant is guided by the type of melancholic features present and the side-effect profile, aiming for side effects to be therapeutic or otherwise minimised. Sedating medications such as mirtazapine are effective if insomnia is a prominent feature, for example.

Antidepressants with serotonergic effects carry a risk of serotonin syndrome in overdose, clinically marked by rigidity, delirium, autonomic instability, hyperthermia, altered conscious state and potentially death.

Antidepressant classes include:

- selective serotonin reuptake inhibitors (SSRIs)
- selective noradrenaline reuptake inhibitors (SNRIs)
- selective serotonin and noradrenaline reuptake inhibitors (SSNRIs)
- tricyclic antidepressants (TCAs)
- monoamine oxidase inhibitors (MAOIs)
- atypical antidepressants, e.g. mirtazapine, agomelatine.

Management of BPAD can be broken down into acute and maintenance treatment phases. Mood stabilisers are the mainstay of both treatment phases.

- Mood stabilisers include lithium (first-line for BPAD type 1 if side effects are tolerable) and three anticonvulsants: valproate (most commonly used if lithium is not indicated), carbamazepine, and lamotrigine (effective for bipolar depression but less so for mania). Unlike antipsychotics, they do not blunt mood, but instead treat and help prevent development of its bipolar extremes.
- Antipsychotics are often used as an adjunct to help address psychotic, behavioural and cognitive symptoms during acute episodes. Several antipsychotics have been shown to be effective adjuncts, although olanzapine and quetiapine are the most commonly prescribed in BPAD.

ELECTROCONVULSIVE THERAPY (ECT)

The induction of a seizure under controlled conditions via the application of a gentle electrical current to the cranium is referred to as ECT. It is indicated as an acute therapy in BPAD type 1 episodes and melancholic depression, including psychotic depression; and as a weekly, fortnightly or monthly maintenance therapy following severe episodes if preferred by the patient. Modern ECT is safe, effective, well-tolerated, and often results in rapid recovery. A link to a video depicting the procedure is included in the resources section at the end of this chapter. Approximately 30% of those receiving ECT have a significant improvement in mental state after one treatment; well over 90% respond within six treatments. Treatments are administered by a psychiatrist up to three times a week, typically for six to 12 treatments, under anaesthesia. Side effects include anterograde and retrograde amnesia, which typically and gradually resolve on cessation of treatment; headache, jaw pain, or muscular pains from the muscle contractions during the seizure (managed with administration of an anaesthetic muscle relaxant); and potential complications of anaesthesia, such as aspiration. While modern ECT is a gentle, effective and efficient treatment, stigma remains prevalent due to ongoing pop cultural depictions of 'unmodified ECT' – the first form of ECT that did not include anaesthesia or careful dose calibration. Patients and their families should be fully involved when considering this treatment. It can also be provided compulsorily under the various Mental Health Acts when the patient cannot provide consent, often due to the presence of mood-congruent delusions, dysexecutive symptoms such as impulsivity, thought disorder and cognitive impairment precluding comprehension of the procedure, or a loss of reality testing. In these circumstances, ECT is likely to be approved if failure to provide it would be life-threatening, or expose the patient to unnecessary suffering.

TRANSCRANIAL MAGNETIC STIMULATION (TMS)

Similar to ECT, TMS involves the application of magnetic stimuli to the cranium, but without anaesthesia. It may be effective in milder forms of melancholic depression. Severe depressions often require alternate treatments, such as ECT. It is currently not covered under the Pharmaceutical Benefits Scheme, and so is administered in private practice only.

DEEP BRAIN STIMULATION (DBS)

Indicated for severe, treatment-refractory melancholic depression and very rarely performed, DBS involves placement of electrodes via neurosurgery and connection of these to an implanted neurostimulator. Its use is governed by the Mental Health Acts, requires approval by a psychosurgery review board, and is only available with informed consent. Some evidence has suggested those undergoing DBS who present with suicidal ideation are at high risk; their treating psychiatrist and neurologist should be contacted as a matter of priority.

SUPPORT NETWORKS

Similar to the ongoing provision of holistic lifestyle advice and encouragement of positive coping strategies (refer to the above section under pre-hospital approaches to treatment), social supports such as family, communities, friends, support networks and groups are key buffers that can bolster a person's capacity to cope with adversity. They can provide pooled resources, advice, positive modelled behaviour, meaning, practical assistance and emotional availability to help a person recontextualise their difficulties, problem solve with greater confidence, enrich their sense of self-worth and identity, and adapt. Higher-quality – more-intimate and meaningful – relationships are more protective than a higher number of less-meaningful and superficial connections. Bolstering support networks is a simple and effective intervention in the pre-hospital setting for many patients presenting with mood disturbances. Mobilising a patient's social supports is a core component of long-term, holistic recovery and relapse prevention for patients presenting with a mood disorder.

Patients who present in crisis, hypomanic or depressed, and do not require transport to hospital can be directed to seek further support via:

- their GP
- a counsellor, psychologist, or psychiatrist, if they have one
- local counselling or psychology services (which may require a Mental Health Care Plan from their GP to obtain Medicare rebates)
- a psychiatrist, via referral from their GP
- non-governmental organisations (NGOs)
- patient information websites
- crisis support hotlines and teams.

Some crisis, NGO and online supports are listed in the resources section at the end of this chapter.

CARING FOR THE CARERS
FAMILY AND SIGNIFICANT OTHERS

The loved ones of someone presenting in crisis, depressed or manic are likely to be heavily impacted by stress, the transference of emotion from the patient and the burden of care. Distressed family and friends may also exhibit high-expressed emotion, potentially exacerbating a patient's own distress. Managing this distress can help manage the pre-hospital scene, allowing for a comprehensive assessment and the safety of those in attendance. Furthermore, a strong support network is instrumental in helping a patient recover, bolsters their resilience and reduces the chance of relapse.

Family and other carers at the scene should be advised that attending to their own wellbeing is important, and that seeking support from their own support networks, including friends, family and their own GP, is crucial while their loved one is unwell. Several healthcare services offer carers' support services. They can also be directed to online services such as Carers Australia and Mental Health Carers Australia, formerly the Association of Relatives and Friends of the Mentally Ill.

LOOKING OUT FOR YOUR PEERS, AND LOOKING AFTER YOURSELF

While this topic is covered more extensively in other chapters, it is an important point to address. People presenting with mood disorders often communicate their affect well, which may lead to assessors feeling empty, miserable, angry or jubilant. These strong emotional responses are both common and natural. It is important to recognise them; this assists diagnostically, helps prevent boundary violations and helps prevent 'emotional burnout', which itself can be considered a subclinical form of non-melancholic depression. Having opportunities to debrief following critical incidents can help identify and address your own or peers' distress (Porter, 2013). It is important to have a regular opportunity to debrief with peers and a supervisor as a matter of routine so that distressing or impactful events can be discussed, even if their impact is not immediately apparent. Resilience, while important to wellbeing, is not a passive phenomenon; it requires time and effort to cultivate, and to identify what gives you energy and a sense of purpose. Paramedicine can prove an emotionally volatile and rewarding career; seeking support from friends, family and your own GP is paramount for long-term wellbeing.

CONCLUSION

Mood disorders are a leading global cause of disability and suffering. Mood disturbance presentations to emergency services are common and require careful assessment to elucidate potential differential diagnoses, likely comorbidities, and underlying biological, social and psychological factors triggering the episode. Mood disorders can be broadly categorised under the headings of non-melancholic depression, melancholic depression and bipolar affective disorder. Acute presentations of each have different natural histories and acute treatments, necessitating careful listening, observing and interacting with patients in diagnosis and effective management. Interpersonal interaction during the pre-hospital assessment process is itself a potentially powerful therapeutic intervention.

LINKS AND RESOURCES

- The Royal College of Australian and New Zealand Psychiatrists clinical practice guidelines for mood disorders: https://www.ranzcp.org/Files/Resources/Publications/CPG/Clinician/Mood-Disorders-CPG.aspx
- 'ECT in Modern Psychiatry': https://www.youtube.com/watch?v=9L2-B-aluCE St George's, University of London & South West London & St George's Mental Health NHS Trust, 2011

Crisis support can be found via:

- Local area mental health services' triage numbers
- Lifeline Australia (13 11 14)
- Beyond Blue (1300 22 4636)
- Kids Helpline (1800 55 1800)
- MensLine Australia (1300 78 99 78)
- Suicide Call Back Service (1300 659 467)
- Veterans and Veterans' Families Counselling Service (1800 011 046)
- Emergency services (000).

Online support for patients and carers can be found at:

- Your Health in Mind, an information site curated by the Royal Australian and New Zealand College of Psychiatrists: https://www.yourhealthinmind.org/
- SANE Australia: https://www.sane.org/
- The Black Dog Institute: https://www.blackdoginstitute.org.au/getting-help
- Beyond Blue: https://www.beyondblue.org.au
- Conversations Matter, a website for resources for discussing suicide: http://www.conversationsmatter.com.au/
- Headspace and eheadspace: https://www.eheadspace.org.au/
- Australian Men's Shed Association: https://mensshed.org/
- Carer Support: https://carersupport.org.au/
- Carers Australia: http://www.carersaustralia.com.au/
- Mental Health Carers Australia: http://www.mentalhealthcarersaustralia.org.au/

REFERENCES

American Psychiatric Association (APA), 2013. Diagnostic and statistical manual of mental disorders, 5th edn. APA, Washington, DC. (DSM-5).

Bloom, D., Cafiero, E., Jané-Llopis, E., et al., 2011. The global economic burden of non-communicable diseases. World Economic Forum, Geneva.

Bromet, E., Andrade, L., Hwang, I., et al., 2011. Cross-national epidemiology of DSM-IV major depressive episode. BMC Med. 9, 90.

Kernberg, O., Yeomans, F., 2013. Borderline personality disorder, bipolar disorder, depression, attention deficit/hyperactivity disorder, and narcissistic personality disorder: practical differential diagnosis. Bull. Menninger Clin. 77 (1), 1–22.

Klein, M., 1935. A contribution to the psychogenesis of manic-depressive states. Int. J. Psychoanal. 16, 145–174.

Porter, S., 2013. An exploration of the support needs of Ambulance Paramedics. Victoria University, Melbourne.

Royal Australian and New Zealand College of Psychiatrists (RANZCP), 2015. Royal Australian and New Zealand College of Psychiatrists clinical practice guidelines for mood disorders. Aust. N. Z. J. Psychiatry 49 (12), 1–185.

Royal Australian and New Zealand College of Psychiatrists (RANZCP), 2016. Royal Australian and New Zealand College of Psychiatrists clinical practice guidelines for the management of schizophrenia and related disorders. Aust. N. Z. J. Psychiatry 50 (5), 1–117.

Thornicroft, G., Rose, D., Kassam, A., 2017. Discrimination in health care against people with mental illness. Int. Rev. Psychiatry 19 (2), 113–122.

Whiteford, H., Ferrari, A., Degenhardt, L., et al., 2015. The global burden of mental, neurological and substance use disorders: an analysis from the Global Burden of Disease Study 2010. PLoS ONE 10 (2), e0116820.

World Health Organization (WHO), 2011. Global status report on non-communicable diseases 2010. WHO, Geneva.

Managing risk, suicidal ideation and suicide attempt

Conrad Newman

LEARNING OUTCOMES

The aim of this chapter is to equip paramedics (and paramedic students) with knowledge and skills relating to assessment and treatment of patients in the pre-hospital setting who are suicidal. The topics which will be covered are:

- The extent of suicide globally and in Australia
- Risk factors, warning signs and their utility
- Protective factors
- Suicide assessment
- Access to means
- Collaboration with carers
- Safety planning.

INTRODUCTION

Paramedics are at the front line of health service delivery in Australia. Decreasing lengths of psychiatric inpatient admissions and the move towards community-based care have led to an increase in the acuity of mental health presentations in the community. This impacts on the nature of paramedics' work and the skill set they must have to meet the needs of individuals in a mental health crisis.

Paramedics must be mindful that the initial contact and evaluation with a suicidal patient can have considerable impact on whether a patient decides to continue in care, and provides a foundation for subsequent interactions (Rudd, 2012). Every contact with a suicidal individual is an opportunity for intervention to help prevent an individual from going on to die by suicide (Cole-King & Platt, 2017).

It is emotionally demanding assessing individuals who are contemplating suicide or those who have attempted suicide. It is important to consider every intervention with a suicidal individual as an opportunity to help the person find their way through a suicidal crisis. While many individuals are accepting of help at times, others will be challenging, not wanting to accept any interventions. Physical trauma, family members (including children) who have witnessed events, or if the individual is evading assessment all serve to increase the competing demands a paramedic experiences in these situations. It is common to experience significant anxiety when the decision is to leave an individual at home rather than convey them to hospital, even when this is the most prudent decision.

BACKGROUND AND PREVALENCE

Suicide is a significant global health problem. Over 800,000 people per year die from suicide worldwide, which equates to one death every 40 seconds. Suicide attempts and ideation are far more common than suicide deaths. The number of people who attempt to die by suicide is believed to be up to 20 times the number of suicide deaths. The number of lives lost each year through suicide exceeds the number of deaths due to homicide and war combined (World Health Organization [WHO], 2016).

According to Slade and colleagues (2009), 13.3% of Australians aged 16–85 years have experienced suicidal ideation, 4.0% have made suicide plans and 3.3% have attempted suicide at some point in their life, which is equivalent to over 2.1 million Australians having thought about taking their own life, over 600,000 making a suicide plan and some 500,000 individuals making a suicide attempt. There are approximately 65,000 suicide attempts in Australia each year (Slade et al., 2009).

In 2016 there were a total of 2866 deaths by suicide (age-specific suicide rate 11.8 per 100,000) – 2151 males (17.9 per 100,000) and 715 females (5.9 per 100,000). This equates to an average of 7.85 deaths by suicide in Australia each day.

For those of Aboriginal and Torres Strait Islander descent in New South Wales, Queensland, South Australia, Western Australia and the Northern Territory, suicide was the fifth most common cause of death. For New South Wales, Queensland, South Australia, Western Australia and the Northern Territory, the standardised death rate for Aboriginal and Torres Strait Islander People (23.8 per 100,000) was approximately twice the rate of non-Indigenous (11.4 per 100,000).

For males, the highest age-specific suicide rate in 2016 was observed in the 85+ age group (34.0 per 100,000), which is significantly higher than the age-specific suicide rate observed in all other age groups. The next highest age-specific suicide rates were the 30–34, 40–44 and 35–39 year age groups (27.5, 27.2 and 24.8 per 100,000, respectively). For females, however, the highest age-specific suicide rate in 2016 was observed in the 50–54 age group (10.4 per 100,000).

Over the past 10 years, the number of suicide deaths was approximately three times higher in males than females. In 2016, 75.1% of people who died by suicide were male. The most common method of suicide is hanging (males 57.8%, females 47.4%), followed by poisoning by drugs (males 9.8%, females 28.1%) (Mindframe, 2018).

For every suicide, at least six close relatives or friends are bereaved. These people have an increased risk of developing depression and also of suicide (Bolton et al., 2015).

There is a substantially higher risk of suicide in people with mental illness compared with the general population. The rate is highest in people with comorbidity and a history of self-harm. There are two notable periods when suicide risk is high: during the first few months after diagnosis, and in the first weeks after discharge from psychiatric admission. Patients who are admitted to hospital with a suicide attempt are an especially high risk for suicide after discharge (Bolton et al., 2015).

CASE STUDY

Michael

You are dispatched to a 35-year-old male who has attempted to hang himself in the back yard. He was discovered by his parents who have called for an ambulance. Dispatch time: 23.40.

You arrive at the house and are greeted by Michael's mother, who looks distressed. She takes you to the rear of the house and into the shed where you meet Michael and his father. Michael initially seems annoyed by your presence, saying, 'You didn't have to call them … I'm all right … I just want to go to bed.' His father tells you that they were awakened at 23.15 by the sound of a loud crash coming from their shed. Michael's parents went to investigate and found him on the floor crying with a noose hanging from a ceiling beam and a broken chair next to him. There were several empty beer bottles around him. Michael told his father, 'I tried to do it but the chair broke.' Michael's parents are shaken and tell you he has been withdrawing from family, with whom he was usually close. They noted he had seemed 'on edge' the past week. He had told his parents in the past few days that his life seemed pointless, he 'may as well be dead' and he was a 'problem they don't need'. Michael repeatedly tells you he just wants to go to bed, and walks back in the house. His mother follows him. Michael does not appear to have any injuries but is walking with an unsteady gait and a slight limp.

His father tells you that Michael is 35 years old and has been living with his parents since he separated from his wife eight months ago. She had told him she could no longer tolerate his alcohol abuse and that he had changed so much from the man he was two years before. They have three children, a son aged 7 and two daughters aged 5 and 3. Michael had worked as a car salesman for the past 10 years and won several awards for his sales records. His work performance has deteriorated significantly in the past two years. He has had frequent absences from work and has received several warnings. His employment was terminated when he arrived at work intoxicated one morning 10 months ago and phoned a customer slurring his words. He lost his licence nine months ago for driving under the influence of alcohol. The loss of his licence has made it difficult for him to find employment. A week ago, his wife told him she had consulted a lawyer to begin divorce proceedings and she was going to limit his access to the children, as he is frequently intoxicated when he visits them. Michael has no formal history of mental illness and is not prescribed any medication.

You go back into the house and are told by his mother that Michael is in his bedroom and has locked the door. There is no noise in the room, but the mum thought it sounded like he got into bed. You knock on the door but Michael does not reply.

CRITICAL REFLECTION

Given that Michael has no injury, no history of mental illness and has gone to bed, discuss your role as a paramedic.
- Do you have any reason to continue with attempting an assessment?
- If Michael was not intoxicated, would any of your thoughts/decisions change?
- Under local legislation, do you have reasonable grounds and an ability to force your way into Michael's room? Identify the legislation that may or may not allow you to do this.

- Your colleague suggests that you should call the police and ask them to force entry into the room. You are not so sure. Consider why calling the police may be helpful, or why they may be a hindrance to your assessment.

ASSESSING AN INDIVIDUAL IN A SUICIDAL CRISIS
ASKING ABOUT SUICIDAL THOUGHTS

As Berman and Silverman (2017) describe, more than a dozen papers published over a 16-year period to 2017 all concluded that asking patients about suicidal ideation does not lead to an increase in suicidal ideation. Asking about suicide may decrease rather than increase suicidal ideation through an empathic, non-judgmental and confident approach (Dazzi et al., 2014). An awareness of your body language and that of the patients is important. For the paramedic, attention to rapport, demonstrating an acceptance of the patient, and attempting to engender hope whenever possible will help build engagement. Try to elicit intent to suicide by starting with open questions followed by specific closed questions. Useful information can be gained from third parties, such as other first responders, family and friends, in addition to any objective evidence. Making plans or preparations for suicide, attempts to avoid discovery, choice of method, a written note or electronic communication and developing a will are all examples of objective evidence (Cole-King & Platt, 2017; Morriss et al., 2013).

SUICIDE RISK ASSESSMENT

Assessing a patient at risk of suicide requires a full biopsychosocial assessment; however, due to time restraints the paramedic may be limited in the amount of information that they can obtain. In time-limited situations, priority should be given to establishing details of the patient's suicidal thoughts, intent and plans, personal and demographic information, and a mental state examination, in order to create a safe plan or environment for the person. It is vital to identify *treatable* and *modifiable* risks, and *protective factors,* as these will be required to guide the patient's management (Simon, 2011). Conducting a suicide risk assessment in a systematic manner decreases the chance of overlooking important risk and protective factors.

Unfortunately in clinical practice the assessment often consists of only asking the patient *'Are you thinking about suicide today?'* with documentation indicating 'no SI' if no ideation is expressed, or if when asked it is denied. The assumption is that the absence of suicidal ideation equates to the absence of any suicide risk, which is not the case. Unfortunately, the assessment too often stops at this point (Silverman & Berman, 2014).

Almost 80% of patients deny suicidal ideation or intent as their last communication (Busch et al., 2003). Asking a patient at risk of suicide about the presence of suicidal ideation, suicide intent and a suicide plan and receiving a denial cannot be relied on by itself.

Denying suicidal ideation may occur for several reasons, including beliefs that suicide is a sign of weakness, that nobody can help (hopelessness) or an intent to die and a wish not to be thwarted (Silverman & Berman, 2014).

HIGH AND LOW RISK

Currently no method of suicide risk assessment can reliably identify who will die by suicide (sensitivity) and who will not (specificity). Any attempt to divide patients into high-risk and low-risk categories is unhelpful and can prevent access to appropriate psychiatric care. Therefore, paramedics need to ensure all patients receive the treatment they require, not based on concepts of a risk categorisation. Do not dismiss any patient who raises concerns of suicide as being low risk (Busch et al., 2003; Cole-King & Platt, 2017; Hawgood & De Leo, 2016; Large & Ryan, 2014a; Large & Ryan, 2014b; Large et al., 2017; Mulder et al., 2016; Ryan et al., 2013; Simon, 2012).

The critical issue is to identify, treat and manage the acute risk factors driving the patient's suicidal crisis rather than the impossible task of trying to predict whether a suicide attempt may occur (Simon, 2012).

Given the difficulties inherent in risk categorisation, there has been a conceptual shift from a *predictive* to a *preventive risk formulation*.

RISK FORMULATION

Risk formulation is defined as 'a concise synthesis of empirically based suicide risk information regarding a patient's immediate distress and resources at a specific time and place' (Pisani et al., 2016, p. 625). To do this we must promote communication and collaboration among professionals, patients and families, rather than attempt to predict behaviour. The goal of assessing the current risk state is not to improve prediction but to determine the interventions required to decrease the acute suicide risk. However, suicide risk can be fluid in nature. Risk formulation can capture the variation in suicide risk of an individual, how the person's current risk compares with their risk at previous points in time, and how risk and situations may change in response to future events (Pisani et al., 2016). Risk formulation should guide and inform intervention from the paramedics and other services.

Most frameworks for approaching suicide risk formulation are generally consistent, collecting details of previous suicide attempts/actions, current thoughts and plans, hopelessness, stressors, the MSE (mental state examination, which looks for the presence of symptoms of possible mental illness), difficulties with impulsivity and self-control, ready access to highly lethal methods, and protective factors (Bolton et al., 2015). In out-of-hospital settings it is important to collect as much information as possible from as many sources as possible, as this helps build a picture of the person and their current difficulties. This should be used to inform further formulation and decision making. Equally important is capturing these factors in documentation to ensure subsequent clinicians/teams are aware of the potential for risk to change over time.

Table 11.1 Demographic and Social Factors Associated With Suicide

Male (age 25–64 and over 75)

Marital status (separated has higher rates than first year after separation, followed by divorced, widowed and married)

Living in a rural area

Aboriginal or Torres Strait Islander

Immigrants, refugees, asylum seekers (victims of torture and trauma, older immigrants from non-English-speaking backgrounds, immigrants from Northern and Eastern Europe)

People with sexual identity conflicts

Lack of social networks (social isolation, living alone, losing a spouse through death or divorce, recent loss of attachments, perception of lack of social support /confidants, homelessness, single occupant of a prison cell)

Major relationship instability

Loss of status

Access to lethal means (firearms, frequently used locations, access due to profession or hobbies)

Victims of domestic violence

People in prison or police custody

Profession (mining and construction workers, truck drivers, doctors (female doctors and anaesthetists), pharmacists, dentists, law enforcement personnel, veterinary surgeons, female nurses and frontline emergency service personnel)

RISK FACTORS

Paramedics should be familiar with established risk factors for suicide at a population level (as detailed in Tables 11.1–11.3), but should not solely rely on this knowledge of demographic risks when assessing risk of specific individuals. A person may be at risk of suicide even though they do not meet many risk factors (Cole-King & Platt, 2017).

Ryan and colleagues (2013) argue the clinician should not be conducting 'comprehensive suicide risk assessments' which focus solely on population-based risk factors. They should be conducting comprehensive clinical assessments of each patient's situations and needs. Risk factors like depression, hopelessness and substance misuse are far too common and non-specific to be useful indicators of suicide risk, but they can be seen as symptoms of mental illness and important pieces of a patient's inner life that, taken together, give us a better understanding of the individual and what needs attention and discussion. They suggest we must gather a comprehensive picture of each individual and use this to tailor optimal management for patients and families. Bolstering family or social support, restricting access to lethal methods of suicide, and making a crisis plan are steps that should be taken for all patients in a psychological crisis.

A focus of research in suicidology to date has been on identifying the risk factors associated with suicide. A representative list of such factors is listed in Tables 11.1–11.3. While these factors are useful at a population level and when

Table 11.2 Background Factors to Consider in History Taking

Previous suicide attempt (significantly more at risk of suicidal behaviour, however the absence of suicide attempts should not be taken as diminishing risk, 60–70% of those who die by suicide do so on the first known attempt; presence of multiple previous attempts, especially if a prior attempt had high medical lethality)

Previous self-harm (recent increasing intent of self-harm, risk of a person dying by suicide after an episode of self-harm is 100 times greater than the general population risk, within 5–10 years, 7% of those who self-harm will die by suicide)

History of a mental illness (depression, bipolar disorder, schizophrenia, other psychotic illness, anorexia nervosa, anxiety disorders, chronic PTSD, personality disorder)

Comorbidity (comorbid disorders, such as substance abuse and schizophrenia)

History of emotional, sexual, physical abuse or neglect (no memory of being special to any adult, bullying)

Chronic physical illness or disability (**pain**, malignancy, dialysis, gastrointestinal disease, cardiovascular disease, tinnitus, epilepsy, multiple sclerosis, dementia, HIV-AIDS, amyotrophic lateral sclerosis)

Repeated relapses of mental illness

Recent admission or discharge from a psychiatric inpatient unit (suicide risk on the first four weeks after discharge increases to 100–200 times greater than normal, and the risk remains for at least 5–10 years after last discharge)

Postpartum (women with a psychiatric disorder, substance use disorder or both, have a significantly increased risk of a postpartum suicide attempt, particularly in the first year after giving birth)

Recent increase in frequency of GP appointments and /or several changes to medication

Alcohol and other substance abuse

Personality traits (impulsivity, aggression, recklessness, risk taking, lability of mood)

Family history (mental illness, suicide, alcohol abuse, bipolar disorder)

Poor work history in the past four years (peak age 40–60)

Relative and peers who have died by suicide (recent suicide or suicide attempt by a relative or peer)

Experienced military combat

---

determining whether an individual is a member of a risk group, they have limited utility when considering an individual's potential for suicide. Paramedics can use these risk factors as considerations within their assessment, however the overall focus is on mitigation rather than prediction; responding to the needs of the individual, not trying to predict subsequent suicidal behaviour (Hawgood & De Leo, 2016).

The low base rate of suicide makes it difficult to accurately predict suicide risk. To identify suicidal individuals, empirically based risk factors for suicide inform longer-term vulnerability, however the acute and fluctuating state of suicidality cannot be understood in the same way. Therefore, the aim of risk assessment should be focused on mitigation of risk and informing effective and personalised care for an individual (Hawgood & De Leo, 2016; McDowell et al., 2011).

Table 11.3 Recent and Current Factors to Consider in History Taking and MSE

Current state

Recent relapse in a mental illness

Hopelessness (perception of the future as persistently negative, particularly worrying if severe, e.g. only able to see 1–2 hours into the future, 'nothing to live for', no sense of purpose; duration of hopelessness)

No reason for living or no sense of purpose in life

Increasing alcohol or drug use

Negative thoughts, helplessness, guilt ('I'm a burden' – perceived burdensomeness)

Intense emotional pain (sense of being trapped, unable to escape the emotional pain)

Sense of shame (especially if severe and /or in conflict with underlying religious, spiritual or cultural beliefs)

Agitation

Anxiety

Being unable to sleep or sleeping all the time

Anger or rage

Psychotic phenomena (persecutory delusions, nihilistic delusions, command hallucinations)

Suicidal ideation (especially if pervasive and compelling, recent worsening and associated with distress, unable to distract from thoughts, inability to generate any optimism, talking or writing about death)

Suicide plans/preparations (talking or writing about death, dying or suicide, preparing will, writing social media posts, note, texts, emails, internet search, looking for ways to suicide, lethality of method chosen, access to means, plans to die with family members)

Cognitive function (low IQ, delirium, previous high premorbid functioning and fear of deterioration)

Recent interpersonal crisis (especially rejection, humiliation)

Recent major loss or trauma or anniversary

Recent loss of attachment, or perception of lack of social supports or confidants

Substance use (increasing use, particularly when precipitated by loss of relationships, alcohol intoxication, drug withdrawal)

Impending legal prosecution

Family breakdown (including child custody issues)

Family conflict (familial stress, perception of being a burden on one's family)

Difficulty accessing help (language barriers, lack of information or support, negative experiences with mental health services prior to immigration)

Withdrawing from friends, family or society

Acting recklessly or engaging in risky activities

Unwillingness to accept help

Seeking revenge

Feeling trapped

Tables adapted from Cole-King & Platt, 2017; Department of Health Victoria, 2010; NSW Department of Health, 2004; Rudd et al., 2012; Van Orden et al., 2010

Psychological autopsies of people who have died by suicide, find that more than 90% have a psychiatric disorder. Patients with more than one mental illness are at particularly higher risk, especially those with both depressive disorders and substance use disorders (McDowell et al., 2011). It is important for a paramedic to screen for both mental illness and substance abuse.

There are some individuals who meet many risk factors and have never contemplated suicide, while there are others who meet none of the risk factors who have a significant potential for suicide. Of the risk factors, one stands out in comparison with the others – a history of a suicide attempt. It is the strongest risk factor predicting suicide and suicide-related behaviour. Suicide attempts that are medically serious have a strong association with an increased risk of mortality and repeated suicide attempts. Fowler, reporting on a five-year follow-up study in 2012, found individuals who made a single suicide attempt are 48 times more likely to die by suicide than the average person (Fowler, 2012). In one sample 60% of individuals died on their first attempt, with more than 80% of deaths by suicide occurring within a year of the initial attempt. This indicates that a history of suicide attempt is a far more lethal risk factor for death by suicide than previously thought (Bostwick et al., 2016). Between 7% and 12% of patients who have attempted suicide will die by suicide within 10 years. The risk of death by suicide is highest during the first year after the attempt. This points to the importance of paramedics asking about and identifying previous attempts, including 'close calls', where a person had planned but did not go through with the attempt. The questioning around intent, prior thoughts and attempts needs to be approached sensitively but directly.

WARNING SIGNS

Risk factors have limited utility for immediate intervention. A patient's age and sex are risk factors that have limited implications for immediate clinical decision making. A risk factor elevates the long-term probability of a suicidal crisis, whereas warning signs are indicative of an active suicidal crisis (Rudd et al., 2012).

Warning signs are specific symptoms or behaviours, which can be acute or subacute in nature, that should be identified and explored in detail (McDowell et al., 2011). Critical suicide warning signs include anxiety and agitation. Anxiety disorders and acute anxiety states can greatly influence suicidal behaviour, as individuals with disorders characterised by significant anxiety, agitation or poor impulse control are more likely to transition from thinking about suicide to making a plan or an attempt (McDowell et al., 2011).

Warning signs are indicated in bold in Tables 11.1–11.3. These are drawn from multiple sources.

PROTECTIVE FACTORS

Protective factors offer a degree of resilience against suicidal behaviours. Notable protective factors include religious affiliations and beliefs, reasons for living, marriage (except in situations of a higher conflict or violent relationship), children in the home (except in the cases of teen pregnancy, extreme economic hardship and postpartum mood or psychotic disorders), supportive social networks, therapeutic contacts, problem-solving skills and a sense of responsibility for others. The evidence base for protective factors is generally weak; however, the relative importance of these factors can be great. Protective factors can vary greatly between individuals. Protective factors may not be fully effective until the patient's suicide potential is reduced, but it is important for paramedics and other first responders to attempt to discuss and highlight possible protective factors at the earliest opportunity. The following types of questions may assist:

- *'Michael, it sounds like things have been pretty bad for a while now, but tell me what is it that has stopped you from attempting to take your life?'*
- *'Is that enough to keep you going?'*
- *'Michael, if you were to die, who would be the most upset?'*
- *'Michael, if you were to die, what would be the thing that you would miss the most?'* (Alternatively, *'who would be the person that you would miss the most?'*)

Clinicians need to be vigilant about a loss of, or change in, protective factors, as this could indicate an increased risk for the patient (Fowler, 2012; Sinclair & Leach, 2017). In the case study of Michael, his wife has filed for divorce and he has been threatened with decreased access to his children. Until this point, his children are likely to have been his greatest protective factor.

A significantly elevated potential for suicide associated with severe mental illness may nullify protective factors (Simon, 2012). In an acute situation with multiple risk factors, particularly with unfamiliar patients, the ability of protective factors to decrease risk should not be overestimated. Protective factors may be easily overwhelmed in a crisis and not available to draw upon, especially in an intoxicated, impulsive or otherwise disinhibited patient (McDowell et al., 2011; Pisani et al., 2016).

EMERGING FRAMEWORKS

Emerging frameworks for risk assessment and management include the Collaborative Assessment and Management of Suicidality (CAMS) (Jobes, 2012), the Connecting with People suicide mitigation approach (Cole-King & Lepping, 2010; Cole-King et al., 2013) and the Screening Tool for Assessing Risk of Suicide (STARS) (Hawgood & De Leo, 2015). These frameworks integrate the identification of risk factors with a collaborative encounter with the patient that recognises the importance of therapeutic engagement. The reader is encouraged to examine these frameworks through the references provided.

INTENT

Shea (2009) conceptualises the suicidal intent of a patient with the following equation:

Real suicidal intent = Stated intent + Reflected intent + Withheld intent

The stated intent is what the person directly tells the clinician about their suicidal intent. The reflected intent is the amount of thinking, planning or actions taken on suicidal ideation that may reflect the intensity of their suicidal intent. This information may be provided by the person, or alternatively by assessment of the environment or through discussion with other people involved. The withheld intent is that which is unconsciously or purposely withheld. The extent, thoroughness and time the patient spends on suicide planning may better reflect the seriousness of their intent, and the proximity of their desire to act on that intent, than their actual stated intent (Shea, 2012). Suicidal persons do not always share their true intentions. The intent to die may not be revealed even in the presence of deep clinical engagement (Hawgood & De Leo, 2016).

It can be challenging for the paramedic to discuss reflected intent when a patient is withholding their intent. Rudd (2006, p. 10) provides an example of how to frame this discussion:

'You've told me you really don't want to die but all of your behavior over the last few days suggests otherwise. You've been drinking heavily, you've written a letter to your husband saying you want to die, and several weeks ago you took an overdose when you knew no one would be home and waited 3 days to tell me about it. I need you to help me make sense of this contradiction. It almost seems like you're telling me one thing and doing another. Frankly, I'm more inclined to consider your behavior as the more important variable here, particularly since I'm very concerned about your safety and well being.'

Identification and understanding of intent can be challenging for the paramedic when clouded by factors such as intoxication, sedation or emotion. It is therefore important to view the assessment as incomplete and err on the side of caution until further information can be obtained.

In the case of Michael, assessment of intent would be difficult given that he is reluctant to talk to paramedics. It is already known that he has attempted to hang himself, and he has admitted this to his father. It is unclear if this was a planned action, or if this was an impulsive act (perhaps in part due to the alcohol intoxication). The amount of detail that he is willing to provide will likely change when he is no longer intoxicated, or with the development of a stronger therapeutic relationship. The paramedic will need to be cautious with their decision making, and in this instance rely primarily on his behaviour as the important variable rather than what he might report.

LANGUAGE

It is important to use clear, unambiguous language combined with good eye contact when asking difficult questions. Terms such as *'thinking of killing yourself'* and *'thoughts of suicide'* are more easily understood than ambiguous terms such as *'You don't want to harm yourself, do you?'*, *'You're not thinking about doing anything silly are you?'* or *'Can you guarantee your safety?'* Relying on no-harm contracts, such as asking a patient to guarantee their safety, have no validity.

HIERARCHICAL APPROACH TO A SUICIDE RISK ASSESSMENT

Rudd (2012) describes a hierarchical approach to assessment which is adapted below for the pre-hospital setting. Take care to ask single questions and not compound questions containing multiple options.

> **Probe for a precipitant:** *Has something happened recently that started you thinking about suicide?*
>
> **Symptomatic presentation:** *How have you been feeling lately? Have you been feeling anxious [nervous, or panicky] or depressed [low or down] lately? Have you had any trouble sleeping or eating? [Explore for additional symptoms of depression and anxiety.]*
>
> **Hopelessness:** *Do you ever feel so bad that it makes you think that it will never get any better?*
>
> **Morbid ruminations:** *When people feel depressed and hopeless they sometimes have a lot of thoughts about death and dying. Do you ever have thoughts about death or dying?*
>
> **Suicidal thinking:** *Sometimes when things are really bad and people think about death, they sometimes think about taking their own life. Have you ever had thoughts about that?*

Step 1: Is the patient having suicidal thoughts? The assessment must identify the patient's perspective, and differentiate between suicidal thoughts (wanting to kill oneself), self-harm (emotion regulation as the primary goal), and morbid ruminations (thoughts of death, dying, or wanting to be dead, but not active thoughts of killing oneself). If required, define the terms for the patient. Document carefully, using direct quotes.

Yes – Obtain more specific information about their thoughts and plans. Get a direct quote from the patient without providing prompts. This provides a means to assess the specificity of the patient's thinking, one marker of intent. Explore each individual method separately. Always question for multiple methods.

No – Document that the person has denied having acute suicidal thoughts. Provide specific quotes of any morbid thoughts; for example, *'I've been thinking a lot about what it would be like for my family if I were gone'*, *'I hope I develop a terminal illness'* or *'I hope I go to sleep and don't wake up'*. Further assessment should be undertaken when the patient reports passive suicidal ideation, for example (Simon, 2012). Passive ideation can rapidly become active, and therefore a mitigating response is still required. It is possible that passive suicidal ideation is equally as high a risk to future suicidal behaviour when compared with active ideation (Menon, 2013).

Step 2: The paramedic must work towards reducing anxiety and resistance by helping the patient become more comfortable with the general topic of suicide.

Start with general and easy-to-answer questions before focusing on specifics; for example, *'How do you feel now that I am here?' 'Has this sort of thing ever happened before? Tell me what happened then.'* Once you can see the person is more comfortable with talking about suicidal thoughts, you could then ask them more specific questions.

Step 3: Assess their recent and current suicidal thoughts, including frequency, intensity and duration (and access to means to suicide). *'OK, we've talked about some of the previous times, but can I ask you more about today and recent times? How much have you been thinking about killing yourself? How often do you have such thoughts? How long do the thoughts last? Do you have access to things that you could use to die? Have you thought about other ways to die? Have you thought about when you would kill yourself or where you would do it?'* The paramedic may have to gently enquire in an inquisitive fashion in order to obtain the required information without damaging the therapeutic engagement that you are trying to build.

Step 4: Assess the person's intent, including their reasons for dying. *'Why do you want to die? How strong is the feeling of acting on your thoughts? Can you rate the strength of these feelings on a scale of 1 to 10, with 1 being "no, not very strong" and 10 being "too strong to resist"?'* The clinician must consider intent not just the patient's behaviour. A patient who takes 10 aspirin tablets in the belief that it will result in death demonstrates high intent (Simon, 2012).

Step 5: *'Have you done any preparation to carry out your suicidal thoughts? Have you done anything in preparation for your death (e.g. life insurance, letters or electronic communications to loved ones, research on the internet)? Have you in any way rehearsed your suicide? In other words, have you gotten your [method] out and gone through the steps of what you do to kill yourself?'*

Step 6: Assess protective factors, including reasons for living. *'How have you made it this far? What keeps you going? Are you hopeful about the future? What would need to happen or need to be different to help you to be more hopeful about the future? Who is it that you call on or rely on during difficult times? What things have been helpful for you in the past? Are there people or things that you need to avoid when you're feeling like this?'*

CORROBORATIVE HISTORY

Patients who are determined to end their lives by suicide may withhold vital information from professionals; however, this information can possibly be obtained from other sources such as friends and family members (Ryan et al., 2015). Additional sources of information include other clinicians who are immediately involved, such as other paramedics, mental health triage services (or similar) and police officers. Interviewing any people who are present with the person to determine the circumstances of their recent behaviour and any previous history is important. Consider contacting other relevant people, such as the person's general practitioner, family members, close friends, significant others, care coordinators/case managers, treating psychiatrist or psychologist, school counsellors and other relevant health and welfare services who know the person. Where possible, previous documentation about the person should be accessed; for example, through the mental health triage service. Corroboration can also provide an opportunity to assess the family or support person's response to the situation and their willingness and capacity to care for and provide a protective environment for the person (NSW Department of Health, 2004).

It can be difficult when a patient does not allow a clinician to contact significant others. One way to circumvent this is to listen to the concerns of significant others without divulging information about the patient. In many jurisdictions concern about the risk to a patient outweighs confidentiality. Familiarity with the provisions of the Mental Health Act in regard to confidentiality is important.

SAFETY OF OTHERS

It is also important to determine whether the person's thoughts include homicide, infanticide or suicide with someone else. Ask the person if they have a partner or children, and have they thought of dying with them? This is particularly important where there are issues of custody or financial concerns, and in instances of postnatal depression or postnatal psychosis. Individuals who are psychotic should be asked about delusional beliefs regarding their children or other family members. For example, a patient with paranoid delusional beliefs that their family may be killed may decide it is preferable to kill their family before this occurs. In these instances, collaborative history is important to shed light on concerns the person may not raise in an interview.

INTOXICATION

Intoxication impedes a valid immediate assessment. If the potential for suicide is raised in an intoxicated person, they should be cared for in an appropriate and safe setting until a full assessment can be conducted (NSW Department of Health, 2004; Ravindranath et al., 2012). At times acute intoxication may be the primary cause of suicidal ideation, but at other times the intoxication will be a result of a suicide attempt (for example, a person consumes alcohol in order to build the 'courage' to complete the act). It is likely that some of the history gained when a patient is intoxicated will be inaccurate, as intoxicants have significant transient effects on a person's mental state that can interfere with an accurate assessment (Ryan et al., 2015).

SAFETY PLANNING

Safety planning is a prioritised list of strategies and sources of support that people can use to alleviate a suicidal crisis (Cole-King & Platt, 2017; Stanley & Brown, 2012). The main components of a safety plan include: reasons for living, recognising distress triggers and warning signs of an impending suicidal crisis; employing internal coping strategies (such as activities to lift their mood or calm or distract them); utilising social contacts in social settings as a means of distraction from suicidal thoughts; utilising family members or friends to help resolve the crisis; contacting mental health professionals or agencies; and restricting access to lethal means with a plan to create a safe environment.

The provision of a safety plan has become a key component of the approach to the suicidal person. The fundamental aim is to help a person in suicidal crisis *live with* being suicidal rather than *die from* being suicidal. Electronic versions are available as a web-based tool and as an app for smartphones (Beyond Blue). Safety planning is not a no-suicide contract with a patient (such as asking a patient to 'guarantee their safety'). It is erroneous to believe that such an action can actually prevent the patient from killing themselves. Health professionals may have a false sense of relief regarding a patient's suicide risk when they use a no-suicide contract. This may lower their vigilance with these patients. The use of such contracts may reflect clinicians' attempts to control the anxiety often experienced when treating patients at risk for suicide (Matarazzo et al., 2014).

With the increasing use of safety plans in the community, a paramedic may be able to discuss a pre-existing safety plan, or work on a new plan with the patient in order to co-create an effective way of managing the situation at that time (refer to the Beyond Blue safety app in the resource section of this chapter).

MEANS RESTRICTION

Access to lethal means of suicide is a significant risk factor across all age groups. Interventions that minimise the access to these means remain the most important form of primary prevention against suicide (Weber et al., 2017). If the means for suicide were less readily available, then suicidal individuals would be less able to make lethal impulsive suicide attempts (Lester, 2012). Restriction of lethal suicide methods is one of the most well-accepted interventions to reduce suicide. It should be addressed with every individual irrespective of perceptions of suicide risk (Large et al., 2017). Method substitution (using a different method other than the preferred) is rare. Suicidal crises are often shortlived and time-limited, so reducing access to lethal means (even temporarily) may prevent suicidal behaviour. Most individuals with suicidal ideation who are prevented from using their preferred method do not die by suicide (Ribeiro et al., 2013).

Medication should be prescribed in non-lethal quantities, and significant others, or the patient's pharmacy, family or carers, should be enlisted to help manage the amount of medication a suicidal individual has access to. Clinicians should always enquire as to the presence or access to firearms, and ask for police assistance in removing them from the home or preventing access at other locations. Awareness of local legislation regarding access to firearms is important. If a patient has made a suicide attempt by hanging or overdose, it is prudent to enlist the support of significant others to remove these means. The paramedic can play an important role in ensuring means have been removed, and this act alone may play a significant part in risk mitigation if considering a decision to leave someone at home.

MANAGEMENT

Having assessed an individual in a suicidal crisis, there are several options available to a paramedic. It is important to refer to the guidelines for the service you work within. Whenever in doubt it is important to discuss the case with colleagues or with supervisors.

1. **The individual is assessed to be able to remain at home** – This can occur when the patient's suicidal ideation does not involve planning, they are able to articulate reasons for living, they do not have any of the warning signs described, and collateral information does not indicate any planning or preparation to suicide or concerns that the individual is minimising their suicidal ideation. The individual has support that is readily available. If it is within working hours, consultation with the patient's general practitioner and any other healthcare providers (such as psychiatrist or psychologist) does not raise concerns. There should be a plan for how and when the individual will next access mental health assistance through their general practitioner or other healthcare provider (e.g. the next day). A safety plan should be completed with the individual.

2. **The individual is assessed as being able to remain in the care of a responsible adult** – The individual may have developed a plan but has not acquired the means and does not want to act on the plan. The points raised above also apply in this instance. The responsible adult should be made aware of how closely they are to monitor the individual, what action to take should they have any concerns (such as contacting emergency services, mental health crisis lines or taking the individual to an emergency department). As above, a safety plan should be completed with the individual and the responsible adult.

3. **The individual needs to be taken somewhere for care or further assessment** – The individual has suicidal ideation with a plan and has access to means, they are ambivalent about living or dying, they have few, or no, supports (or their supports do not feel able to provide care), they have prominent depression, hopelessness, helplessness, loneliness, feelings of being trapped, perceive themselves as a burden on others, or exhibit other warning signs. In this instance the individual requires further assessment by specialist mental health services. The least restrictive option should be considered, such as conveying the individual to an emergency department as a voluntary patient. Where the patient refuses further assessment, and there is concern about their potential for suicide, then conveying them under the local Mental Health Act should be considered. Australian jurisdictions have provisions for paramedics to transport individuals for further assessment in these instances. Familiarity with the Mental Health Act is important for paramedics.

CONCLUSION

Paramedics play a vital role in the assessment of individuals in a suicidal crisis in the community. An assessment is an opportunity to build therapeutic engagement and demonstrate compassion. It is important to take the individual's perspective about the lethality of their attempt or plan. The goal is to understand the circumstances that led to their suicidal crisis, the nature of their suicidal thoughts, their perception of the future, the degree of planning and preparation they have undertaken, and their ability to resist their suicidal thoughts. When in doubt about what action to take, it is useful to consult a superior or a local mental health crisis line. It is important to remember every assessment has the potential to save a life.

LINKS AND RESOURCES

- Suicide call-back service – free counselling for suicide prevention and mental health via telephone, online and video for anyone affected by suicidal thoughts, 24/7: https://www.suicidecallbackservice.org.au/
- Lifeline is a national charity providing all Australians experiencing a personal crisis with access to 24-hour crisis support and suicide prevention services: https://www.lifeline.org.au/
- Mensline provides free 24/7 help, support, referrals and counselling services for men via telephone, online and video: https://mensline.org.au/
- beyond blue support service: https://www.beyondblue.org.au/get-support/get-immediate-support
- beyond blue safety planning app Beyond Now: https://www.beyondblue.org.au/get-support/beyondnow-suicide-safety-planning

REFERENCES

Berman, A., Silverman, M., 2017. How to ask about suicide? A question in need of an empirical answer. Crisis 38 (4), 213–216.

Bolton, J., Gunnell, D., Turecki, G., 2015. Suicide risk assessment and intervention in people with mental illness. BMJ 351.

Bostwick, J., Pabbati, C., Geske, J., et al., 2016. Suicide attempt as a risk factor for completed suicide: even more lethal than we knew. Am. J. Psychiatry 173 (11), 1094–1100.

Busch, K., Fawcett, J., Jacobs, D., 2003. Clinical correlates of inpatient suicide. J. Clin. Psychiatry 64 (1), 14.

Cole-King, A., Lepping, P., 2010. Suicide mitigation: time for a more realistic approach. Br. J. Gen. Pract. 60 (570), e1–e3.

Cole-King, A., Platt, S., 2017. Suicide prevention for physicians: identification, intervention and mitigation of risk. Medicine (Baltimore) 45 (3), 131–134.

Cole-King, A., Green, G., Gask, L., et al., 2013. Suicide mitigation: a compassionate approach to suicide prevention. Adv. Psychiatr. Treat. 19 (4), 276–283.

Dazzi, T., Gribble, R., Wessely, S., et al., 2014. Does asking about suicide and related behaviours induce suicidal ideation? What is the evidence? Psychol. Med. 44 (16), 3361–3363.

Department of Health Victoria, 2010. Working With the Suicidal Person: Clinical practice guidelines for emergency departments and Mental Health Services. Mental Health, Drugs and Regions Branch, Victorian Government Department of Health, Melbourne.

Fowler, J., 2012. Suicide risk assessment in clinical practice: pragmatic guidelines for imperfect assessments. Psychotherapy (Chic.) 49 (1), 81.

Hawgood, J., De Leo, D., 2015. STARS: Screening Tool for Assessing Risk of Suicide. Griffith University, Brisbane.

Hawgood, J., De Leo, D., 2016. Suicide prediction – a shift in paradigm is needed. Crisis 37 (4), 251–255.

Jobes, D.A., 2012. The Collaborative Assessment and Management of Suicidality (CAMS): an evolving evidence-based clinical approach to suicidal risk. Suicide Life Threat. Behav. 42 (6), 640–653.

Large, M., Ryan, C., 2014a. Suicide risk assessment: myth and reality. Int. J. Clin. Pract. 68 (6), 679–681.

Large, M., Ryan, C., 2014b. Suicide risk categorisation of psychiatric inpatients: what it might mean and why it is of no use. Australas. Psychiatry 22 (4), 390–392.

Large, M., Ryan, C., Carter, G., et al., 2017. Can we usefully stratify patients according to suicide risk? BMJ 359.

Lester, D., 2012. Suicide prevention by lethal means restriction. In: Simon, R., Hales, R. (Eds.), The American Psychiatric Publishing Textbook of Suicide Assessment and Management. American Psychiatric Publishing, Arlington, VA.

Matarazzo, B., Homaifar, B., Wortzel, H., 2014. Therapeutic risk management of the suicidal patient: safety planning. J. Psychiatr. Pract. 20 (3), 220–224.

McDowell, A., Lineberry, T., Bostwick, J., 2011. Practical suicide-risk management for the busy primary care physician. Mayo Clin. Proc. 86 (8), 792–800.

Menon, V., 2013. Suicide risk assessment and formulation: an update. Asian J. Psychiatr. 6 (5), 430–435.

Mindframe, 2018. Facts and stats about suicide in Australia. Online. Available: http://www.mindframe-media.info/for-media/reporting-suicide/facts-and-stats 30 August 2018.

Morriss, R., Kapur, N., Byng, R., 2013. Assessing risk of suicide or self harm in adults. BMJ 347.

Mulder, R., Newton-Howes, G., Coid, J., 2016. The futility of risk prediction in psychiatry. Br. J. Psychiatry 209 (4), 271–272.

NSW Department of Health, 2004. Framework for Suicide Assessment and Management for NSW Health Staff. NSW Department of Health, North Sydney.

Pisani, A., Murrie, D., Silverman, M., 2016. Reformulating suicide risk formulation: from prediction to prevention. Acad. Psychiatry 40 (4), 623–629.

Ravindranath, D., Deneke, D., Riba, M., 2012. Emergency services. In: Simon, R., Hales, R. (Eds.), American Psychiatric Publishing Textbook of Suicide Assessment and Management. American Psychiatric Publishing, Arlington, VA.

Ribeiro, J., Bodell, L., Hames, J., et al., 2013. An empirically based approach to the assessment and management of suicidal behavior. J. Psychother. Integr. 23 (3), 207.

Rudd, M., 2006. The Assessment and Management of Suicidality. Professional Resource Press/Professional Resource Exchange, Florida.

Rudd, M., 2012. The clinical risk assessment interview. In: Simon, R., Hales, R. (Eds.), American Psychiatric Publishing Textbook of Suicide Assessment and Management. American Psychiatric Publishing, Arlington, VA.

Rudd, M., Berman, A., Joiner, T., et al., 2012. Warning signs for suicide. In: Shrivastava, A., Kimbrell, M., Lester, D. (Eds.), Suicide From a Global Perspective: Risk assessment and management. Nova Science Publishers, Hauppauge, NY.

Ryan, C., Large, M., Callaghan, S., 2013. Suicide risk assessment: where are we now? Med. J. Aust. 199 (8), 534.

Ryan, C., Large, M., Gribble, R., et al., 2015. Assessing and managing suicidal patients in the emergency department. Australas. Psychiatry 23 (5), 513–516.

Shea, S., 2009. Suicide assessment. Psychiatr. Times 26 (12), 1–6.

Shea, S., 2012. The interpersonal art of suicide assessment. In: Simon, R.R., Hales, R.E. (Eds.), The American Psychiatric Publishing Textbook of Suicide Assessment and Management. American Psychiatric Association, Arlington, VA.

Silverman, M., Berman, A., 2014. Suicide risk assessment and risk formulation part I: a focus on suicide ideation in assessing suicide risk. Suicide Life Threat. Behav. 44 (4), 420–431.

Simon, R., 2011. Preventing Patient Suicide: Clinical assessment and management. American Psychiatric Association, Washington DC.

Simon, R., 2012. Suicide risk assessment: gateway to treatment and management. In: Simon, R., Hales, R. (Eds.), American Psychiatric Publishing Textbook of Suicide Assessment and Management. American Psychiatric Association, Arlington, VA.

Sinclair, L., Leach, R., 2017. Exploring thoughts of suicide. BMJ 356, j1128.

Slade, T., Johnston, A., Teesson, M., et al., 2009. Mental Health of Australians 2: Report of the 2007 National Survey of Mental Health and Wellbeing. Department of Health and Ageing, Canberra.

Stanley, B., Brown, G., 2012. Safety planning intervention: a brief intervention to mitigate suicide risk. Cogn. Behav. Pract. 19 (2), 256–264.

Van Orden, K., Witte, T., Cukrowicz, K., et al., 2010. The interpersonal theory of suicide. Psychol. Rev. 117 (2), 575.

Weber, A., Michail, M., Thompson, A., et al., 2017. Psychiatric emergencies: assessing and managing suicidal ideation. Med. Clin. 101 (3), 553–571.

World Health Organization (WHO), 2016. Preventing Suicide: A global imperative. WHO, Geneva.

Caring for a person who has self-harmed

12

Lyza R. Helps

LEARNING OUTCOMES

By the end of this chapter you will:

- develop an understanding of the characteristics of non-suicidal self-injury (NSSI) and its management in the pre-hospital setting
- develop an understanding of the similarities and the differences between NSSI and intentional and suicidal self-harm (ISSH)
- explore and challenge common misconceptions about NSSI
- develop and explore knowledge in relation to the current treatments and therapies for people who self-harm
- explore and develop an understanding of risk assessments and management in the pre-hospital setting for people who self-harm
- explore and develop in the pre-hospital setting a plan for managing workplace stress, in relation to managing people who self-harm.

INTRODUCTION

'There are times when I look at my scars and see something else: I see a girl, just a girl, someone who was trying to cope with something horrible … something that should never have occurred. My scars show pain and suffering, but they also show my will to survive.'

Sophie

One of the key challenges in managing self-harm is the often problematic definitions of self-harm, and the complex relationship between non-suicidal self-injury (NSSI) and intentional and suicidal self-harm (ISSH). The main distinguishing factor is 'intent'; that is, injuries inflicted without an 'intent' to die. Non-suicidal self-harm can be amongst the most debilitating conditions, posing great challenges and great rewards with effective early intervention by workers in the pre-hospital setting. People who engage in NSSI experience significant stigma and possibly damaging responses from health professionals and the wider community (Robinson et al., 2016). The consequential harm from uncompassionate, unhelpful and often trivialising responses can be more damaging than the original injury, leading to 'an aversion to care seeking' and an increase in the risk of further, possibly lethal, self-harm. Individuals who inflict NSSI often also exhibit ISSH, which further complicates the picture, especially for emergency workers in the pre-hospital setting (Robinson et al., 2016).

Self-harm can refer to a range of behaviours an individual does to themselves to cause harm, regardless of motive or if there was suicidal intent (Robinson et al., 2016). Studies such as the Non-Suicidal Self-Injury Disorder Scale (NSSIDS), used by Victor and colleagues (2016) indicate that specific measures of the characteristics of non-suicidal self-harm can be ascertained, and do occur independently of 'other' types of disorder (Victor et al., 2016). While the reasons behind self-harm can be complex and are often diverse, the behaviour often occurs in response to intense emotional pain, psychological and emotional distress, overwhelming negative feelings and thoughts, and a sense of hopelessness (Robinson et al., 2016). While self-harm can be accompanied by suicidal thoughts, often there will be no suicidal intent.

Significant changes occur in adolescence, including biological, neurological and emotional, coupled with emerging experiences of independence, work, and romantic and sexual relationships. Adolescence is a time of significant tension, increased independence and additional responsibilities which may overwhelm, especially where affect regulation and poor coping skills or previous abuse are present (Shaffer & Jacobson, 2009, cited in Robinson et al., 2016). Adolescence is also a peak period of first onset for mental illness and an increase in risk-taking behaviours (AIHW, 2018b). Self-harming behaviours often begin or co-occur with these significant events (Robinson et al., 2016).

Negative events, trauma or other stressors experienced over time may lead to engaging in self-harming behaviours where more helpful coping skills are unavailable (Robinson et al., 2016).

A 2013 Australian survey of 13,600 people aged 15–19 years found 71% of those with a 'diagnosable mental illness' and 29% of those without a diagnosable mental illness, identified 'coping with stress' as their number one health concern (Ivancic et al., 2014). Further analysis of the survey data found that young people with a probable serious mental illness were two-and-a-half times more likely to indicate that coping with stress was a major factor in leading to NSSI (Ivancic et al., 2014). Self-harm often correlates with a range of mental health problems in later life (Klonsky et al., 2015), with Robinson and others finding that '11–16-year-olds who engaged in self-poisoning were much more likely to be diagnosed with a mental illness in adulthood' (2016, p. 6). In another study this correlation showed an almost 'fourfold risk of being diagnosed with major depression, and three times the risk of being diagnosed with an anxiety disorder' (Goldman-Mellor et al., 2014, p. 121). Early research (Favazza, 1996) suggested that for some people self-harming may have an addictive element that could be related to an endorphin release. Later this led to additional research that tended to support these findings (Bresin & Gordon, 2013).

Robinson and colleagues (2016) reported that young people who engaged in self-harm have higher levels of systemic inflammation, an older 'heart age' than those that do not self-harm, and are twice as likely to meet diagnostic criteria for a metabolic syndrome colleagues. Self-harm may also be associated with motor vehicle accidents. Robinson and colleagues (2016) also reported on studies that have shown that among newly licensed drivers, those who self-harmed were significantly more likely to be involved in a serious vehicle crash early in their driving life. Self-harm occurs in all age groups, transcending socio-economic conditions, educational achievement and gender. NSSI is often not the problem, but rather an insight into other severe emotional distress.

CASE STUDY
Sophie

You are dispatched at 10.00 p.m. to a residential address for a 17-year-old female who has a cut to her left foreman, the actual extent of the injury not known at this time. Sophie and her one-year-old daughter (Taylah) have been staying with a cousin (Maree, also 17), who made the call to emergency services, at the government housing commission home they share. According to Maree, Sophie had her boyfriend stay over the previous night and they were all drinking heavily and having 'a good time', but earlier in the evening today, around 7.00 p.m., a fight broke out between Sophie and her boyfriend, leading to yelling, screaming and eventually items being broken. The argument appeared to be about 'money'. The boyfriend left the house at the time, saying '*I won't be back*' and that he was '*tired of all of this*'. The dispatcher could not ascertain from Maree either the extent of the injury or the whereabouts of the one-year-old child.

At 10.25 p.m., you arrive at the residence and note that the front door is wide open. There are lights on throughout the house, and a neighbour reports they have called the police. They also say they saw Maree put the infant in a car seat and leave less than five minutes ago. On entering the property, which is quiet, there are multiple items spread on the floors throughout, including children's toys, nappies, various items of clothing and several empty and broken bottles. To the left is the dining room, and you can see a mattress without bedding against a wall. Sophie is sitting against the lounge suite nearby with her head in her hands, crying uncontrollably. There is a pair of scissors next to her and a small amount of blood dripping down her arm. There appears to be no one else in the house. The crew attempt to engage Sophie to find out what has occurred, but Sophie is not responding and continues to cry, muttering to herself between sobs. After 10 minutes of observing and trying to talk to Sophie, she eventually responds, saying '*I cut myself with these*', handing the scissors next to her to the paramedic without any aggression. You note that there are multiple, horizontal 'old scars' on her arms and thighs. Sophie continues to talk and allows the crew to examine her arm: there is evidence of continued small pulsing blood loss from a vertical cut that extends from her wrist to the middle section of her forearm, approximately 4 cm long.

Vital signs
- Glasgow Coma Score: 15
- Oxygen saturations: 96%
- Respiratory rate: 26
- Heart rate: 110 strong/regular/pounding
- Blood pressure: 95/50
- Electrocardiograph: Sinus tachycardia
- Blood sugar level: 4.1 mmol
- Pain score: 3/10

Wound assessment

4 cm 'superficial' vertical laceration extends from mid-left forearm to 3 cm above the wrist.
    Evidence of active minor bleeding (non-arterial >30 ml, approx.)

Other observations

Evidence of multiple, horizontal scars (fully healed) likely from previous self-harm.

At 10.55 p.m. the police arrive and inform you that they have spoken with Maree, who has gone to stay at a friend's house with the infant. They have heard from another crew that the boyfriend has been located at his own home and was asleep when they arrived. Upon questioning, the boyfriend reported to police that *'she does this all the time, I'm sick of it. Her dad used to beat and molest her, and she ran away and lived on the streets'*. He also reports he *'can't do this anymore'* and won't be returning. The police are satisfied that Sophie is willing to receive support from the paramedics, that the situation is under control, and there are no safety risks to the crew. The police leave the residence after confirming that Sophie has agreed to go to hospital.

MISCONCEPTIONS ABOUT SELF-HARM

'People who self-harm only do so to get attention'

The Australian National Epidemiological Study of Self-Injury (Martin et al., 2010, in the 'ANESSI Report') states that 83% of the respondents who self-injured in the four weeks prior to the survey did not receive or seek medical or psychological attention. The lack of help seeking reflects the secrecy of the behaviour, and suggests that the belief that people self-injure to get attention and manipulate others is a clear fallacy (Martin et al., 2010). Evidence from the Australian Institue for Health and Welfare suggests that 6–8% of young people aged 15–24 years engage in self-harm in any 12-month period (AIHW, 2014). Lifetime prevalence rates of self-harm have been estimated at 17% of females and 12% of males aged 15–19 years, and 24% of females and 18% of males aged 20–24, although it is acknowledged that under-reporting is common, with many never seeking help (AIHW, 2017).

'It's no big deal, the injuries are not that serious anyway, it wastes hospital resources'

Headspace (n.d.) and the ABS (2016) estimate that only 13% of young people who self-harm will present for hospital treatment. Suicide and self-harm combined account for considerable levels of mortality and morbidity among young people (Martin et al., 2010). In young people, self-harm is the seventh-leading disease burden in Australia, which may lead to premature death, substantial disability and interruptions to healthy life years (ABS, 2016; Headspace, n.d.).

PREVALENCE OF SELF-HARM

To understand NSSI, one must also understand just how widespread NSSI is in the community. People who engage in NSSI and then report the injury are thought to be only a small proportion of the total numbers of people who engage in self-harm. Statistics specifically for NSSI are also difficult to extrapolate as a single data group, as the data often remains embedded with ISSH and suicide data. Other factors affecting a comprehensive understanding of the problem is that many people who self-harm never seek treatment, or the nature of the injuries are not recorded as self-harm. The case study 'Sophie' highlights this fact, with Sophie not previously reporting her numerous self-injuries.

Additionally, self-harm by misadventure always remains a controversial addition to NSSI, as it often occurs during a time when inappropriate risk taking may be enmeshed with developmental milestones such as the adolescent period. Having stated these limitations, we will begin by exploring the global prevalence rates, followed by the Australian picture.

KEY POINTS

- There is limited accurate data on NSSI, hence there is a huge variation in reported data.
- NSSI is under-reported, and there is difficulty separating NSSI data from trauma and overdose records at the emergency department triage.
- Reluctance to seek help for self-harm delays treatment and early intervention.
- Stigma and misunderstanding of NSSI contributes to delays in care and support for those who self-harm.

GLOBAL PREVALENCE RATES

Global prevalence rates of NSSI reported in various samples indicate ranges from 11% to 38% in samples of university students (Dudgeon et al., 2014; Taliaferro & Muehlenkamp, 2017) and from 13.2% to 46.5% in samples of high-school students (Baetens et al., 2014; Taliaferro & Muehlenkamp, 2017), although these authors acknowledge that these rates are very likely to be a 'gross underestimation' of the actual rates in the community. The case study 'Sophie' highlights this problem, with the crew identifying a *significant number* of previous cuts that until that night had gone unreported.

AUSTRALIAN PREVALENCE RATES

In Australia, prevalence rates are also difficult to cite due to the collection of self-harm data being embedded with those of suicide and suicidal self-harm rates, and the under-reporting of self-harm in the community. Data is also difficult to extrapolate from hospital records, as the person's presentation may be recorded as adult trauma, general mental health related or suicide attempt, leading to the ongoing confusion that exists between NSSI and ISSH (ABS, 2016). Martin and others (2010) found that lifetime data rates the overall prevalence of self-injury as 8.1% in the community; that is, approximately 200,000 people each year. Higher prevalence rates were seen in females (8.9%) than males (7.3%). The study identified that the four most common methods of self-injury were cutting, scratching, hitting the body or a part of the body on a hard surface, and punching or hitting oneself. Over 50% of respondents claimed that they were driven by a desire to manage emotions, and over 25% self-injured to punish themselves for perceived wrongdoing (Martin et al., 2010). What the studies do suggest, though, is agreement in the literature that high prevalence rates for self-harming behaviours need to be further explored and understood (Victor et al., 2016).

ECONOMIC AND PERSONAL COSTS OF SELF-HARM

NSSI can have a significant effect on social engagement, friendships and intimate relationships, as well as on education and employment, while loss of income via unemployment and stigma is also a considerable personal cost (Long, 2018). A report for the Australian Federal Government (Mendoza, 2009) cited that along with devastating personal losses to the person, there were significant economic costs to the national health budget, estimated to be in the range of $133.3 million annually. According to hospital admission/separation data in the Australian public health system, the cost for every admission was on average $3542 for each patient (AIHW, 2017).

SELF-HARM AND CONTAGION

Contact with others who engage in acts of self-harm (friends or family) is known to lead to an increase in the risk of self-harm to others in the group, especially in young people (Hawton et al., 2012; Taliaferro & Muehlenkamp, 2017). Family members and friends who self-harm can at times have an almost cult-like following with younger people. With hundreds of websites discussing new methods, ideas for beginners, and similar activities, younger and younger children are engaging with the notion of a sense of 'community' within these followings, with many falling prey to contagion (Davis & Pimpleton-Gray, 2017; Hawton et al., 2012).

DEFINING AND ASSESSING NON-SUICIDAL SELF-HARM

The term 'self-harm' is usually taken to mean an act of deliberate but non-suicidal harm, inflicted upon the self to regulate affective (emotional) distress. Previously thought to be associated almost exclusively with borderline personality disorder, it is now generally accepted that self-harm occurs in a much wider context (Zetterqvist, 2015). The *Diagnostic and Statistical Manual of Mental Disorders* (American Psychiatric Association, 2013) currently outlines the potential criteria for non-suicidal self-injury disorder (NSSID) to be defined as a 'disorder' that requires further study (Shaffer & Jacobson, 2009; Zetterqvist, 2015). Table 12.3 details the criteria that will be included in the *DSM-5* update and almost certainly in the *DSM-6* (Albión et al., 2013; Zetterqvist, 2015). This table discusses the proposed diagnostic criteria for non-suicidal self-injury disorder (NSSID), of note the criteria include an ongoing preoccupation with self-harm (which would be an important addition to screening questions in pre-hospital assessment) and that the self-harm is utilised to manage emotional states, as per the case study of 'Sophie', supporting previous findings from research (American Psychiatric Association, 2013; Zetterqvist, 2015).

Tables 12.1, 12.2 and 12.3 highlight considerations for assessing self-harm to determine whether it is likely to be ISSH rather than NSSI. It is important to note that this assessment forms a small part of the overall clinical presentation and does not indicate a permanent or fixed state, so it is vital for the paramedic to continue a dynamic (continual) assessment.

FACTORS CONTRIBUTING TO SELF-HARM

Sociological and psychological factors in NSSI are diverse and complicated. There is a lack of literature that examines the sociological and functional factors that relate to NSSI. Though requiring more intensive research, two consistent themes do emerge across the literature: those of 'intrapersonal' factors (occurring within the person) and 'interpersonal' factors (occurring within the community/people around the person).

Table 12.1 Self-harm – Common Presentations

Examples of Self-harm (Adapted From Finkelstein et al., 2015)

- Cutting (e.g. scratching with sharp objects, knives, ice picks, shards of glass)
- Burning (e.g. gas stoves, fires, cigarettes and cigarette lighters)
- Inserting objects (e.g. pins, needles, splinters of wood)
- Ingestion of foreign bodies (e.g. razor blades)
- Rubbing against objects or surfaces (e.g. glass, wood or sharp surfaces)
- Hair pulling (e.g. twisting and pulling out clumps)
- Asphyxiation (e.g. use of rope progressively tightened, or lamp cords, belts, etc., with no intention to die)
- Suffocating/asphyxiating
- Interfering with wound healing, pulling off scabs or rubbing household cleaners into the wound
- Banging the head against objects
- Self-drowning, holding face under water
- Deliberate self-neglect
- Deliberate starvation (not associated with anorexia nervosa or body image/body dysmorphia)
- Withholding medication or other treatments

Continued ...

Table 12.1 Self-harm – Common Presentations *continued*

Self-harm by 'Misadventure'

Debate is widespread about whether to include deliberate risk taking where self-harm is often an 'expected' outcome. Reasons often cited for this debate relate to the development of human behaviour through what would be considered 'normal young person's development'. This is where increased risk taking is often embedded within the expectations of developmental milestones, as an effort to increase self-direction, conflict with parental (authority) figures and a desire to express individuality.

- Substance abuse – ingestion of alcohol or other substances that are either knowingly causing harm or believed to be likely to lead to self-injury
- Non-culturally-based body modifications, e.g. tattoos, piercings and deliberate scarring, often performed under unhygienic conditions
- Driving dangerously
- Sexual promiscuity
- Withholding or overuse of medications or other treatments
- Engaged in fighting or other aggressive activities with the intention of getting hurt

Key Points

- Assess for more than one type of self-harm and consider indirect injuries and misadventure.
- It is possible that you cannot see some injuries, with their either being covered by clothing, or perhaps being internal.
- Self-harm may not actually be physical, but could be an action to deliberately harm their reputation.
- Assess the 'motivation' to self-harm.
- Misadventure could be a deliberate attempt at self-harm or increasing the likelihood/risk of harm.
- Misadventure could be caused by other factors, e.g. mania or psychosis.

Example Questions

'Sophie, besides the cutting that you have told us about, are there any other ways you have hurt yourself in the past? How often have you done that?'

'Are there times when you do dangerous or risky things that might cause harm to you but where you just don't care?'

'Sophie, can you tell me about what you think might be the reasons you do these things?'

Adapted from: Hawton et al., 2012 and Whitlock et al., 2014

Table 12.2 Characteristics of Non-suicidal Self-harm and Suicidal Self-harm

Characteristics	Self-harm Behaviour	Suicidal Behaviour
Intention	To relieve emotional pain; to live and feel better Clearly state that they weren't intending to kill themselves, or that they just want the pain to stop Likely to be less severe injury	To put an end to unbearable pain; to die Clearly express they want to die, anger at being interrupted Likely to be more severe injury
Method	Thought to be non-lethal, i.e. shallow cutting, burning, etc. Haemodynamically stable Superficial injury (though may inadvertently injure themselves more seriously)	Lethal or thought to be lethal, e.g. hanging or large ingestion May be haemodynamically unstable May be more severe or a more potentially lethal method
Potential to be fatal	Unlikely to be fatal and perceived by the person as non-fatal Usually state they didn't intend to harm themselves to a point where the potential for irreversible harm or death is the outcome, no intent	Highly likely or seen by the person as likely to be fatal Chose this method as a direct intent to die
Frequency	Frequent, repeated multiple small scars evident, multiple healing small cuts, burns, etc. States they have done this many times, no expectation of death or serious harm	Most likely to be a single or occasional attempt Expected to die, states intent clearly, more lethal attempt
Discovery	NSSI is often secretive and planned so that it doesn't come to someone's attention Other NSSI is very public, where a person wants to make their distress known in a very public way	Often suicide attempts are planned in a way to avoid being discovered; however, others may be impulsive and not well thought out Note also that people can change their mind after an attempt and notify someone, but this does not mean that they did not have suicidal intent at the time

Adapted from: Government of Western Australia, 2017

Table 12.3 Criteria for Non-suicidal Self-injury Disorder

Diagnostic Criteria for NSSI	Pre-hospital Assessment/ History Taking
Criterion A In the last year, the individual has, on five or more days, engaged in intentional self-inflicted damage to the surface of their body of a sort likely to induce bleeding, bruising or pain (e.g. cutting, burning, stabbing, hitting and excessive rubbing), with the expectation that the injury will lead to only minor or moderate physical harm (i.e. there is no suicidal intent). Note: The absence of suicidal intent has either been stated by the individual or can be inferred by the individual's repeated engagement in a behaviour that the individual knows, or has learned, is not likely to result in death.	**Key points** Assess for suicidal intent **Example questions** *'Sophie, what did you think would happen when you were cutting yourself? Were you trying to kill yourself tonight?'* *'Sophie, I've/we've noticed some scars on your arms, have you cut yourself before?'*
Criterion B The individual engages in the self-injurious behaviour with one or more of the following expectations: (1) to obtain relief from a negative feeling or cognitive state (2) to resolve an interpersonal difficulty (3) to induce a positive feeling state. Note: The desired relief or response is experienced during or shortly after the self-injury, and the individual may display patterns of behaviour, suggesting a dependence on repeatedly engaging in it.	**Key points** Assess desired response from the NSSI **Example questions** *'Sophie, what was going through your mind, just before you cut yourself?'* (assessing antecedents, triggers) *'Sophie, after you cut yourself, what did you feel?'* (assessing effect) *'Sophie, can you tell me about why you have cut yourself?'* (assessing for purpose and outcome)
Criterion C The intentional self-injury is associated with at least one of the following: (1) interpersonal difficulties or negative feelings or thoughts, such as depression, anxiety, tension, anger, generalised distress, or self-criticism, occurring in the period immediately prior to the self-injurious act (2) prior to engaging in the act, a period of preoccupation with the intended behaviour that is difficult to control (3) thinking about self-injury that occurs frequently, even when it is not acted upon.	**Key points** Assess triggers, cognitions (thoughts), frequency **Example questions** *'Sophie, how often do you think about hurting yourself?'* *'Are there times when you think about hurting yourself but don't actually do it?'* *'Sophie, are there emotions that you feel overwhelmed by? Do you have other ways of coping with these?'*

Table 12.3 Criteria for Non-Suicidal Self-Injury Disorder *continued*

Diagnostic Criteria for NSSI	Pre-hospital Assessment/History Taking
Criterion D The behaviour is not socially sanctioned (e.g. body piercing, tattooing, part of a religious or cultural ritual) and is not restricted to picking a scab or nail biting.	
Criterion E The behaviour or its consequences cause clinically significant distress or interference in interpersonal, academic or other important areas of functioning.	**Key points** Assess level of distress and social impact **Example question** 'Sophie, does hurting yourself prevent you from doing other things, like going to work or doing social activities?'
Criterion F The behaviour does not occur exclusively during psychotic episodes, delirium, substance intoxication or substance withdrawal. In individuals with a neurodevelopmental disorder, the behaviour is not part of a pattern of repetitive stereotypes. The behaviour is not better explained by another mental disorder or medical condition, e.g. psychotic disorder, autism spectrum disorder or intellectual disability.	**Key points** Assess for depression, suicidal intent and other possible disorders.

Adapted from DSM-5 (American Psychiatric Association, 2013)

Intrapersonal factors that have been connected to NSSI include emotional (affect) dys-regulation and anti-dissociation (that is, NSSI is used as a strategy to avoid dissociative feelings), while interpersonal factors include interpersonal influences (e.g. family and social relationships) and peer bonding. Individuals with impaired intrapersonal functions, such as impaired emotional regulation, low self-esteem, and lowered resilience and self-efficacy are more likely to benefit from interventions that focus on affect regulation, often requiring intensive treatment and significant risk management. These individuals are significantly more likely to progress from NSSI to ISSH in the future. Individuals for whom interpersonal factors are prominent may benefit from interventions that focus on developing effective interpersonal skills (Klonsky et al., 2015).

CRITICAL REFLECTION

Reflecting on the case study of 'Sophie', examine the evidence for:
- interpersonal factors (occurring around the person)
- intrapersonal factors (occurring within the person).

Which factors appear to feature more prominently?

What questions might you like to ask Sophie in order to clarify or explore these factors?

Further studies (Hawton et al., 2012; Klonsky et al., 2013) indicate that sociological factors and stressors that are known to be associated with NSSI include:

- family breakdown or conflict (interpersonal)
- relationship problems (intra- and interpersonal)
- family/friends' history of self-harm, contagion effect (inter- and intrapersonal)
- disempowering and invalidating relationships (interpersonal)
- being bullied (interpersonal)
- school or work problems (interpersonal)
- alcohol and drug abuse (intra- and interpersonal)
- past trauma, neglect and/or physical, emotional or sexual abuse (intra- and interpersonal)
- homelessness (intra- and interpersonal)
- disconnection from society (intra- and interpersonal)
- lacking supportive networks/sense of belonging (interpersonal)
- domestic violence in the home (interpersonal) (AIHW, 2018b)
- poor responses by health professionals (interpersonal).

Hawton and colleagues (2012) go on to discuss psychological factors, which they found included:

- tendency towards aggression and/or violence as a primary means of solving conflict
- low self-esteem
- impulsivity, particularly with alcohol consumption
- poor coping skills
- poor problem-solving skills
- emotion dysregulation
- a previous history of self-harm, in the context of psychological distress with low tolerance traits, and affect dysregulation
- existing/emerging mental illness
- poor ability to express or name emotions
- perfectionism traits.

While self-harm remains a significant problem in the general population, within younger populations there are particular high-risk groups:

- people with a mental illness (including personality disorders)
- people of Aboriginal and Torres Strait Islander (ATSI) backgrounds
- young people in immigration or juvenile detention
- young people in out-of-home care
- people living in rural and remote areas
- young people who are lesbian, gay, bisexual, transgender, queer or intersex (LGBTQI).

CRITICAL REFLECTION

Reflecting upon the case study of 'Sophie', examine the evidence for:
- sociological factors
- psychological factors.

How would this information assist workers in the pre-hospital setting?
How would the accurate documentation and handover of this information assist the staff in the emergency department?

CRITICAL REFLECTION

Using the case study 'Sophie', detail your mental state assessment, with a particular focus on the presenting symptoms /presentation and the biological, sociological and psychological factors you would note to hand over at triage.

From your assessment, write your patient care record (PCR). Include your primary and secondary assessment and the key points you would consider for handover at the emergency department.

PRESENTATIONS OF SELF-HARM

Table 12.1 presents some of the more common presentations of self-harm likely to come to the attention of pre-hospital workers, along with some of the less common methods for consideration.

Clinically, self-harm occurs in a range of mental illnesses (Klonsky et al., 2013); however, in this context self-harm can be seen as an indicator of the level of distress, or of the potential severity of the illness, as opposed to the central feature of the disorder (Klonsky et al., 2015). Glazebrook and others (2015) found that self-harm may be used:

- to deal with negative emotions, pain, tension, loneliness
- as a punishment, either for real events or where they perceived to be at fault
- to feel *alive* or *real*, i.e to combat feelings of numbness/dissociation
- to have a sense of control of their life when they don't otherwise feel in control
- to attempt to attract care and support when they are unable to use words.

CRITICAL REFLECTION

You have identified several behaviours in a patient who you are concerned might be extreme risk taking as an act of self-harm (e.g. reckless driving, sexual promiscuity). How would you differentiate between self-harm caused by mania, psychosis or misadventure (as an act of harm)?

PROTECTIVE FACTORS THAT MAY POTENTIALLY REDUCE THE RISK OF SELF-HARM

Societal protective factors:

- secure parental attachment and warmth (Glazebrook et al., 2015)
- social connectedness or a sense of belonging (Taliaferro & Muehlenkamp, 2017)
- cultural identification and connection (Robinson et al., 2016).

Personal/individual protective factors:

- emotional intelligence (Glazebrook et al., 2015)
- a problem/solution focus rather than emotion-oriented coping style (McMahon et al., 2013)
- personality factors, including an understanding and acknowledgment of personal strengths, hope, future plans
- team sports and connections to community.

CRITICAL REFLECTION

Utilising the case study 'Sophie':
- what is the importance of assessing for protective factors in the person, even after the self-harm has occurred?
- what are the identifiable protective factors in the case study?

ASSESSMENT AND HISTORY TAKING – AN OVERVIEW

This section of the chapter brings together key points to consider when arriving on scene, and, along with your previous reflective exercises, brings together professional knowledge (theory) with professional practice (clinical activities). A mental health assessment by paramedics is multifaceted and should include the following:

- scene awareness, presence of blood, other persons, exits
- danger – initial impressions, observations of behaviour/body language/conversation and how the person is relating to the world
- pause and plan – look, listen and watch as you approach
- response
- airway
- breathing
- circulation
- disability
- treatment and intervention
- dynamic risk assessment – a core component of any attendance considers 1. the workers, 2. any children present, 3. the person, and 4. other people

- mental state examination
- collateral information (from witnesses, support people, other agencies)
- transporting the person (if required)
- documentation.

On attending a scene such as the one above, there are occasions where it may be difficult to assess whether the presenting symptom of 'self-harm' may be only the surface reaction to a deeper issue/illness or assault. It is not uncommon to receive the call-out for self-harm only to find out the person has been assaulted (AIHW, 2018a), or is acutely floridly psychotic, profoundly depressed or otherwise seriously unwell. It is *vital* not to assume that it is a simple case of self-harm, with a minor injury.

QUESTIONS TO CONSIDER WHEN FIRST ATTENDING AN NSSI CASE

- Does the patient look unwell? Are they breathing? Is there any cyanosis? Excessive bleeding? Is there a threat to the limb due to severed arteries, veins or nerves? Consider and review what you see. Rapidly determine whether the formal primary survey is required. If unsure, it is always best to assume that the patient requires a primary survey.
- Is the person responding? Do they answer questions? Are they crying, upset, angry? If they are talking, crying or responding, then airway is intact?
- Are they seated, pacing or lying down?
- What is the colour of the injured limb?

(Adapted from Ambulance Victoria, 2018)

Pause-and-plan moment

When people are distressed (crying and not responding directly to you), continue to talk quietly to the person, use rapport-building questions and actions.

> '*Sophie, we would like to help you, can we offer you a blanket?*' (may decrease anxiety, protect dignity).
> '*Sophie, we are concerned, you look really upset, can we come in? We would like to help*' (ask for permission to approach as this builds rapport).
> '*Sophie, we are just wondering about your daughter: is she being taken care of tonight? What is her name? How old is she?*' (assessing the safety of others, builds rapport, may place the focus of conversation on a protective factor rather than the stress).

Pausing and taking time on approach (where immediate loss of life is not likely), provides an opportunity for workers in the pre-hospital setting to discuss likely treatment scenarios and establish a plan of action. Ideally, these discussions should be openly held in front of the patient to allow their input. Possible suggestions for this discussion include:

'Sophie, we are just talking about how best to help you tonight. We would like to come over there and have a closer look at your arm, and we would like to think about taking you to hospital so you can receive additional help – what are your thoughts about this?' (rapport-building skill).

Ambulance Victoria's (2018) clinical practice guidelines suggest that during the pause-and-plan moment, paramedics should consider and discuss differential diagnoses. This is helpful to prevent possible errors in the plan of action by incorrectly focusing on one diagnosis to the exclusion of all others.

General principles during assessment of self-harm include:

- Establish a therapeutic relationship using empathy, openness, acceptance and avoiding prejudice.
- Assess the extent of the injury and initiate treatment.
- Encourage a sense of hope for the future.
- Explore the reasons and meanings of the self-harm, including intent.
- Clarify current stressors (acute and chronic).
- Assess the mental state.
- Obtain a thorough history where possible, including collateral information.
- Monitor and record 'dynamic risk'.
- Complete a primary survey.

Specifically, as part of the primary/initial survey, assess the severity of the self-harm and if there is any risk to airway, breathing or circulation. Assess for hypovolemic shock and possible changes in consciousness. Be aware of any hidden injuries or internal injuries that the person may have. The establishment of rapport and the approach is essential to be able to gain vital sign observations and to obtain the history, which will assist with assessing for hidden or internal injuries and the level of risk and intent behind the self-harm.

Mental state examination

(Referring to the case of 'Sophie', and providing general considerations in cases of self-harm.)

Appearance: Describe what they are wearing, how they look: unkempt, clean, dirty? Do they look their stated age? Does the clothing seem appropriate to the weather? (Note, it is not uncommon for people who self-harm to wear clothing that hides their scars or injuries.) Describe also the environment in your broader assessment: while this is not their actual 'mental state', the environment will provide a lot of clues to Sophie's behaviour (examples include a disorganised environment, poor evidence of self-care, diminished resources, chaotic environment, all of which are evident in the case study).

Behaviour: Explore what Sophie is 'actually' doing. Describe what you see, but don't try to interpret at this point, e.g. sitting on the floor, knees drawn up to the chest, crying and sobbing, not responding to questions (initial). People who self-harm may be agitated, pacing and threatening (more likely in suicidal ideation), or withdrawn and upset (more likely in NSSI).

Conversation: Include thought flow and content, general themes.

Affect: Do they appear, happy, sad, depressed, anxious? Describe *your impression* of their emotional state, their mood.

Mood: What do they state their mood is? Describe what the patient says it is. In the case of self-harm, the person is often upset, crying or distressed by a specific preceding event.

Perception: Are they reporting hallucinations? Do they appear to be responding to someone that you can't see? Are they saying odd things? Are they expressing delusional content, etc.? Does their language/speech make sense? Can you follow it?

Cognition: Orientation to time/place, place/person. (Note if they are talking and responding to questions approximately, if the information makes sense – there is no need at this point to ask formal questions.) You may need to defer when the person fails to respond. Be clear: say you are unable to assess if they don't respond.

Insight: In the case of Sophie, insight is not present. People who deliberately self-harm rarely have insight about the potential complications of their actions, e.g. are often oblivious to the risks of infection, tetanus, accidental severing of main arteries and veins, or nerve damage. Note: if they are aware of these, it is likely that the injury is related to intentional suicidal thoughts – consider as a suicidal act.

Judgment: Always impaired if alcohol or other drugs are involved. High levels of stress and emotion can also impair one's judgment. (Examples in Sophie's case, evidence of alcohol, broken beer bottles, third-party confirmation of drinking and arguing.)

Engagement/Rapport: May be superficial (e.g. they cooperate), or perhaps may be well established when the person provides more personal/intimate information, talks freely and agrees with treatment plan.

DIFFERENTIAL DIAGNOSES

Suicide attempt

See the prior discussion on the difference between non-suicidal self-harm and suicidal ideation and attempt. If in doubt or the patient will not engage, assume it is a suicide attempt and manage the primary life-threatening concerns and the management of the emotional distress associated with a suicide attempt.

Other mental health presentations

When considering differential diagnosis or co-occurring conditions, other defined mental illnesses need to be considered when assessing someone who has self-harmed. For example, the incidence of depression and anxiety in association or as a prime cause of non-suicidal self-harm is significant, and the person may show signs which need to be acknowledged and are critical to your risk assessment as a pre-hospital clinician. Other mental illnesses which can be the basis for self-harming behaviour are personality disorders, psychosis and substance use.

Medical or organic causes

Delirium can lead to the incidence of self-harm and often can be associated with marked changes in cognition and behaviour (see Chapter 8, Part 2).

Family violence/assault or rape

It is not uncommon that NSSI is a visible demonstration of a much larger issue, distress or illness. It is important to consider whether there is a history or current issue with family violence. It is not uncommon for younger women and men to deny that the current presenting injury is related to family violence (AIHW, 2018a).

Sexual assaults, likewise, may be initially denied, and self-injury may be a response to sexual assault, particularly when a known person was involved (AIHW, 2018a).

ASSESSMENT OF RISK

Dynamic risk assessment in people who self-harm

Recognising the dynamic (constantly changing) level of risk at a scene where someone has self-harmed requires the crew to be vigilant for 'red flags'. These are signs that the person's situation or actions are more likely to lead to intentional suicide attempts or higher lethality attempts (Whitlock et al., 2014). These 'red flags' could include:

- previous self-harm incidents, particularly when the injuries are becoming more serious
- younger age
- suicidal ideation
- family violence, sexual or physical abuse
- poor engagement with services or family
- homelessness
- drug and alcohol abuse, which increases impulsivity
- impulse control disorders
- diagnosis of comorbid mental illness.

Ask, observe, check!

- **Means:** Do they have available means (over-the-counter medication, prescribed medication, cutting implements, etc.)? Ask: *'Sophie, do you have any medications? Other drugs? What have you used in the past to cut yourself?'*
- **Methods:** How do they intend to do harm to themselves? With what? When? How many times have they done this before? Ask: *'Sophie, how have you hurt yourself before? How often do you do this?'*

- **Plans:** How advanced is the planning? Have they gathered the needed means? Have they given away personal items?
- **Intent:** Did they intend to kill themselves? What were they doing this for?
- **Thoughts:** Note any odd or bizarre thoughts, identify antecedents (triggers or pre-existing situations that may be the basis for the self-harming or associated emotional pain). Did something happen just before they harmed themselves?
- **Support:** Who do they live with? Do they consider this person supportive? What services are they involved with?
- **History:** Have they harmed themselves before? How often? What with? Were they taken to hospital before? How many times?
- **Impulsivity:** Do they have conduct disorders (younger age)? Frequent impulsive injuries? Do they state an inability to control their self-harm?
- **Drug and alcohol factors:** Essential to check: have they been drinking, smoking cannabis or taking other illicit drugs?
- **Protective factors:** '*Sophie, have there been times when you have thought about harming (or killing) yourself but you didn't? What stopped you?*'

Adapted from (Whitlock et al., 2014)

CRITICAL REFLECTION

Reflect on the case study 'Sophie':
- Make notes about each identifiable risk factor, using the above points.
- Identify the priorities in managing the scene.
- Define 'dynamic risk assessment'. Why is this important in the pre-hospital setting?

TRANSPORTING THE PERSON WITH SELF-HARM, FAMILY VIOLENCE OR SEXUAL ASSAULT

- Assess the injury and attend as needed to the dressing of the wound, remain vigilant but matter-of-fact. Focus on the person, don't over-focus on the injury (if it is superficial). Talk more directly to the person, continue using rapport-building skills and assessments.
- Cover the person with a blanket, while maintaining a view of the injury, and, using an even tone of voice, ask questions about the person's situation.
- If there are concerns of imminent risk of danger to the person or someone else, including the crew, and this risk cannot be mitigated by the crew, notify police.
- In the case of sexual assault, transport the patient to a hospital with the required forensic facilities if possible. Where possible, any potential forensic

evidence (e.g. items of patient clothing) should be placed in a bag and transported with the patient.

- If there are any possible police charges, be aware that the area is potentially a crime scene. Maintain the integrity of the scene as much as possible.
- Continue dynamic risk assessment and MSE en-route.

(Ambulance Victoria, 2018)

ALTERNATIVES TO TRANSPORT

In the event that the person refuses care and/or transport, and assessment has indicated that there is no imminent threat (i.e. assessments indicate that the person is unlikely to self-harm in the immediate future), crews may provide details of available supports and contact numbers for crisis services, and reiterate that the person may call back at any time. The following issues must be clearly addressed if transporting the person is either refused or not required.

- Check they are medically stable, any injury is minor (e.g. superficial scratch or cut).
- Safety contracting – they agree to seek immediate help if anything changes, and guarantee that they will not harm themselves again. (Note, if intoxicated with substances, the possibility of safety contracting is invalidated due to impaired judgment and this contract cannot be accepted.)
- Good supports available – there is another person (not intoxicated) who agrees or can stay with the person and assist them to contact community services. Or has a stable and good rapport with a local GP, or community worker or mental health case manager, who agrees to see the person promptly.
- There is a family member or friend who agrees to stay with the person and help them to contact support services.

DOCUMENTATION

The importance of thorough and objective documentation when attending a scene where a person has self-harmed cannot be underestimated, as this information both adds additional guidance for assessments in ED, and provides a comprehensive picture of strengths the patient may have and the potential limitations that may exist within an environment. Along with risk assessments, mental state examination and medical condition (primary and secondary survey) provide in-depth information to the mental health and healthcare team. Examples of additional information can include home situation, others living at the address, living standards, supports available to the person, evidence of self-care, children living in the environment, or other at-risk situations such as unstable accommodation or domestic violence.

CURRENT APPROACHES TO CARE AND TREATMENT

Communicating effectively with someone exhibiting suicidal ideation or self-harm involves the use of supportive and *human-level* communication, which cannot be underestimated at the point of contact. Pre-hospital workers are in a unique position to engage the person, build rapport and demonstrate help with their self-harm. How the communication begins, how engaged the client feels or how seriously they feel their concerns are addressed, often determines whether they will seek help in the future (Muir-Cochrane et al., 2018).

One in 10 young people committing an initial act of self-harm or stated intention to self-harm will eventually go on to harm themselves more seriously, at times leading to death. This link between self-harm, suicide ideation and attempted suicide remains ever-present, with results from research suggesting that NSSI is an especially important risk factor for future suicide. The person who has self-harmed is often in an impaired cognitive and emotional state with a sense of confusion, fears being judged, is feeling pain and desperation, and requires concerted focus and assessments skills (Klonsky et al., 2015).

CRITICAL REFLECTION

Utilising the case study of 'Sophie', consider how you would build rapport, identifying what exact wording you would use to facilitate communication.

PHARMACOLOGICAL THERAPIES

According to the Royal Australian and New Zealand College of Psychiatrists clinical practice guidelines for the management of deliberate self-harm (cited in Carter et al., 2016, p. 941): 'pharmacotherapy is not effective for reducing repetition of DSH and should not be initiated unless otherwise indicated'. Although there are no specific medications for NSSI, clients with self-harm are often diagnosed with comorbid conditions, especially PTSD, depression and anxiety. These comorbid conditions are treated with a variety of medications, including selective serotonin reuptake inhibitor and anxiolytics (Carter et al., 2016).

PSYCHOLOGICAL THERAPIES

Treatments aimed at reducing or eliminating NSSI, are more likely to involve a range of psychological therapies. A brief review in relation to 'Sophie' and how these therapies may be beneficial for people who engage in NSSI are listed below.

DIALECTICAL BEHAVIOUR THERAPY (DBT)

DBT skills training focuses on enhancing clients' capabilities by teaching them behavioural skills (Linehan et al., 1991). Emotion regulation, particularly in relationships, is often a challenge for people with a history of trauma in childhood. Sophie's history suggests both trauma in childhood and current relationship issues.

COGNITIVE BEHAVIOURAL THERAPY (CBT)

CBT is a short- to medium-term psychotherapy, developed initially for people with depression (Beck, 1970). CBT is also now utilised in a variety of contexts, conditions and behavioural-oriented issues. CBT is goal directed, being focused on solving current problems and modifying dysfunction and poor coping by identifying and correcting inaccurate and/or unhelpful thinking and behaviour (Beck, 1970).

ACCEPTANCE AND COMMITMENT THERAPY (ACT)

ACT is a psychological therapy based on mindfulness techniques and present moment awareness. ACT teaches 'acceptance' skills for responding to overwhelming experiences (Hayes et al., 2016).

SOLUTION-FOCUSED BRIEF THERAPY (SFBT)

SFBT is an approach that draws on personal strengths and resources, and studies future hopes rather than the problem (Iveson, 2002). It focuses people's attention on where they want to go to, and then aids the person to map out how to get there.

    The use of SFBT in the emergency setting has proven to be beneficial to the clinician in being able to talk to a patient who has self-harmed (McAllister et al., 2009). The therapy provides a framework for engaging a person and helping them to feel supported, have a positive outlook, and be more optimistic for change. While little has been written about the use of SFBT by paramedics, there is a great deal of literature on the use of SFBT in the emergency setting (Durrant, 2016; McAllister et al., 2009), and therefore there is great potential for paramedics to use this approach in any crisis situation including self-harm.

OTHER TREATMENTS

It is also important to be aware that NSSI is often a complex interplay of sociological circumstances in the person's life. There may well be alternative social supports that are helpful where treatments and interventions are called for to address specific challenges. A list of web resources and community services are added at the end of the chapter, but in brief these circumstances may include:

- Family assessments and counselling in the community, especially where the person is very young, and the approach needs to or should include the whole family.
- Homelessness supports are likewise often necessary where the person may be 'sleeping rough' or couch surfing (where the person sleeps in different homes each night).
- Financial support services can assist with housing, support payments and budgeting, as these stressors can increase the incidence of self-harm due to frustration.
- Vocational rehabilitation can address and support educational and/or employment deficits or support strengths.

CARING FOR THE CARERS

The importance of providing immediate support for carers at the scene by reassuring them that:

1. they did the right thing to seek help for their loved one
2. any mixed feelings about seeking this assistance on behalf of their loved one is normal
3. they have access to contact numbers for the hospital or may choose to ride along with their loved one

is very important. Carers are at an increased risk of isolation, depression and chronic illness without the opportunity to have respite, and without support in the community (Petrie et al., 2018). Assisting carers to prioritise their own well-being, by way of diet, rest, exercise and regular respite has been linked to an overall decrease in health risks (Carer Support Service Australia, 2018). Resources listed at the end of the chapter provide more detailed contacts and support networks.

CONCLUSION

Non-suicidal self-harm can be a significant part of the workload for paramedics. The importance of respectful, supportive and engaging communication cannot be underestimated in responding to self-harm calls. The initial point of care provided by pre-hospital emergency workers may be one of the only times that the person contacts health services to receive assistance. Non-suicidal self-harm may be considered as a desperate communication and as an affect regulation that requires workers in the pre-hospital setting to develop skills not only in communicating effectively, but also in in-depth physical and mental health assessment. This chapter may be considered as the launching point for further analysis of the under-reported dilemma of non-suicidal self-harm.

LINKS AND RESOURCES

- SANE Australia. Self-harm facts and guides. Contains a variety of guides for the person who is self-harming, carers and health professionals: https://www.sane.org/mental-health -and-illness/facts-and-guides/self-harm
- Headspace Australia. Understanding self-harm – for health professionals: https://headspace .org.au/health-professionals/understanding-self-harm-for-health-professionals/
- Health Direct. Provides a variety of Australia-wide resources for health professionals and carers on self-harm: https://www.healthdirect.gov.au/self-harm
- Psychosocial support – Beyond Blue. Offers support and forums for consumers to seek support and advice and assistance for family and carers of people who self-harm: https:// www.beyondblue.org.au/the-facts/self-harm-and-self-injury
- Financial Supports. Australian government site for financial assistance portal: https://www .dss.gov.au/our-responsibilities/communities-and-vulnerable-people/programs-services/ emergency-relief

REFERENCES

Albión, O., Ferrer, M., Calvo, N., et al., 2013. Exploring the validity of borderline personality disorder components. Compr. Psychiatry 54, 34–40. doi:10.1016/j.comppsych .2012.06.004.

Ambulance Victoria, 2018. Clinical practice guidelines for ambulance and MICA paramedics, Version 1.2.1. Ambulance Victoria, Melbourne.

American Psychiatric Association (APA), 2013. Diagnostic and statistical manual of mental disorders, fifth edn. APA, Washington, DC. (DSM-5). Online. Available: https:// dsm.psychiatryonline.org/doi/book/10.1176/appi.books.9780890425596 12 May 2018.

Australian Bureau of Statistics (ABS), 2016. Causes of Death, Australia. Published 8 March.

Australian Institute of Health and Welfare (AIHW), 2014. Falls, self-harm, transport injuries and assault most common causes for hospitalised injury in young. (Media release.) Online. Available: https://www.aihw.gov.au/news-media/media-releases/2014/2014-nov-1/falls-self-harm -transport-injuries-and-assault-m. 20 January 2018.

Australian Institute of Health and Welfare (AIHW), 2017. Admitted patient care data 2015–2016, Health Services Series, No. 75. Cat. no. HSE 185. ABS, Canberra.

Australian Institute of Health and Welfare (AIHW), 2018a. Family, domestic and sexual violence in Australia. Online. Available: https://www.aihw.gov.au/reports-statistics/behaviours-risk -factors/domestic-violence/overview. 7 March 2018.

Australian Institute of Health and Welfare (AIHW), 2018b. Mental health services in Australia. Online. Available: https://www.aihw.gov.au/reports/mental-health-services/mental -health-services-in-australia/classifications-and-technical-notes. 7 March 2018.

Baetens, I., Claes, L., Onghena, P., et al., 2014. Non-suicidal self-injury in adolescence: a longitudinal study of the relationship between NSSI, psychological distress and perceived parenting. J. Adolesc. 37 (6), 817–826.

Beck, A., 1970. Cognitive therapy: nature and relation to behaviour therapy. Behav. Ther. 1, 184–200.

Bresin, K., Gordon, K., 2013. Endogenous opioids and non-suicidal self-injury: a mechanism of affect regulation. Neurosci. Biobehav. Rev. 37 (3), 374–383.

Carer Support Service Australia, 2018. Online. Available: https://carersupport.org.au 10 June 2018.

Carter, G., Page, A., Large, M., et al., 2016. Royal Australian and New Zealand College of Psychiatrists clinical practice guidelines for the management of deliberate self-harm. Aust. N. Z. J. Psychiatry 50 (10), 939–1000.

Davis, S., Pimpleton-Gray, A., 2017. Facebook and social contagion of mental health disorders among college students. IAFOR J. Psychol. Behav. Sci. 3 (2).

Dudgeon, P., Walker, R., Scrine, C., et al., 2014. Effective strategies to strengthen the mental health and wellbeing of Aboriginal and Torres Strait Islander people. Australian Institute of Family Studies, Canberra. Cited in Robinson, J., McCutcheon, L., Browne, V., et al., 2016. Looking The Other Way: Young people and self-harm. Orygen, The National Centre of Excellence in Youth Mental Health, Melbourne.

Durrant, M., 2016. Solution-focused work in the busy emergency department of a large city hospital: an interview with David Hains. J. Solution-Focused Brief Ther. 2 (2), 61–71.

Favazza, A., 1996. Bodies Under Siege: Self-mutilation and body modification in culture and psychiatry. John Hopkins University Press, Baltimore.

Finkelstein, Y., Macdonald, E., Hollands, S., et al., 2015. Long-term outcomes following self-poisoning in adolescents: a population-based cohort study. Lancet Psychiatry 2 (6), 532–539. doi:10.1016/S2215-0366(15)00170-4.

Glazebrook, K., Townsend, E., Sayal, K., 2015. The role of attachment style in predicting repetition of adolescent self-harm: a longitudinal study. Suicide Life Threat. Behav. 45 (6), 664–678.

Goldman-Mellor, S., Caspi, A., Harrington, H., et al., 2014. Suicide attempt in young people: a signal for long-term health care and social needs. JAMA Psychiatry 71, 119–127.

Government of Western Australia, 2017. Guideline: Self-injury (non-suicidal self-injury). Child and Adolescent Health Service, Perth. ((?)) Online. Available: https://ww2.health.wa.gov.au/~/media/Files/Corporate/general%20documents/CACH/CHM/CACH.SH.Selfinjury.pdf. 25 November 2019.

Hawton, K., Saunders, K., O'Connor, R., 2012. Self-harm and suicide in adolescents. Lancet 379 (9834), 2373–2382.

Hayes, S., Strosahl, K., Wilson, K., 2016. Acceptance and Commitment Therapy: The process and practice of mindful change, second ed. Guilford Press, New York.

Headspace Australia, n.d. Understanding self-harm – for health professionals. Online. Available: https://headspace.org.au/health-professionals/understanding-self-harm-for-health-professionals/. 9 September 2018.

Ivancic, L., Perrens, B., Fildes, J., et al., 2014. Youth Mental Health Report. Mission Australia and Black Dog Institute, Australia.

Iveson, C., 2002. Solution-focused brief therapy. Adv. Psychiatr. Treat. 8, 149–157.

Klonsky, E., Glenn, C., Styer, D., et al., 2015. The functions of non-suicidal self-injury: converging evidence for a two-factor structure. Child Adolesc. Psychiatry Ment. Health 9, 44. doi.org/10.1186/s13034-015-0073-4.

Klonsky, E., May, A., Glenn, C., 2013. The relationship between non-suicidal self-injury and attempted suicide: converging evidence from four samples. J. Abnorm. Psychol. 122 (1), 231–237.

Linehan, M., Armstrong, H., Suarez, A., et al., 1991. Cognitive-behavioral treatment of chronically parasuicidal borderline patients. Arch. Gen. Psychiatry 48 (12), 1060–1064. doi:10.1001/archpsyc.1991.01810360024003.

Long, M., 2018. 'We're not monsters … we're just really sad sometimes': hidden self-injury, stigma and help-seeking. Health Sociol. Rev. 27 (1), 89–103. doi:10.1080/14461242.2017.1375862.

Martin, G., Swannell, S., Harrison, J., et al., 2010. The Australian National Epidemiological Study of Self-Injury (ANESSI) report. Centre for Suicide Prevention Studies, Brisbane.

McAllister, M., Moyle, W., Billett, S., et al., 2009. 'I can actually talk to them now': qualitative results of an educational intervention for emergency nurses caring for clients who self-injure. J. Clin. Nurs. 18 (20), 2838.

McMahon, E., Corcoran, P., McAuliffe, C., et al., 2013. Mediating effects of coping style on associations between mental health factors and self-harm among adolescents. Crisis 34 (4), 242–250.

Mendoza, J., 2009. Submission to the Senate Community Affairs Committee Inquiry into Suicide in Australia. ConNetica Consulting, Moffat Beach.

Muir-Cochrane, E., O'Kane, D., Helps, L., 2018. Communication with people who have a mental illness. In: Levett-Jones, T. (Ed.), Critical Conversations for Patient Safety. Pearson, Sydney.

Petrie, K., Gayed, A., Bryan, B., et al., 2018. The importance of manager support for the mental health and well-being of ambulance personnel. PLoS ONE 13 (5), https://doi.org/10.1371/journal.pone.0197802.

Robinson, J., McCutcheon, L., Browne, V., et al., 2016. Looking The Other Way: Young people and self-harm. Orygen, The National Centre of Excellence in Youth Mental Health, Melbourne.

Shaffer, D., Jacobson, C., 2009. Proposal to the DSM-V Childhood Disorder and Mood Disorder Work Groups to include non-suicidal self-injury (NSSI) as a DSM-V disorder. American Psychiatric Association, Washington, DC. Online. Available: http://www.dsm5.org/Proposed%20Revision%20Attachments/APA%20DSM-5%20NSSI%20Proposal.pdf, 10 December 2018, and http://www.dsm5.org/Proposed%20Revision%20Attachments/APA%20DSM-5%20NSSI%20Proposal.pdf, 31 August 2018.

Taliaferro, L., Muehlenkamp, B., 2017. Adversity among children and youth non-suicidal self-injury and suicidality among sexual minority youth: risk factors and protective connectedness factors. Acad. Paediatr. 17 (7), 715–722.

Victor, S., Davis, T., Klonsky, E., 2016. Descriptive characteristics and initial psychometric properties of the Non-Suicidal Self-Injury Disorder Scale. Arch. Suicide Res. 21 (2), 265–278. doi:10.1080/13811118.2016.1193078.

Whitlock, J., Exner-Cortens, D., Purington, A., 2014. Assessment of non-suicidal self-injury: development and initial validation of the Non-Suicidal Self-injury–Assessment Tool (NSSI–AT). Psychol. Assess. 26 (3), 935–946. http://dx.doi.org/10.1037/a0036611.

Zetterqvist, M., 2015. The DSM-5 diagnosis of non-suicidal self-injury disorder: a review of the empirical literature. Child Adolesc. Psychiatry Ment. Health 9 (31), doi:10.1186/s13034-015-0062-7. Published online 28 September 2015.

Caring for a person with psychosis

13

Bonita C. Lloyd and Heidi Newton

LEARNING OUTCOMES

After reading this chapter you will:

- understand what psychosis is
- identify the signs and symptoms of psychosis and possible causes
- know how to approach someone with psychosis
- understand the risk issues relating to psychosis
- begin to understand the reasons for when a person may or may not require transportation to hospital.

INTRODUCTION

In medicine, the term 'psychosis' is used to convey an altered mental state in which a person loses the capacity to distinguish some aspects of what is and is not real (Sadock et al., 2015). During a period of psychosis, a person's thoughts and perceptions can be disturbed such that they make inaccurate inferences about external reality, even despite evidence to the contrary. The term 'psychotic' describes an illness in which someone experiences psychosis. This should not be confused with the use of the word 'psychotic' in the common vernacular, in which it may be used to imply rage or violence. On the contrary, people experiencing psychosis are no more likely to commit homicide than anyone else (Sadock et al., 2015). However, they are more likely to be the victims of violence than people who have intact reality testing (Galletly et al., 2016).

Psychosis can have a number of underlying causes which can be difficult to determine, particularly during a first psychotic episode. The current evidence suggests that psychosis occurs due to a variety of factors in a person's early life which predispose the person to experience psychotic symptoms in the future, particularly with onset during adolescence and early adulthood (Early Psychosis Guidelines Writing Group and EPPIC National Support Program, 2016). Precipitating factors for psychotic episodes include stress, substance use, and medical conditions (Early Psychosis Guidelines Writing Group and EPPIC National Support Program, 2016). It is vital for the paramedic to assess and understand the cause, as there can be many different underlying pathological processes for which the treatments can be very different.

Psychotic symptoms can be caused by the use of – or withdrawal from – alcohol, illicit substances (such as THC, amphetamines or hallucinogens) or medication (such as prednisolone, opiates or certain anti-hypertensives). These episodes of psychosis are termed 'drug-induced' or 'substance-induced', and usually resolve relatively quickly once the offending substance is eliminated or withdrawals are completed (American Psychiatric Association [APA], 2013).

A psychotic episode due to an underlying medical condition is known as 'organic psychosis'. Examples of medical conditions which may manifest in psychosis include head injuries, epilepsy, encephalitis, brain tumours, dementia, or systemic illnesses such as autoimmune disorders or thyroid disease (Sadock et al., 2015).

Psychosis can also be caused by an overwhelming or intensely stressful event or situation, including trauma, abuse or other social factors, in which case it is known as a 'brief psychotic disorder' or a 'brief reactive psychosis' (APA, 2013).

Finally, a number of mental illnesses can cause psychosis. These will be outlined in more detail below, but include brief reactive psychosis, delusional disorder, schizophrenia, schizoaffective disorder, and severe depression or mania (APA, 2013).

HISTORICAL CONTEXT

Throughout history, people with psychosis (due to schizophrenia or other causes) have been subject to stigma and discrimination. Bizarre or potentially unnerving symptoms have often been poorly understood, and this has resulted at times in cruel or barbaric treatments, such as starvation, flogging, exorcisms and trephining (an attempt to expel evil spirits by drilling holes into the skull) (Faria, 2013; Fulford et al., 2013). People with schizophrenia have also historically been incarcerated in institutions in order to keep them segregated from society, which may have been due to beliefs that they posed danger, or because relatives were embarrassed to acknowledge they had a family member with a mental illness.

Over time, there has been a gradual move away from these pejorative approaches, instead embracing the recovery paradigm, which will be outlined later in the chapter. One example specific to people with a lived experience of psychosis is Hearing Voices International: an organisation aimed at supporting those who have experienced voices to live a meaningful life, including methods of coping with distress if the voices experienced are distressing to the person involved (Hearing Voices Network SA, 2018).

CASE STUDY

Jed

You are dispatched at 1.41 p.m. after a call from the housemate of a 28-year-old man who has been behaving bizarrely for the past 24 hours, characterised by hanging towels in the window, recording car licence plates, refusing to go outside, and crying. On arrival, you can see that the front windows have been covered by towels, and there is a computer on the front lawn. You can hear a dog barking in the back yard. The housemate confirms the dog is secured in the yard and cannot come inside, and that no one else is home.

The housemate lets you inside, and you see a man standing in the corner of the living room, looking anxious, with red eyes as though he has recently been crying. You are introduced to Jed. He appears tense and initially declines to sit down. He acknowledges your presence and gives his name and date of birth, but refuses to answer other questions. His clothing is slightly dirty, and he appears not to have showered recently. Jed picks up a notepad, animatedly explaining that this is his record of proof that *'they sent the cars to check on me'*. You notice a baseball bat behind the front door.

His housemate reports that Jed yesterday returned from a weekend away. Since his return Jed has not slept or eaten, and has become increasingly concerned with monitoring passing cars, taking notes. He has been intermittently crying, and put his computer on the lawn, claiming it could be hacked to spy on him. He began keeping the baseball bat by the door *'for protection'*, but has not threatened or harmed anyone. Jed agrees that the housemate can move the bat to another room, and agrees to sit on the couch and have observations taken.

Vital signs
- Glasgow Coma Score: 15
- Oxygen saturations: 99%
- Respiratory rate: 24
- Heart rate: 90 strong / regular / pounding
- Blood pressure: 135/90
- Electrocardiograph: Sinus tachycardia
- Blood sugar level: 4.5 mmol
- Pain score: 1/10
- Mucous membranes appear dry in keeping with mild dehydration.

You explain that your role is to assess his safety and understand his concerns. He appears more comfortable with the housemate present; the housemate stays and also provides verbal reassurance. Jed explains he believes *'people'* are monitoring the property and may want to arrest him. He describes having stayed up all night keeping watch and recording licence plates. He knows *'they'* are coming because the *'dog has been barking in a weird pattern, telling me'*, and because he observed three blue cars in a row pass the house yesterday. He begins sobbing, expressing fear of being imprisoned or kidnapped, but is vague about why he believes *'they'* might want to do this. His eyes dart around the room, and he occasionally stands up, abruptly, when hearing passing traffic, looking fearful.

CRITICAL REFLECTION
Outline your mental state examination of Jed.

The housemate describes this behaviour as highly out of character; he believes Jed was drinking and may have smoked ICE (crystal methamphetamine) while away on the weekend. Jed has a history of binge drinking on weekends, and smoking cannabis approximately once per fortnight. He is not known to have any medical or mental health problems or to take prescribed medications. The housemate is not aware of any family nearby, stating Jed moved in two years ago after relocating from interstate for a job with a landscaping company, and normally works doing this 30 hours per week, but did not go to work today.

Jed asks what the number plate of your ambulance is. He seems to have difficulty concentrating on your questions, often asking you to repeat yourself. He denies having had anything to eat or drink today. He asks for your help to monitor the passing traffic for *'dodgy-looking ones'*. He is orientated to month and year, but not the day, believing it to still be the weekend. He acknowledges having smoked a pipe with friends, but does not know what was in it, only that it *'was different'* to when he *'smokes weed'*. He wonders if this is why *'they'* are after him. He complains of a non-specific headache.

CRITICAL REFLECTION

- What else would you need to know in order to assess whether this is an organic or a primary psychiatric illness?
- What would you need to know to determine whether this is a new psychiatric illness or an acute exacerbation of a previously existing illness?

What else do you want to know?

In addressing initial risks, Jed should be asked whether he has undertaken any measures – other than the bat – to protect himself from the perceived threat. Given his headache, physical signs and acute behavioural change, it would be important to ascertain whether there had been any recent illness or injury, especially any head injury while away or symptoms of infection which could have caused a delirium. It would be prudent to enquire about allergies, and it would be useful to know when the patient last ate or drank (does this explain the clinical dehydration, or, if not, does this suggest there is a further underlying medical cause?). Diagnostically, it would be helpful to ask the patient how long ago he began to have these concerns – does there appear to be a temporal relationship with smoking the unknown substance?

What are the risk issues to consider?

The patient is distressed, fearful and lacking in insight – these factors could contribute to a risk of unpredictable behaviour. The bat inside the door is of concern, as it appears to have been placed there as a potential weapon with which to defend himself from perceived threats in the context of paranoid persecutory beliefs. This means that anyone who might be incorporated into the patient's paranoid delusional system could appear to the patient to pose a threat and thus be at risk of aggression from him. Jed appears unable to look after himself at home – he is not eating, drinking or showering, and he is therefore at risk of neglect. The patient's housemate is very distressed; the patient's behaviour could pose a risk to Jed's reputation and potentially also his future accommodation situation; the housemate could become too frightened to continue living with the patient. If left untreated, there is a risk of further deterioration in mental state, and a corresponding exacerbation in the abovementioned risks. The psychosis is suspected to be related to the reported drug use, but it will be important to assess for other underlying causes and manage these accordingly.

CRITICAL REFLECTION

You explain your concern to Jed that he seems dehydrated, afraid and could be unwell. You advise that he should come to hospital for further assessment, fluids, a health check and to help him feel safe.

Consider the following alternatives to Jed's case:

1. Jed agrees and wants his housemate to accompany him, as he says this helps him feel protected from *'them'* at the moment. He agrees he feels tired, edgy and wants something to help him sleep tonight. He does not usually take medication.
2. Jed becomes agitated, raising his voice, stating *'they'* could get him if he goes to the hospital, and their house would be vulnerable if he's not there to guard it. You explain you need to take him in under the Mental Health Act for assessment. His housemate tries to reassure him that he and the dog will look after the property, and that he is safe. Jed refuses to be transported to

hospital and adamantly refuses any medications, under the belief that he needs to remain home and alert so that he can protect himself.

3. Jed has a history of a similar episode (possibly drug related), and after an overnight admission in the emergency department was prescribed several weeks' oral olanzapine 5 mg at night. He has not taken the medication for the past week and still has seven of the tablets remaining. He appears to understand that things are 'not right' and thinks it may be best to take two of the tablets and go to bed.

For each option above, discuss:

- the possible risk factors (consider short and long term, risks to self and others)
- the possible treatment options (consider hospital or community-based care, short- or long-term medications, likely prognosis)
- how your mental state examination would differ in each of the scenarios.

RECOGNISING PSYCHOSIS – SIGNS AND SYMPTOMS

It is important to understand the spectrum of possible symptoms of psychosis, in order to be able to recognise it. Psychosis can affect the way a person is able to perceive and process information. It can affect their senses, thoughts, reasoning, emotions and communication (National Collaborating Centre for Mental Health, 2014).

Depending on the symptoms a person has, psychosis can present in many different ways (National Collaborating Centre for Mental Health, 2014). It is often preceded by a prodrome, a period of non-specific or low-grade symptoms (Thompson et al., 2016). Symptoms of psychosis due to a schizophreniform illness (such as schizophrenia or schizoaffective disorder) can be classified as either positive or negative symptoms. *Positive symptoms* refer to symptoms which occur in addition to usual experience, such as hallucinations, delusions or disorganised thinking. *Negative symptoms* are those in which usual functioning is diminished or absent; these include social withdrawal, poor self-care and poverty of thought. Negative symptoms are less prominent in other psychotic disorders, but account for a significant burden of morbidity in schizophrenia (APA, 2013). Symptoms of psychosis are explained in further detail below.

HALLUCINATIONS

Hallucinations are a false sensory perception which occurs in the absence of any relevant external stimulation for the sense affected (Sadock et al., 2015). Some hallucinations are more commonly seen in particular underlying pathologies; for example, auditory hallucinations are often due to a primary psychiatric illness, whereas visual, tactile or olfactory hallucinations may be more suggestive of an organic cause (Semple & Smyth, 2013).

Hallucinations can occur in any of the sensory modalities, and are not under voluntary control (APA, 2013):

- *Auditory hallucinations* are noises heard in the absence of a real cause for the sound. For example, a person might hear voices, whispering or banging when no one else is around. In an attempt to understand their experience, a person might then incorrectly attribute the noises to their environment (a delusional belief); for example, they might accuse their neighbours of planting a microphone in their house and speaking through it to cause voices, or interpret banging noises to mean someone is hiding in their ceiling. Sometimes auditory hallucinations can be commanding in nature, giving instructions to a person that they may find hard to ignore. This can include commands to harm themselves or others, causing distress, and an increased risk of harm.

- *Visual hallucinations* are visual experiences that others do not share – for example, seeing visions of someone following, of someone being harmed, or of demons. Note that this is distinct from visual illusions, where a person may think they see something from the corner of their eye, and when they look nothing is there, or when it is getting dark a shadow appears to be in the shape of a person, but on closer inspection it is proven not to be so.
- *Tactile hallucinations* are experiences of touch; for example, the sensation of bugs crawling on or under the skin (*formication*), or of being able to feel what seems to be a device or lump that is not felt by others.
- Hallucinations may also affect taste (*gustatory*) and smell (*olfactory*); these are not to be confused with the memory of taste or smell that might be invoked by trauma.

DELUSIONS

A delusion is a false belief, based on incorrect inference about external reality, and firmly held despite contradictory evidence or proof (Sadock et al., 2015). Belief in a particular concept such as religion, deity or spiritual experience, which is recognised and shared by others within a community, church, family or social group, is not a delusion (Semple & Smyth, 2013). Delusions can be categorised based on their content. They are considered bizarre if they are implausible and do not derive from ordinary life experiences (APA, 2013). Different types of delusions are explained below:

- *Paranoid and persecutory delusions* – beliefs of oneself or others being targeted or persecuted by people or organisations. These are the most commonly occurring type of delusion (APA, 2013).
- *Referential delusions* – inferring something from the environment makes reference to the person; for example, a person believing that news stories on television are about them, or that the computer is sending special messages.
- *Misidentification* – belief that someone or something is not what it appears; this can include beliefs that loved ones have become imposters (Capgras delusions).
- *Somatic* – beliefs about the body, such as having cancer.
- *Nihilistic* – belief that things are unreal, do not exist or will be destroyed.
- *Grandiose* – beliefs of having superpowers, being God, a saviour, invincibility, of wealth and fame.
- Delusions of control (*passivity experiences*) describe a belief that external persons or beings can take control of one's body and actions.

Depending on the individual and their circumstances, the content of delusions can be extremely varied. Some delusions are highly distressing and frightening, while others may be experienced as exciting or reassuring. Those suffering from delusions may go to great lengths to seek to prove or disprove their experiences, which can detrimentally affect their function, relationships and reputation. They may also seek to protect themselves, or escape their experience, which can place them at risk of harm to themselves or others. They may be distrusting and suspicious of others (National Collaborating Centre for Mental Health, 2014).

DISORGANISED THOUGHTS AND BEHAVIOURS

When a person's ability to process and use information is affected by psychosis, it may be apparent in their thoughts, and thus in their communication and speech, or behaviours (APA, 2013). Psychosis can affect cognitive processing, and the ability to reason, make decisions or plan and carry out tasks. This might be apparent in a person displaying odd and disorganised behaviours, or being unable to take care of themselves (and those around them) in their usual way. They may find it difficult to complete tasks and function in their daily lives. For example, not being able to problem-solve when cooking, paying bills or cleaning, losing items, neglecting self-care and hygiene, or becoming vague and incoherent without necessarily being aware of the problems.

- Disorder of the form of thought (*thought disorder*) is usually apparent in a person's communication, most often in their speech. Assessing the severity of impairment can be more complicated if the person you are assessing comes from a different linguistic background (APA, 2013). As a result of their thought processes being affected by psychosis, a person may have difficulty expressing themselves in a way that is understood by others, with speech that is stilted, unusually fast or slow, vague or lacking in content, or rambling and incoherent, jumping from topic to topic in a disorganised manner.
- A person suffering from psychosis may also experience thought-tampering phenomena, some common forms of which are outlined in Table 13.1 (Sadock et al., 2015).
  As with verbal communication, psychosis can also affect a person's ability to use and respond to non-verbal cues, as well as their memory and concentration (National Collaborating Centre for Mental Health, 2014). They may display incongruent emotional reactions or expressions, and have difficulty comprehending and retaining information. This may include altered ability to follow instructions or respond to questions (National Collaborating Centre for Mental Health, 2014).

Depending on the person, psychosis may present with one or a combination of the above symptoms. For example, a person who is well presented, with unaffected speech and communication skills may have paranoid delusions about being

Table 13.1 Thought Tampering

Thought broadcast	An experience of having others read or know one's thoughts
Thought echo	Believing others can repeat one's thoughts
Thought insertion	Believing others can insert thoughts into one's mind that are not one's own
Thought blocking/withdrawal	A thought is stopped or removed in its midst – this is often apparent in conversation

Adapted from Sadock et al., 2015

persecuted by 'bikies' or government agencies, causing them to stay up all night guarding their home, and writing letters to law enforcement. A person with psychosis may not describe any delusional beliefs or hallucinations, but might have a progressive decline in their self-care, as evidenced by not showering, cooking, eating, or taking care of their pets, or beginning to wander their neighbourhood in their pyjamas. Someone with tactile hallucinations of bugs crawling under their skin may begin thinking of using a kitchen knife to remove them.

CAUSES OF PSYCHOSIS

Psychosis can be due to a number of different underlying illnesses. It may be precipitated by sleep deprivation, stress, substance use, an infective illness or other medical condition, or be due to an underlying psychotic disorder such as schizophrenia. It may be brief and a one-off experience, or an episode of a recurring or chronic psychiatric disorder (National Collaborating Centre for Mental Health, 2014).

Often it is not possible to determine the cause of psychosis at a brief potentially one-off interaction, making assessment difficult in the pre-hospital setting. Diagnosing the underlying cause can require further assessments, investigations and collateral information about the person's symptoms and circumstances over time. The nature of the hallucinations, delusions and disorganised thought should be taken into account when approaching the patient in order to conduct a pre-hospital examination. If the patient is experiencing paranoid persecutory ideation, for example, they may be too frightened to engage in a comprehensive pre-hospital examination. In this circumstance, priority should be given to obtaining vital signs and excluding any medical emergencies, with detailed documentation of any relevant mental state features that are impacting on your ability to complete your examination, and the gathering of as much collateral history as possible.

Causal factors for psychosis can be considered as biological, psychological and socio-cultural.

BIOLOGICAL CAUSES

Biological causes include physical, genetic and organic precipitants, such as the following.

- Increased genetic vulnerability to psychosis due to a family history of schizophrenia or bipolar affective disorder. This is explored in more detail later in this chapter.
- Vulnerability to psychosis due to developmental problems (such as those related to premature birth or serious neonatal illness), brain injury or seizure disorder, sleep deprivation, pregnancy or postpartum period.
- Psychosis due to serious infections (including sepsis and encephalitis), delirium, or metabolic or endocrine diseases.
- Intoxication with or withdrawal from drugs and alcohol, overdoses, analgesics and side effects of prescribed treatments, including stimulant medications, steroids and cytotoxic medications (APA, 2013).

PSYCHOLOGICAL FACTORS

Psychological factors can include:

- past and/or recent trauma, which may include experiences of abuse (physical, emotional, sexual) or neglect, or life-threatening experiences
- current and recent stressors in the person's life, which can include – but are not limited to – relationship breakdown, bereavement or grief and loss, occupational conflict or loss of employment, or the change or loss of a role within the family or community.

SOCIO-CULTURAL FACTORS

Socio-cultural factors may include financial hardship, social isolation, legal or forensic problems, a change in a person's supports, relocation or emigration. In industrialised countries, the incidence of schizophrenia is higher in urban areas than rural areas (Sadock et al., 2015).

CRITICAL REFLECTION

In relation to 'Jed's' case:
- identify any hallucinations that may be present
- identify any delusions that may be present
- identify any social or cultural factors that may need to be considered in Jed's assessment, treatment and recovery.

ASSESSMENT AND HISTORY TAKING

There are a number of different psychotic disorders which may underlie an acute episode of psychosis. These can be differentiated by their duration, speed of onset, severity and symptoms (APA, 2013).

Brief psychotic episodes may occur unexpectedly, often in response to a stressful life event, and in the absence of another underlying psychotic disorder. Longer-term disorders may have chronic or episodic psychotic symptoms.

Schizophrenia and schizoaffective disorder typically begin in late adolescence or early adulthood, preceded by a period of non-specific functional decline (*prodromal period*), although they can also begin later in life. Schizophrenia is equally prevalent in men and women, although the age of onset is typically earlier in men (Sadock et al., 2015). Exacerbations of these disorders may be characterised by psychotic symptoms and decline in functioning. The 'affective' part of schizoaffective disorder refers to the presence of psychosis plus significant mood disturbance, including depressive, manic or mixed mood symptoms. The epidemiology of schizophrenia and schizoaffective disorder varies, but the prevalence in Australia is in the vicinity of 1–2.37% (Galletly et al., 2016).

There are a number of proposed aetiologies for schizophrenia. The 'dopamine hypothesis' suggests psychosis is associated with increased activity of dopamine in the brain; however, whether this relates to the amount of dopamine, its action at receptor sites, or the number or action of receptor sites remains unclear, and a number of other neurotransmitters have also been implicated, including – but not limited to – serotonin, norepinephrine (noradrenaline), gamma-Aminobutyric acid (GABA) and glutamate (Sadock et al., 2015). While it is recognised that there is a genetic component to the illness, modes of genetic transmission of schizophrenia are not known, with many genes proposed to confer increased vulnerability to developing schizophrenia, including DISC-1, Catechol-O-Methyltransferase (COMT), and alpha-7-nicotinic receptors (Sadock et al., 2015). It is also recognised that there is an increased incidence of schizophrenia in babies of mothers who suffer prenatal infection, for example with influenza and rubella, and research exploring possible autoimmune theories is ongoing (Sadock et al., 2015).

Exacerbations of psychosis in a person with a psychotic disorder may occur in the context of the biopsychosocio-cultural factors described above, changes in treatment or changes in following recommended prescribed treatment, or without an identified precipitant.

Drug-induced episodes of psychosis are often distinguished by the temporal relationship between recreational or prescribed drug-use and the emergence of symptoms, however this can be variable for different substances, and between individuals. For example, use of cocaine, amphetamine or other sympathomimetic agents can rapidly induce psychotic symptoms (APA, 2013), whereas psychosis induced by alcohol or other sedatives may occur after days or weeks of use. Substance-induced psychosis is generally self-limiting, with symptoms resolving once the substance is cleared from the body (APA, 2013). However, in individuals with an underlying primary psychotic illness, drug use may precipitate a more prolonged exacerbation of psychosis.

INITIAL (PRE-HOSPITAL) ASSESSMENT

The principles of initial assessment for the person suffering from psychosis are the same as those for other mental health presentations. However, it is particularly important to observe the environment, and the way the person interacts with people and the environment around them.

- **Scene awareness:** Look at the environment: who is on scene and what are their relationships to the person needing care? Did the affected person or someone else call for help, and is the person aware of the referral?

  Are there any indications that police should also be requested to attend, if not already flagged within the operational communications centre (such as prior knowledge of the address or persons present being associated with threats or aggression, weapons at the residence, pets that might need to be restrained)?

  What is the layout of the property/location? Are there exit points? Is there a risk of being trapped or locked in?
- **Primary assessment:** Where is the person? How do they appear? How are they interacting and communicating with others?
- **Danger:** Include initial impressions/observations of behaviour/body language/conversation and how the person is relating to the world and people around them. LOOK, LISTEN AND WATCH as you approach.

Regarding the management of acute agitation, the Royal Australian and New Zealand College of Psychiatrists (RANZCP) guidelines for schizophrenia by Galletly and colleagues (2016) advise on page 44:

> *The management of the acutely disturbed psychotic person requires calm strategies that protect the safety and dignity of all concerned. The first step should be to try to engage the person and understand what is driving their agitation. Sometimes simple measures such as orienting and explaining what is happening can be enough to defuse the situation. Attention should be paid to the physical environment, such that stimulation is reduced and safety ensured. Objects that might be thrown or used as weapons should be removed, where possible.*

- **Response** – include acknowledgement of you and your role (considering that hallucinations and delusions may inhibit their understanding)
- **Airway**
- **Breathing**
- **Circulation**
- **Disability**

While psychotic symptoms may be prominent, consider that the cause may be related to organic/medical factors. Address what needs to be managed that is life threatening, including consideration of differential diagnosis and comorbidities – this includes initial considerations of the possible causes of apparent psychosis, including any signs of head injury, infection, medical illness or drug use, and discerning whether there is a known history of mental illness and treatment for this. It is also important to remember that patients with chronic mental illness suffer poorer physical health outcomes and shorter life expectancy than the general population (Galletly et al., 2016), and the person with psychosis can still be experiencing an acute myocardial infarction, stroke, pulmonary embolism, gastrointestinal bleed, or other physical issues which should not be overlooked. Other potential medical issues of which to be aware in patients with psychosis include clozapine toxicity (especially if a patient has ceased smoking cigarettes abruptly), neuroleptic malignant syndrome (NMS), or catatonia. (See Chapter 7 and the case study of 'Anthony'.)

Mental state assessment

The mental state assessment will be of particular importance for the initial and also ongoing assessments of the person, acting as a source for comparison. (Refer to Chapter 5 for further details.)

- **Appearance:** Are they dressed appropriately for the weather? Is there evidence of poor self-care? Is there any evidence of deliberate self-harm? Are they holding anything? Do they look physically well?
- **Behaviour:** Are there abnormal motor movements (such as signs of medication side effects) or eye contact? Do they appear agitated or hypervigilant? Is their behaviour disorganised?
- **Conversation:** (including thought flow and content): Is speech fast or slow? Do they speak spontaneously or only in response to questions? Do their responses make sense? Can they convey meaning and communicate their needs and views? What are the themes of conversation? Do they describe any delusions or hallucinations?
- **Affect:** What do you observe of how they are feeling? Is it congruent to the situation? Does it markedly fluctuate (is it 'labile'), or is there diminished reactivity ('blunted')? Do they appear depressed or manic?
- **Mood:** What do they state about how they are feeling?
- **Perception:** Does the person appear to be responding to hallucinations or stating delusional beliefs? How do they view the world around them? Do they feel safe?
- **Cognition:** Are they oriented to person, place and time? Does their memory or concentration seem impaired?
- **Insight:** What is their understanding of what is occurring? Do they believe they could be unwell? Do they understand your role? Do they understand the concerns of others about their situation?
- **Judgment:** Are they behaving in a way that is safe for them and those around them? Are they acting in response to delusions or hallucinations, thereby placing themselves or others at risk?

- **Engagement/rapport:** What is the person's response and engagement with you (or others present)? Are you able to establish a therapeutic alliance with the person? Have they incorporated you into their delusions (e.g. accusing you of being part of the conspiracy to harm them, controlled by their family)?

When to transport, and alternative care pathways

Following assessment, if a patient appears to be psychotic but they are not medically compromised, the next decision relates to whether or not they should be transferred to hospital. This decision is generally informed by assessment of risk rather than the presence or absence of psychotic features, as some patients have chronic psychotic symptoms which do not warrant acute hospital care. Factors indicating the patient should be transferred to hospital include suicidal ideation (either in terms of an attempt, thoughts which are difficult to resist, command hallucinations, intent or plan – including thoughts of committing suicide in order to evade capture by perceived persecutors), thoughts or plans to harm others (including the carrying of weapons to defend against perceived attack), new or worsening perceptual disturbance, cognitive impairment which is not usual for the patient, or other significant distress. Other aspects of the patient's presentation which may prompt a decision to transport to hospital include evidence that the patient is unable to care for themself, such as squalid living conditions, disorganised behaviour or poor oral intake. This includes dehydration, which may occur in drug-induced psychoses, psychosis due to medical illness or in primary psychiatric illnesses, all of which may require intravenous fluids pre-hospital or in the hospital setting.

An assessment of their medical and social supports is also required to assist your decision-making process. If the patient has psychotic symptoms but does not meet the criteria above, other alternative care pathways may be more appropriate. These include contacting any existing mental health practitioner (care coordinator, psychologist, psychiatrist), or contacting the patient's general practitioner to arrange an appointment to discuss a mental healthcare plan or ongoing assessment. Most areas have a mental health crisis assessment team ('CAT' or similar), or an emergency mental health triage number which can be used to facilitate further assessment and/or follow-up. Assessment should also include the level of engagement that the person has with the community supports. Finally, contacting a family member or friend may be appropriate, both in terms of verifying that they do not have any concerns that might indicate hospital assessment is required, and to arrange provision of ongoing support for the patient.

Legal and ethical considerations

If you believe the patient requires further assessment and/or treatment in hospital but they are refusing this, consideration may be given to the implementation of the relevant Mental Health Act (MHA). Most MHAs can only be used to enforce treatment if a patient lacks capacity to make decisions about their care, and because of this poses a risk to themselves or others. An example of this might be that the patient in the vignette above refuses to be conveyed to hospital because he believes the paramedics are part of the conspiracy against him, because he is hearing an auditory hallucination that is advising him not to cooperate, or because his thoughts are so muddled that he is unable to understand what is going on or to plan what to do about it. It is important to note that not all patients with psychosis lack capacity, and that capacity is decision-specific. This means that a patient may be experiencing auditory hallucinations but still be able to make reasoned, informed decisions regarding their healthcare; in such a case, enforcing further assessment/treatment via the MHA may be legally and ethically dubious. In keeping with the recovery paradigm, patients should be empowered to be involved in decisions pertaining to their care, on a voluntary basis, unless the psychosis renders them unable to safely do so.

CRITICAL REFLECTION

- If (as stated above) not all psychotic patients lack capacity, how would you assess capacity for someone with psychosis?
- At what point does a person with psychosis stop having the right to self-determination?

APPROACHES TO TREATMENT

The key general principles in approaching someone who is experiencing psychosis are to be present, listen, communicate and educate.

Approach the person suffering from psychosis as you would any other patient – with curiosity, kindness and without judgment, being mindful of the risk concerns described above. Avoid cornering the patient, or placing yourself in a position where you might be cornered.

COMMUNICATING WITH SOMEONE WHO IS EXPERIENCING PSYCHOSIS

Psychosis can interfere with a person's ability to understand and communicate with others. Speak in a calm tone, speak slowly, and use plain language and short, clear sentences. It may be beneficial to repeat information, and confirm the person understands. Allow them time to process and respond to information.

Someone experiencing hallucinations may have trouble listening or concentrating on what you are saying. In some cases, those with auditory hallucinations may experience voices commenting on your instructions or questions. They may appear distracted, and have difficulty retaining any information provided. A person suffering from delusions may seek your opinion or advice about their beliefs. It is important not to collude or confirm with their delusional beliefs or manipulate them, but to remain non-judgmental. Challenging their beliefs can be perceived as confrontational. It is recommended to acknowledge their beliefs and distress, and attempt to clarify common concerns (e.g., acknowledging that a person believes they have a chip implanted in their body, and that this is causing them to feel anxious, not sleep, and be distressed, and that distress is what you are concerned about and would like to help them with, rather than agreeing or disagreeing with them about the presence of the chip).

This is further outlined on page 44 of the RANZCP's guideline regarding the management of the acutely agitated patient (Galletly et al., 2016):

> *One person should communicate with the agitated individual in a clear even voice. The individual should be offered reassurance that they are safe and that the intent is to ensure the safety of all concerned. Interventions need to be carefully explained and a rationale provided. Always try to defuse the situation by careful negotiation. The following techniques can be useful:*
>
> * *Ventilation: allowing the opportunity to express fears, frustration, anger*
> * *Redirection: exploring solutions to allow the person to gain control*
> * *Time out: where possible, offer the person a low stimulus environment to assist them to gain control.*

Communication from the paramedic, both verbal and non-verbal, remains the key to a good therapeutic relationship even with a person experiencing psychosis.

CLINICAL HANDOVER

Information garnered by paramedics at an initial interaction can be extremely useful for staff later involved in the patient's care, including for diagnostic assistance and in assessing the severity of illness, likely time course and associated risks. Documentation and handover should include your assessment and mental state examination, and any collateral information obtained from others present, especially if the patient is thought-disordered or otherwise unable to communicate meaningfully. Other useful observations include the presence of drugs or drug paraphernalia, the state of the patient's abode (for example, if their house is in squalor, which could indicate poor self-care for a significant period of time), and any environmental clues that the patient might be experiencing psychosis (such as doors being barricaded or windows covered).

It is also significant to document and hand over any recognised triggers gained through conversation and observation that appear to increase the person's distress or increase their sense of feeling unsafe. Alternatively, it is also useful for further care to document what appears to work in decreasing the person's distress, or if their level of distress changes during the period of contact with them.

Ensure you hand over any known medical history, allergies and known medications. If possible, bring the medications with the patient to hospital. If it has been necessary to administer any medications to the patient prior to or during transport, please record and hand over the indication for administration, the name, dose and route of administration, and any observed response. Where possible, do not administer sedating medications that may limit further assessments of a person's mental state, unless it is required for safety reasons (such as to manage acute agitation or distress that has not responded to other interventions).

BIOPSYCHOSOCIAL APPROACHES TO CARE
SHORT-TERM CARE

While it may not be possible to determine the cause of a person's psychosis at initial contact with them, gathering information about possible causes will help guide any treatment required. Psychotic disorders are heterogeneous, and the severity of symptoms can predict aspects of the illness, such as the degree of cognitive impairment (APA, 2013). The early detection and treatment of psychotic disorders, such as schizophrenia, are associated with improved outcomes (Galletly et al., 2016).

Initial assessment and collateral information are very important in guiding short-term care. Enquire about recent stressors, any substance use, illness, if the person has a diagnosis of mental illness, is on or recently changed or ceased medications, and whether they have a history of previous episodes (Byrne, 2007). Where possible, record the names and doses of any prescribed medications, and the contact details of any treating health providers. Noting the relevant mental state features, including the person's self-care, behaviours and content of delusions or hallucinations, will assist as a point of comparison for further assessments.

Obtaining information from any collateral sources present is also very valuable. Make the above enquiries of any friends or family present, and record their contact details if possible.

Initial assessments, tests and information gathering will aim to identify any contributing infection, medical condition, intoxication, psychosocial stressors and underlying psychiatric disorder.

Short-term treatment has the aim of decreasing distress, decreasing risk, stabilising and decreasing symptoms, stabilising the social situation, and linking with social supports (Early Psychosis Guidelines Writing Group and EPPIC National Support Program, 2016).

LONG-TERM CARE

Longer-term treatment of psychosis will involve containing risks, and providing the safest but least-restrictive possible setting for ongoing assessments and treatment, considering the biopsychosocial factors relevant to the individual. This can range from voluntary follow-up with a general practitioner (GP), to specialist community mental health service, or to involuntary hospital care under the relevant state or territory's Mental Health Act.

Treatments will vary depending on the identified cause, but may include one, all, or a combination of:

- antipsychotic medications (commencing a new medication, or optimising or restarting existing treatments)
- supportive counselling and psychoeducation
- psychotherapy
- support from health service providers (GP, mental health units or community teams, mental health nurses, pharmacists, social workers, occupational therapists, non-government organisations including support groups) to engage the person in ongoing treatment, follow-up and to maintain their best level of function, including assistance with social relationships, employment, finances and housing.

Antipsychotics

Antipsychotics are a group of medications shown to be effective in managing psychotic symptoms and acute agitation. They can be used both short- and long-term, depending on the presentation of symptoms and underlying psychotic disorder. Antipsychotics are broadly categorised as 'typical' or 'first-generation' medications, or 'atypical' or 'second-generation' medications (see Chapter 18 for further details). First-generation antipsychotics have high-affinity antagonism of dopamine, and have been in use longer, whereas second-generation medications, which are newer in comparison, have lower-affinity antagonism of serotonin and dopamine, or partial dopamine agonism (Sadock et al., 2015). Long-term use of 'typical' medications is more associated with sedation and stiffness, whereas 'atypical' medications can be more likely to cause metabolic changes and weight gain, but are considered more effective for negative symptoms of schizophrenia, associated depressed mood, and cognitive deficits (Sadock et al., 2015).

All antipsychotics can cause side effects. In the acute-care setting, it is important to consider the possibility of sedation, cardiovascular changes (QTc prolongation and postural hypotension), and risk of extra-pyramidal side effects (EPSEs). EPSEs describe a group of symptoms arising from the action of these medications on certain neuromuscular pathways in the body, causing restlessness, muscle cramps, joint stiffness, involuntary movements and dystonia or muscle spasms. In rare cases, the muscles of the eyes, mouth or throat can be affected by dystonia, and can lead to airway compromise. The risk of EPSEs can be mitigated with use of the lowest effective dose of antipsychotics, avoiding polypharmacy, and if they occur, administration of benztropine (an anticholinergic agent which can relieve EPSEs) orally or by intramuscular injection, and benzodiazepines.

Antipsychotics, including their different side-effect profiles and indications, are explored further in Chapter 18.

Psychological therapies

Increasingly, psychological therapies and psychosocial strategies are proving to be of benefit in people with psychosis. The current recommendations are that these should be used as an adjunct to antipsychotic medications, and that they are an integral part of person-centred, recovery-focused care (National Collaborating Centre for Mental Health, 2014).

Evidence-based therapies which may be useful include cognitive behavioural therapy for psychotic symptoms (such as meta-cognitive therapy, or 'thinking about thinking'), social skills training, and therapies aimed at assisting with some of the losses and trauma often associated with psychotic illnesses, including experiences of stigma, rejection and social isolation (Galletly et al., 2016). Other therapies, such as acceptance and commitment therapy (ACT) or mindfulness-based therapies, may also be of use.

Other therapies and requirements for recovery

As advances have been made in the understanding of psychosis, there have been corresponding refinements in treatment and approaches to treatment. Shifts have been made to increase community-based care and early-intervention services, and to aim to reduce the need for hospitalisation (National Collaborating Centre for Mental Health, 2014). Thought has been given to the common barriers for this group in terms of social and economic disadvantage, and how health services can best assist people experiencing psychosis in negotiating these.

The recovery paradigm (see Chapter 2) heavily informs current clinical practice when working with people who have schizophrenia or experience psychosis due to other causes. Rather than focusing merely on symptomatic recovery, outcomes should now be considered in a manner that includes the subjective views and values of the person experiencing psychosis. Slade (2009) differentiates between clinical recovery (symptom reduction; the traditional focus of treatment), functional recovery and personal recovery. Personal recovery involves adapting to the limitations of illness in order to have a meaningful life. When goals for recovery are considered more broadly in this way, and with the person experiencing the illness at the centre of care planning, people are treated holistically and with dignity. The 'hearing voices' or 'Maastricht approach' is one example of how the recovery paradigm can be utilised to inform the provision of individualised care (Hearing Voices Network South Australia, 2018).

CARING FOR THE CARERS

Family psychoeducation is also of benefit, and should be offered as part of routine care of patients with schizophrenia. Minimising the distress and burden for family members has been shown to have positive effects on the individual's recovery.

Carers, family and friends of people who experience psychosis can suffer significant grief and distress. It is important to communicate with family and significant others on scene in order to keep them informed about what is happening and how you are going to provide care for their loved one. Carers, family and friends can provide useful collateral information and can at times assist to reassure the patient, particularly if the patient is suspicious of new people in the context of paranoid persecutory ideation. You can assist family and friends on scene by communicating clearly, providing support and suggesting resources they may wish to consult in future (see the list at the end of this chapter for examples).

Finally, it is important to recognise and manage your own emotional response to the patient with psychosis. Some people may find interacting with patients with these kinds of difficulties emotionally draining and anxiety-provoking, especially if they are highly distressed or agitated on scene, or if the patient incorporates you into their delusional system. These emotional responses are understandable, but it is important to be aware of them so that they do not unduly influence how you interact with the patient. Debriefing with a co-worker or trusted colleague can be invaluable, and can help you to continue to provide quality care into the future. Another important strategy that can assist in keeping responses and interactions with a patient who is suffering from psychosis as constructive as possible is to try to imagine what it might be like for them, given their perceptual disturbances and distorted sense of reality. Patients suffering from psychosis are often frightened, confused, distressed or a combination of these, and keeping this in mind can help to mitigate unintentionally unhelpful responses.

CONCLUSION

People experiencing psychosis can present in a variety of different ways, often with medical comorbidities, and can be challenging but ultimately highly rewarding to assess and manage in the community. Paramedics play an important role in establishing engagement, managing risks to the patient and others, gathering information (which may not be available to other healthcare providers that can assist with diagnosis and treatment), utilising medication judiciously, making decisions regarding when hospital care may be required, and providing support and reassurance to the patient and their loved ones in what is often a frightening and distressing experience.

LINKS AND RESOURCES
For further reading for health professionals
- Royal Australian and New Zealand College of Psychiatrists (RANZCP). Clinical Practice Guidelines (health professionals): https://www.ranzcp.org/Publications/Guidelines-and-resources-for-practice/Schizophrenia-CPG-and-associated-resources

Information for your patients and their carers
- Your Health In Mind: https://www.yourhealthinmind.org/
- Mental Illness Fellowship of Australia Inc.: www.mifa.org.au/en/
- SANE Australia: https://www.sane.org/
- Headspace, a Youth Mental Health Foundation: https://headspace.org.au/
- Orygen, youth mental health: https://www.orygen.org.au/

- TED talk – Eleanor Longden 'The voices in my head': https://www.youtube.com/watch?v=syjEN3peCJw&vl=en
- 2012 National Report Card on Mental Health and Suicide Prevention – videos:
- Ausmentalhealth – https://www.youtube.com/channel/UC6pWbzRT5EAFbtAH5buUaVw
- John – https://www.youtube.com/watch?v=pI-iz36ciM8&index=38&list=UU6pWbzRT5EAFbtAH5buUaVw
- Pat and Keith – https://www.youtube.com/watch?v=PcvsJFdvTh8&list=UU6pWbzRT5EAFbtAH5buUaVw&index=41

REFERENCES

American Psychiatric Association (APA), 2013. Diagnostic and Statistical Manual of Mental Disorders, fifth ed. American Psychiatric Publishing, Washington, DC. (DSM-5).

Byrne, P., 2007. Managing the acute psychotic episode. BMJ 334 (7595), 686–692.

Early Psychosis Guidelines Writing Group and EPPIC National Support Program, 2016. Australian Clinical Guidelines for Early Psychosis, second ed. Orygen, The National Centre of Excellence in Youth Mental Health, Melbourne.

Faria, M., 2013. Violence, mental illness and the brain – a brief history of psychosurgery: part 1 – from trephination to lobotomy. Surg. Neurol. Int. 4, 49.

Fulford, K., Davies, M., Gipps, R., et al., 2013. The Oxford Handbook of Philosophy and Psychiatry. Oxford University Press, Oxford.

Galletly, C., Castle, D., Dark, F., et al., 2016. Royal Australia and New Zealand College of Psychiatrists clinical practice guidelines for the management of schizophrenia and related disorders. Aust. N. Z. J. Psychiatry 50 (5), 1–117.

Hearing Voices Network South Australia, 2018. Online. Available: https://hvnsa.org.au/about-the-hearing-voices-movement-approach/. 20 June 2018.

National Collaborating Centre for Mental Health, 2014. Psychosis and schizophrenia in adults: the NICE guideline on treatment and management, updated ed. Online. Available: https://www.nice.org.uk/guidance/cg178/evidence/full-guideline-490503565

Sadock, B., Sadock, V., Ruiz, P., 2015. Kaplan & Sadock's Synopsis of Psychiatry, eleventh ed. Wolters Kluwer, Philadelphia. electronic book.

Semple, D., Smyth, R., 2013. The Oxford Handbook of Psychiatry, third ed. Oxford University Press, New York.

Slade, M., 2009. The contribution of mental health services to recovery. J. Ment. Health 18, 367–371.

Thompson, A., Marwaha, S., Broome, M., 2016. At risk mental state for psychosis: identification and current treatment approaches. Br. J. Psych. Adv. 22 (3), 186–193.

Caring for a person with substance use and mental health concerns

Michael Baigent

LEARNING OUTCOMES

The material in this chapter will assist the paramedic to:

- understand the effects that substances of abuse can have on the mental state and behaviour
- decide on the likely cause of the patient's presentation in terms of it being intoxication, withdrawal, substance induced or related to their substance use disorder
- determine the severity of the substance use disorder (whether the patient is likely to be dependent or not)
- appreciate the risks involved in the substance-related presentation
- consider the best location to manage the person based on their presentation and needs.

INTRODUCTION

This chapter focuses on the behavioural and mental health problems that are encountered by paramedics amongst those who use alcohol and other drugs. Drugs of abuse (licit and illicit) and alcohol are collectively termed substances in the *Diagnostic and Statistical Manual of Mental Disorders* (5th ed.) (*DSM-5*) (American Psychiatric Association [APA], 2013). Users of substances can present with alterations in behaviour, mood and thinking that is the result of intoxication, withdrawal, chemically induced psychiatric symptoms or disorders, or a consequence of addiction. The problems can be the outcome of substance use combined with a pre-existing mental disorder. Commonly more than one substance is consumed at a time. Understanding the variety of effects of the substances and typical patterns of use gives the clinician confidence when confronted with what can be difficult situations in the pre-hospital settings. The crisis encounter may tip the person's resolve to finally avoid or cease substance use, or it may be one of the many in the chronic problem of dependence. For the paramedic, every interaction that they have with a person with substance-related problems can be a chance to intervene with treatment or education. Substance use disorders are associated with predictable physical problems which may cause medical emergencies and complicate the presentation. Although medical complications should always be assessed in parallel with the mental and behavioural consequences, they are not the subject of this chapter.

CASE STUDY
Martin

You have been dispatched at 8.35 a.m. to a residential address at the request of police, who have attended to a call from an elderly resident who reported that she found a man in her house. On arrival, you are introduced to Martin, a 57-year-old male. Martin is sitting at the kitchen table with the police and drinking a cup of tea that has been made by the female resident (Elsie). Police tell you that Elsie awoke to find Martin in her laundry. While she was initially shocked, she quickly realised that Martin posed no threat to her; however, she was concerned because Martin believed that he was actually in his own house. Elsie called the police and then turned on the kettle.

Police have identified Martin, and advise that he lives alone in a unit in a neighbouring suburb. He has no police record.

On interview, Martin tells you that he is 37 years old and lives in this house with his wife and three daughters (aged 3, 5 and 7). Martin points at photos on the wall and says that they are various family members. You can see Elsie in the photos, but you cannot see Martin.

On examination of Martin's mental state, you note the following:

Appearance: Martin appears to be in his mid-sixties. He is thin, unshaven and has uncombed hair. He is wearing casual clothes and slippers. While slightly dishevelled, he appears basically clean. There are heavy nicotine stains on his left hand. No signs of trauma or injury.

Behaviour: Martin is sitting on the chair and repetitively appears to pick up something small from the table and roll it between his fingers. There is noticeable tremor. He has a distressed restlessness to his demeanour.

Conversation: He speaks without slurring, but answers the questions with some effort. His speech is generally goal directed.

Affect: Martin appears perplexed, anxious and on edge, but says that his mood is 'OK'.

Perception: He denies hearing or seeing things, but he cannot explain what he is picking up from the table.

Cognition: He is disorientated to the date and place. He seems to think it is 20 years ago.

Vital signs
- Glasgow Coma Score: 14
- Respiratory rate: 17
- Heart rate: 125
- Blood pressure: 155/90
- Temperature: 37.3
- Blood sugar level: 4.8

CRITICAL REFLECTION
- What conclusion would you draw from Martin's mental state, particularly his disorientation?
- What could explain his odd behaviour?
- Would you consider that he is psychotic?
- What would be vital to know at this point?
- How could this information be obtained?

Police Communications provide the phone number for one of Martin's daughters. You learn from her that her parents divorced 15 years ago. Before the divorce, the family lived in the house now owned by Elsie. The daughter lives interstate and has not seen her father for 18 months.

CRITICAL REFLECTION

• What else would you like to know from Martin's daughter?

Martin refuses to go to the hospital.

CRITICAL REFLECTION

• Martin does not appear to be suicidal or violent. Under what circumstances can you transport Martin against his will?
• Consider your local legislation and identify which laws or sections apply.
• What might happen if he is not transported?
• What treatment will he receive at hospital?

CRITICAL REFLECTION

• During his hospitalisation, Martin discloses that he has been a heavy alcohol user for most of his adult life. Hospital records confirm this. Staff try to reinforce the seriousness of his condition and the risk he poses to himself if he continues to drink. He says that he thinks he might stop for a bit. He is discharged with no follow-up arrangements. How confident would you feel about this situation?

HOW COMMON IS DRUG USE?

Nearly 5% of all deaths in Australia are from alcohol (3.4%) and illicit drug use (Australian Institute of Health and Welfare [AIHW], 2018a). Alcohol remains the most commonly used substance in the Australian population; approximately 5000 die annually because of its use. Seventeen per cent reported consuming it over the previous month at a 'risky' level (on average more than two standard drinks per day) (AIHW, 2017a). The percentage of Australians who reported drug use in the previous 12 months per drug type is shown in Table 14.1. Those aged 20–29 years have the highest prevalence rates for use of nearly every substance. Cannabis remains the most commonly used illicit substance in Australia, followed by pharmaceuticals, e.g. sleeping pills, tranquillisers, codeine products, oxycodone (Endone, oxycodone), tramadol, morphine, gabapentinoids (gabapentin and pregabalin) and fentanyl. The data gathered pre-dates codeine preparations in over-the-counter products being rescheduled to prescription only, which hopefully stemmed what had been regarded as a growing problem.

There was a decline in the use of methamphetamines reported over the past 12 months over the 2013–2016 period (from 2.1% to 1.4%); however, the overall rate at which crystalline form ('ice') was used rose from 0.4% to 0.8% of the population.

The latest Australian data on presentations to the emergency department by diagnosis reveals that mental and behavioural disorders due to psychoactive substance use account for 27% of mental health presentations, whereas mood disorders and psychotic illnesses together accounted for only 23% (AIHW, 2018b). The Northern Territory recorded 57% of their presentations to the ED as due to a mental and

Table 14.1 Recent Drug Use, People Aged 14 or Older, 2016 (%)

	Recent Use (Last 12 Months)
Alcohol	77.5
Cannabis	10.4
Ecstasy	2.2
Meth/amphetamine (speed)	1.4
Cocaine	2.5
Hallucinogens	1.0
Inhalants	1.0
Heroin	0.2
Ketamine	0.4
GHB	0.1
New psychoactive	0.3
Pharmaceuticals (excludes OTC such as paracetamol, aspirin and other non-opioid pain killers)	4.8
Illicit use of any drug	**15.6**

Adapted from Table 2.1. National Drug Strategy Household Survey, 2016: detailed findings. Australian Institute of Health and Welfare (AIHW, 2017a)

behavioural disorder due to substance use, over twice the national average. Despite the drama and excitement associated with many methamphetamine presentations, Australian ambulance officers have estimated that 20% of their call-outs are a result of alcohol consumption (Lynagh et al., 2010). Drug-induced deaths are more likely to be due to prescription drugs than illicit drugs (AIHW, 2017b).

Use of more than one drug is commonplace; for example, the majority of those who reported recent (previous 12 months) illicit drug use, also smoked, used other drugs and reported 'risky' levels of drinking (AIHW, 2017a) (see Fig. 14.1). The exception is people who misuse pharmaceutical drugs are less likely to use other illicit drugs (Fig. 14.1).

WHY PEOPLE USE

Genetic heritability is thought to account for 40–60% of the variation between individuals' likelihood of being diagnosed with a drug or alcohol use problem (Yu & McClellan, 2016). However, the focus of this research evidence has been on alcohol.

Addiction to a substance is the outcome of social, psychological and biological processes. Access, expectations and the social setting in which use occurs are important factors contributing to the emergence and maintenance of problematic use. The 'reward circuit' refers to areas of the brain involved with addictive drug effects. This circuit is activated during intoxication, and rewards the user with the pleasant feelings (Koob & Volkow, 2016; Kwako & Koob, 2017). Through positive

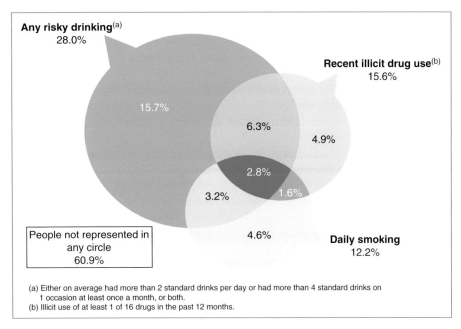

FIGURE 14.1

Source: AIHW, 2017a, Figure 2.1

reinforcement there is more frequent use. Classical conditioning links reward experiences with cues associated with the drug, and causes strong cravings to arise when in a situation in which drug use has previously occurred. Not all keep using, but continuous use with ensuing neuro-adaption leads to a withdrawal/negative affect state. In this state, using is driven by the need to alleviate unpleasant feelings (negative reinforcement) as well as in pursuit of its rewarding experiences. In the state of addiction, sources of reward narrow to those related to the drug, such that there is preoccupation with it. Priority is given to the drug and its consumption over health and other areas of life. Insight is often impaired.

In clinical settings, dependence is often synonymous with 'addicted'. The term 'addiction' is generally not used in clinical settings, as for some it has critical or judgmental connotations. 'Abuse' is used to refer to regular use which is problematic but does not have features of dependence, such as tolerance and withdrawal. Severe problems can and do nevertheless result from regular abuse of a substance, but it is not necessarily a precursor to addiction (Hasin et al., 2013). Terminology has evolved so that in the *DSM-5* (APA, 2013) a patient who abuses a substance to their detriment, but is not 'addicted', can be diagnosed with substance use disorder. The patient who is dependent or addicted is diagnosed as having a substance use disorder, with the specifier as 'severe'. Single episodes of substance use can of course result in severe mental and behavioural disturbance, related to intoxication or high levels of intake leading to toxicity.

The features used for diagnosis of a substance use disorder, under the *DSM-5* are summarised below (APA, 2013):

A. A cluster of symptoms and behaviours reflecting impaired control over substance use:
  1. using more or for longer than intended
  2. unsuccessful in controlling use, despite a desire to reduce or stop
  3. a great deal of time is spent taking, obtaining or recovering from the substance
  4. strong urges or cravings to use that can completely preoccupy
B. Symptoms that are due to social impairment:
  5. repeated use leads to failing to meet obligations at work, home or school
  6. continued use despite social or interpersonal problems as a result of substance use
  7. important activities in social, family, work, or recreational areas are reduced because of substance use
C. Risky use
  8. using in situations that are physically hazardous
  9. continuing use, despite physical or psychological problems exacerbated or caused by the substance
D. Neuro-adaption
  10. emergence of tolerance (need more for the same effect)
  11. withdrawal symptoms emerge as the substance levels begin to diminish (in the regular user).

The problematic pattern of use needs to have been present for at least 12 months. Specifiers are used to denote the severity of the disorder, with *mild* cases having two to three symptoms, *moderate* four to five, and *severe* six or more. Reflecting the nature of severe substance use disorders as chronic relapsing, remitting conditions, *in early remission* is applied when the person has stopped or reduced their intake and the criteria would no longer be met for between three and 12 months. For periods of greater than 12 months, *in sustained remission* can be used. Moderate or severe substance use disorder reflects dependence on the substance.

INTOXICATION, WITHDRAWAL AND SUBSTANCE-INDUCED SYMPTOMS OF A MENTAL DISORDER

Alteration in mental state can occur during intoxication, withdrawal and because of the substance-inducing symptoms that simulate a mental disorder. Suicide and suicidal ideation and behaviour are consistently associated with all substances of abuse (Breet et al., 2018).

Intoxication is sought by the user to enhance experiences or suppress a feeling. The effects are drug specific and dose dependent, and are influenced by the expectations of the user as well as the setting in which they are taken. A regular user is less sensitive to the effect of the drug than someone who has never taken it. Having a lower threshold for reacting to the drug, the naïve or infrequent user may experience undesired sequelae of intoxication or toxicity at lower doses compared with the experienced user. At the extremes, the user loses insight and is no longer aware that the substance taken is the cause of their experiences. The effects of excessive dosing can be seen even in experienced users if they consume enough. These are summarised below according to broad classes. Impaired judgment is seen in all with intoxication.

Regular users establish tolerance because the relevant receptors adapt to the constant action of the substance. Larger doses are required to achieve intoxication, and for many who are dependent the drug is taken to prevent or alleviate symptoms of withdrawal as well as in the hope of experiencing the desired feeling of intoxication. Withdrawal syndromes are measurable physiologically in alcohol, opioids and sedative hypnotics. For amphetamine-type stimulants and cannabis they can emerge, but there are no measurable findings on physical examination. Hallucinogens and inhalants are not associated with withdrawal syndromes.

Substance-induced mental disorders are distinguished from the behavioural and emotional disturbances that accompany dependent, entrenched or recurrent substance use, e.g. distress due to use. They are temporary mental disorders that are caused by the chemical effects of the substance. The type and nature vary according to the action of the drug. Once again, the *DSM-5* criteria provide a useful description that helps its identification.

SUBSTANCE/MEDICATION-INDUCED MENTAL DISORDER

1. Features of a mental disorder.
2. Evidence from the history (including from other sources), physical examination or laboratory findings that:
   a. the disorder begins within a month of taking the substance or withdrawal
   b. the substance involved can cause the mental disorder.
3. The disorder is not better explained by an independent mental disorder, which is suggested by the presence of the independent mental disorder prior to using the substance, or the symptoms lasting more than a month after the substance was stopped.
4. It is not better explained by delirium.
5. The disorder causes significant impairment or distress.

Although substance-induced mental disorders should not persist more than a month after use is stopped, there are exceptions: substance-associated neuro-cognitive disorders due to the effects of alcohol or inhalants (because of neurotoxicity), or sedative-hypnotic-anxiolytics (because of long half-life medications); and hallucinogen persisting perception disorder.

Substance-induced mental disorders can lead to clinically significant presentations that warrant treatment like any other mental disorder. The stigma associated

Table 14.2 Unwanted Effects of Intoxication That May Alter Mental State

Drug action/type	Mental and behavioural problems associated with high levels of intoxication
Stimulants	Inability to sleep, anxiety, agitation, emotional lability, excessive talkativeness, irritability, rage, altered perceptual experiences from illusions to hallucinations, delusions (typically persecutory, jealousy, referential, parasitic infestation), stereotypy and eventually delirium
Substances which are sedative	Disinhibition, aggression, sedation, impaired attention, reduced alertness, impaired cognitive functioning, disorientation, delirium
Hallucinogens	Frightening perceptual experiences and mood alteration, dissociation, hallucinations and delusions and delirium (particularly with the anticholinergics)
Dissociative hallucinogens	Sedation, dreamlike state, depersonalisation and derealisation, reduced physical awareness (e.g. of pain), delusions, hallucinations and delirium, coma

Effects are listed in order of dose effect. Physical effects are not listed but are highly likely to accompany excessive dosing with the substances.

with people who have substance use disorders can result in resistance in the health-care setting to provide adequate care. A substance-induced psychosis, which at presentation can be indistinguishable from schizophrenia (Ali et al., 2010), requires treatment in a similar fashion to an exacerbation of schizophrenia. This is given in the same way that a person with a myocardial infarction receives the same treatment, whether they are a smoker, obese or not.

Substances can be grouped together according to their main actions. Problems that arise in excessive dose of each group are outlined in Table 14.2.

SEDATING SUBSTANCES – DEPRESSANTS

Alcohol, benzodiazepines, and gamma-hydroxybutyrate (GHB)

The predominant action of alcohol, benzodiazepines and gamma-hydroxybutyrate (GHB) is to slow down or sedate. People often utilise this to depress or to reduce feelings of anxiety. Alcohol stimulates $GABA_A$ receptors (along with inhibition of glutamate and NMDA receptors) and benzodiazepines particularly act by stimulating the $GABA_A$ receptors. Alcohol brings about mild mood elevation, relaxation and subtle disinhibition. Cannabis has similar mood effects, but will also create the sense of time slowing. Benzodiazepines are often taken to augment the effects of other substances. GHB affects performance and behaviour within 30 minutes of consumption and lasts for up to six hours depending on the dose. An initial stimulation effect is followed by sedation and potentially coma in higher doses (Kamal et al., 2017).

PROBLEMS COMMONLY SEEN WITH ALCOHOL, BENZODIAZEPINES AND GHB

Alcohol and benzodiazepines can produce prominent depressive disorders during intoxication. Considering the high and sustained blood alcohol levels maintained by many with moderate to severe alcohol use disorders, this mood disorder can continue as long as the person is drinking. Inhibitions are relaxed while intoxicated, so this combination has been found in many attempted and completed suicides. Anxiety is a feature of withdrawals from sedative substances, and may occur daily. Alcohol and benzodiazepine intoxication can increase aggressive behaviour.

Alcohol withdrawal

This is common and only seen in the alcohol dependent. When there is a history of chronic heavy intake, withdrawals can be life threatening, and complicated by delirium or seizures. The most severe withdrawals are seen in those who have consumed large amounts over many years. Withdrawals may arise in alcohol-dependent people consuming more than eight standard drinks for males, and six standard drinks for women. Early symptoms and signs begin 6–24 hours after the last drink.

Symptoms and signs include:

- anxiety and depressed mood
- insomnia
- increased heart rate and blood pressure
- tremor
- sweating
- agitation
- seizures (usually within the first two days of withdrawals)
- hallucinations (usually accompanies severe withdrawal)
- confusion as part of delirium (begins usually between two and six days).

Alcohol withdrawal can be managed at home under safe conditions, provided the person can be regularly reviewed and have close medical monitoring if medication is prescribed.

The medication management of withdrawals involves time-limited symptom control with diazepam (unless the patient has impaired liver functioning or has respiratory compromise, in which case lorazepam is used). Not all people need medication for their alcohol withdrawals; however, if there is a history of needing medication for withdrawals or of complicated withdrawals (delirium or seizures), medication will be required. The Clinical Institute Withdrawal Assessment for Alcohol – revised version (CIWA-Ar) is used in most settings to monitor withdrawals (Sullivan et al., 1989). It is a standardised measure with a score of 8–10 interpreted as the point at which benzodiazepines are required (see below) (Haber et al., 2009). While the paramedic would not normally complete a full alcohol withdrawal assessment using a CIWA-Ar (or similar) tool, it is useful for them to note the main criteria for assessing alcohol withdrawal symptoms (see Fig. 14.2).

Addiction Research Foundation Clinical Institute Withdrawal Assessment for Alcohol (CIWA-Ar)

Patient_____ Date |__|__|__| Time ____:____
                         y m d   (24 hour clock, midnight=00:00)

Pulse or heart rate, taken for one minute:_____ Blood pressure: _____/_____

NAUSEA AND VOMITING—AS "Do you feel sick to your stomach? Have you vomited?" Observation.

0 no nausea and no vomiting
1 mild nausea with no vomiting
2
3
4 intermittent nausea with dry heaves
5
6
7 constant nausea, frequent dry heaves and vomiting

TREMOR—Arms extended and fingers spread apart. Observation.

0 no tremor
1 not visible, but can be felt fingertip to fingertip
2
3
4 moderate, with patient's arms extended
5
6
7 severe, even with arms not extended

PAROXYSMAL SWEATS—Observation.
0 no sweat visible
1 barely perceptible sweating, palms moist
2
3
4 beads of sweat obvious on forehead
5
6
7 drenching sweats

ANXIETY—Ask "Do you feel nervous?" Observation

0 no anxiety, at ease
1 mildly anxious
2
3
4 moderately anxious, or guarded, so anxiety is inferred
5
6
7 equivalent to acute panic states as seen in severe delirium or acute schizophrenic reactions

AGITATION—Observation.

0 normal activity
1 somewhat more than normal activity
2
3
4 moderately fidgety and restless
5
6
7 paces back and forth during most of the interview, or constantly thrashes about

TACTILE DISTURBANCES—Ask "Have you any itching, pins and needles sensations, any burning, any numbness or do you feel bugs crawling on or under your skin?" Observation.

0 none
1 very mild itching, pins and needles, burning or numbness
2 mild itching, pins and needles, burning or numbness
3 moderate itching, pins and needles, burning or numbness
4 moderately severe hallucinations
5 severe hallucinations
6 extremely severe hallucinations
7 continuous hallucinations

AUDITORY DISTURBANCES—Ask "Are you more aware of sounds around you? Are they harsh? Do they frighten you? Are you hearing anything that is disturbing to you? Are you hearing things you know are not there?" Observation.

0 not present
1 very mild harshness or ability to frighten
2 mild harshness or ability to frighten
3 moderate harshness or ability to frighten
4 moderately severe hallucinations
5 severe hallucinations
6 extremely severe hallucinations
7 continuous hallucinations

VISUAL DISTURBANCES—Ask "Does the light appear to be too bright? Is its colour different? Does it hurt your eyes? Are you seeing anything that is disturbing to you? Are you seeing things you know are not there?" Observation.

0 not present
1 very mild sensitivity
2 mild sensitivity
3 moderate sensitivity
4 moderately severe hallucinations
5 severe hallucinations
6 extremely severe hallucinations
7 continuous hallucinations

HEADACHE, FULLNESS IN HEAD—Ask "Does your head feel different? Does it feel like there is a band around your head?" Do not rate for dizziness or lightheadedness. Otherwise, rate severity.

0 not present
1 very mild
2 mild
3 moderate
4 moderate severe
5 severe
6 very severe
7 extremely severe

ORIENTATION AND CLOUDING OF SENSORIUM—Ask "What day is this? Where are you? Who am I?"

0 oriented and can do serial additions
1 cannot do serial additions or is uncertain about date
2 disoriented for date by no more than 2 calendar days
3 disoriented for date by more than 2 calendar days
4 disoriented for place and/or person

This scale is not copyrighted and may be used freely.

Total CIWA-A Score_____
Rater's Initials_____
Maximum Possible Score 67

FIGURE 14.2

Addiction Research Foundation Clinical Institute Withdrawal Assessment for Alcohol (CIWA-Ar)

Reproduced from Sullivan et al., 1989

When alcohol withdrawal is associated with poor nutrition or medical problems, an acute thiamine deficiency can develop causing encephalopathy (Wernicke's), characterised by ophthalmoplegia, ataxia and confusion. This is a medical emergency. The patient requires intravenous thiamine and hospitalisation. Avoid intravenous dextrose until recovered. Even with intervention, the surviving patients are at risk of permanent memory impairment: this is known as 'Korsakoff's psychosis', even though it should be noted that it is not actually a psychosis. Overall, this complication of alcohol withdrawal is known as the Wernicke-Korsakoff syndrome.

Withdrawal complicated by delirium is often referred to as delirium tremens. Sweating, agitation, fever and disorientation are severe, and the patient requires hospitalisation. This is more likely in undernourished or medically ill patients.

GHB

Dependence can arise rapidly (within weeks of continuous use), and withdrawals can be abrupt and severe. It operates on GHB_B receptors primarily, so withdrawals are not easily managed with benzodiazepines (Kamal et al., 2017).

OPIOIDS

Morphine, heroin, codeine, oxycodone, methadone, fentanyl, tramadol, Panadeine

Opiates are derived from opium and can be obtained through prescription (such as codeine, morphine, oxycodone, methadone, fentanyl, tramadol), purchased over the counter (such as Panadeine) or obtained illegally (such as heroin). They are sedating but also bring about euphoria. Heroin is favoured by users because of feelings of calmness and relaxation (Lankenau et al., 2010), appealing to people wanting to escape the harsh realities of their lives.

PROBLEMS COMMONLY SEEN WITH OPIOIDS

The mental and behavioural problems associated with use of these substances are far less dramatic than with stimulants or alcohol. The high rates of abuse of benzodiazepines along with heroin places this group at inadvertent risk of overdose death. Otherwise, problematic presentations are seen around drug seeking which can become urgent if the supply is threatened and withdrawals are imminent. Withdrawal symptoms are greatly feared by opioid-dependent patients. Opioid withdrawals are similar for all opioids, but the onset and duration varies between drugs, reflecting their relative half-lives. Heroin withdrawals begin 6–12 hours after last use, and will last up to five days. For drugs with longer half-lives such as methadone or codeine, withdrawals commence after one to two days. Pupil dilation and piloerection are objective signs.

STIMULANT SUBSTANCES

Stimulants such as amphetamine, methamphetamine, cocaine and MDMA (3,4-methylenedioxymethamphetamine; also known as 'ecstasy', which is also hallucinogenic) will enhance energy and stamina and elevate mood. They increase monoamine (noradrenaline, dopamine and serotonin) activity through enhanced release (methamphetamines, amphetamines, MDMA); and reduced reuptake and metabolism of dopamine (amphetamine, methamphetamine). Cocaine inhibits their reuptake (Moszczynska & Callan, 2017). MDMA particularly enhances serotonin activity, thought to be the reason for the sense of closeness its users' value. Cocaine is generally taken nasally, but can be injected. MDMA is typically taken orally. Amphetamines are less commonly used than methamphetamines – both can be taken orally, intranasally or injected intravenously. Methamphetamine ('Meth') in its crystalline form ('ice') is often smoked. Peak effects from methamphetamines are noticed within 15–20 minutes of injecting or smoking, or within 1–3 hours of oral consumption, with the effects lasting up to 12 hours (Cruickshank & Dyer, 2009).

PROBLEMS COMMONLY SEEN WITH METHAMPHETAMINES AND OTHER STIMULANTS

Because the drug is activating, the mental and behavioural disturbances (e.g. agitated psychotic presentations) are often pressing and dramatic, requiring an immediate response. Although methamphetamine users are far fewer in numbers than alcohol-related presentations, their emergency presentations are often more memorable. People who are both intoxicated with methamphetamines and psychotic as a result are amongst the most frightening and behaviourally disturbed presentations seen in the acute setting. Prolonged use causes neurotoxicity and measurable cognitive changes (particularly related to executive functioning) (Cruickshank & Dyer, 2009; Moszczynska & Callan, 2017). These can impair the user's ability to comprehend and retain complex multistage instructions when sober.

In addition to emergency presentations with psychosis, delirium or behavioural problems associated with methamphetamines, users frequently experience symptoms of mental illness: 48% of those using ecstasy and 42% of those using methamphetamines in the previous 12 months reported being diagnosed or treated for a mental illness (compared with 14% of the general population) (AIHW, 2018a). Stimulant drugs elevate mood during intoxication, but in regular users this can be followed by two to six weeks of withdrawal anxiety and depressive symptoms on cessation as part of the withdrawal syndrome. Secondary dysphoria is caused by the problems from the regular drug use, and compounds the drug's direct mood affects. Stimulant-induced depressive disorders and anxiety disorders can occur. The stimulant user is far more likely to seek help for symptoms of mental illness, but may not disclose their use. This means that many are incorrectly diagnosed with various psychiatric disorders, including bipolar disorder, major depression or attention deficit disorder. Schizophrenia may be difficult to distinguish from someone who continues methamphetamine use despite repeated psychotic episodes.

HALLUCINOGENIC SUBSTANCES (HALLUCINOGENS)

LSD (D-lysergic acid diethylamide), ayahuasca, mescaline, psilocybin, various botanical compounds (e.g. datura, cannabis), benztropine, dissociative anaesthetics (ketamine and phencyclidine (PCP)) and MDMA ('ecstasy'; n.b. also a stimulant)

'PSYCHEDELICS'

LSD (d-lysergic acid diethylamide), ayahuasca, mescaline, angel's trumpet, datura, magic mushrooms (psilocybin) and benztropine alter perceptual experiences, consciousness and mood. Research is returning to explore the potential therapeutic effects of the 'psychedelics' such as LSD, mescaline and psilocybin, which stimulate the $5-HT_{2A}$ receptor (Kyzar et al., 2017). They are, however, known to have the potential to cause psychological disturbance, including psychosis, and at the same time to potentially induce personality changes (e.g. changes to openness to experience). LSD has an onset of action over 20–60 minutes and can last up to 10 hours. These hallucinogens do not have withdrawal syndromes associated with chronic use.

Problems commonly seen with 'psychedelic' hallucinogens

A 'bad trip' is a distressing experience from intoxication, but rarely leads the user to seek intervention as insight that it is a drug effect is usually retained. An hallucinogen-induced psychosis can be considered when insight is absent. Symptoms should abate quite quickly once the drug is cleared. A relatively rare disorder called hallucinogen persisting perception disorder can follow hallucinogen use, and is characterised by persistent and recurrent 'flashbacks' (re-experiencing aspects of their experience in an instance of intoxication). This disorder can persist for longer than a month after last use, and, for some, they persist for years.

CANNABIS

Cannabis is sought for its mood elevation, sedation and perception of time slowing. It can be considered a sedating substance; however, perceptual disturbances are commonplace. Impaired memory and performance of complex tasks also feature. After intake, pupils become bloodshot and appetite increases. Usually smoked, the effects arise within minutes, but may take up to two hours if eaten in prepared food. Intoxication will last for three to four hours. Widely regarded as a 'safe' or 'soft' illicit, harms nevertheless are frequent. It contains multiple chemicals (a variety known as cannabinoids) that exert their effects through binding with the body's endocannabinoid system, which is involved with mediating functions such as memory, emotions, movement and cell functions. Cannabinoid receptors (CB_1)

are located in the central nervous system, and these interact with a variety of other neuro-receptors to produce its effects (Greydanus & Merrick, 2016).

Problems commonly seen with cannabis use

Panic is a common side effect of cannabis abuse, probably mediated through cannabinol. It is not uncommon for a single panic during intoxication to establish a cannabis-induced anxiety disorder whereby fear of recurrence perpetuates the anxiety symptoms. In those predisposed, features of a panic disorder may continue, and cannabis is considered to have precipitated the first episode of panic in this disorder rather than having a cannabis-induced anxiety disorder. At high doses, cannabis, via its psychoactive ingredient tetrahydrocannabinol, can cause psychotic symptoms which recede when the drug effects subside. A 20-year cohort study showed that nearly 50% of those diagnosed with cannabis-induced psychosis in Denmark were later diagnosed with schizophrenia. A consistent association has been found in large cohort studies between adolescent cannabis use and the development of schizophrenia (Zammit et al., 2002). Chronic users develop amotivation, and cognitive performance is affected (Volkow et al., 2016). Cannabis can induce hyperemesis. Dependent users can experience withdrawals during which there is irritability, dysphoria, sleeplessness and appetite loss.

DISSOCIATIVES (DISSOCIATIVE ANAESTHETICS)

Ketamine and phencyclidine (PCP) predominantly relax, disinhibit and affect memory and perception, and at high enough doses, as they are anaesthetics, will impair consciousness. Ketamine's onset is within seconds after intravenous administration, but considerably delayed to up to 30 minutes when taken orally. It is a mild stimulant at low doses, and psychedelic at higher associated with executive function impairment (Sassano-Higgins et al., 2016). Ketamine and PCP act through the NMDA receptor antagonism, but also inhibit reuptake of dopamine, which could account for early interest in it as a model of schizophrenia (Lodge & Mercier, 2015). PCP was a popular drug of abuse in the 1960s and 1970s.

Problems commonly seen with dissociatives

In larger doses both can induce psychosis, to the extent that in the 1960s PCP was regarded as a 'schizomimmetic drug' (Lodge & Mercier, 2015). Delirium can be a severe effect, particularly associated with hallucinations (see Table 14.2).

INHALANTS

Inhalants are volatile hydrocarbons derived from glues, gases and petrol.

These substances are largely used by teenage children, with rates of use dropping significantly thereafter. These are highly neurotoxic substances, and fatalities are not infrequent. A constellation of medical complications accompany their abuse (Tormoehlen et al., 2014). Under intoxication, central nervous system depression produces disinhibition, apathy and impaired judgment along with incoordination. Dependence can arise, and long-term use is associated with neuro-cognitive impairment.

POLYSUBSTANCE USE

Concurrent use of multiple drugs will produce complicated intoxication and withdrawal syndromes, disinhibition and judgment impairment.

SUBSTANCE USE EXACERBATING SYMPTOMS OF MENTAL ILLNESS

People with mental illnesses use substances at higher rates than the general population. Although the 'self-medication' hypothesis has much face validity, it is not generally the core reason for substance use in this group, who have been found to be using substances for the same reasons as the general population. The exception is found in anxiety disorders, where alcohol and other substances are used in self-medication in early adolescence at the onset age of these disorders. Unfortunately, this can lead to substance dependence and worsened outcomes for the anxiety disorder. Similarly, alcohol abuse may begin following a traumatic experience to combat nightmares associated with post-traumatic stress disorder. Helping initiate sleep only, alcohol actually impairs sleep architecture and is likely to worsen the symptoms.

In manic states, driven to pursue pleasurable activities, some patients use large quantities of drugs or alcohol, which can complicate presentations and confound diagnosis. Patients with schizophrenia frequently abuse psychotomimetic drugs, knowingly worsening their psychotic symptoms but valuing the intoxication.

Depressed patients, particularly those who have anxiety, may develop an alcohol use disorder as a result, and in these cases the history of when each condition began will reveal this.

Patients with borderline personality disorder have marked distress intolerance and regularly use substances to attempt self-regulation; however, substance abuse is more often a consequence of their impulsivity. The combination of intoxication and a crisis in such patients can be very dangerous.

APPROACHES TO TREATMENT AND CARE
ASSESSMENT
Approach

Whenever there is the possibility of substance use, the paramedic must consider whether the person is likely to be intoxicated, withdrawing or experiencing symptoms of a mental disorder arising from use. Substance intoxication can also mask underlying conditions (e.g. head injury or sepsis). Increased impulsivity, and judgment impairment, will make their behaviour unpredictable. Substances that impact on the person's attention will impair their ability to remain alert during assessment, as well as their comprehension of questions and recall of events. Approaching the assessment in a non-judgmental way is paramount. Simple language should be used.

Situational awareness

The environment provides valuable insight as to the role that drugs or alcohol are playing in the presentation. Observe for evidence of discarded alcohol containers, injecting paraphernalia, ice pipes or bongs.

Risk

The paramedic must approach the assessment of risk to patient and self, prepared for sudden shifts in focus and affect, as well as the patient's disinhibition and unpredictable behaviour. The various state and territory Mental Health Acts do not generally permit enforcing treatment for intoxication or a substance use disorder. If the person has a substance-induced mental disorder, they may be placed under the state's or territory's Mental Health Act for treatment of that mental illness. Careful assessment for suicidal thinking, behaviour and intentions is required in each presentation, together with the determination about the person's capacity for decision making (see risk assessment in Chapter 11). Dangerous intoxication is generally managed in an emergency department rather than in a mental health setting because of the high risks of medical complications, e.g. death through alcohol intoxication. Intoxication may impair judgment significantly, creating a situation requiring intervention under the Mental Health Act. In some circumstances, a severe substance-induced mental illness following high levels of intoxication in a medically stable individual requires management in a mental health environment, e.g. amphetamine-induced psychosis. In the community, such situations frequently require police involvement.

History: fundamental areas to cover

- *Is the person delirious or psychotic?* (Whatever the cause, this needs to be assessed for as a priority. There is no point attempting to help the person plan to address their substance use under these circumstances.)
- *What substance does the person use, and how is it taken?* (Substance effects vary according to type and mode of intake.)
- *Is the patient dependent on the substance or have a severe substance use disorder?* (Refer to the criteria for substance use disorder.) (If severe, withdrawals will therefore be a possibility, or a substance-induced mental disorder will be more likely, e.g. amphetamine-induced psychosis.)
- *When did they last use?* (This will tell you whether they are likely to be intoxicated, withdrawing, or neither.)

• *Did they have a pre-existing mental illness?* (Because the drug may have caused an acute exacerbation of it.)

Mental state examination

A systematic mental state examination becomes more important as the level of cooperation and ability to provide a history is less. There can be clues as to what has been taken. Under the headings, the following are relevant:

> *Appearance:* Pupillary dilation in stimulant intoxication or opioid withdrawal; pinpoint in opioid intoxication; bloodshot glazed eyes in cannabis use; odours reflecting alcohol or cannabis use; track marks (opioid, stimulant or benzodiazepine).
>
> *Behaviour:* Stereotypy (repetitive purposeless actions), scratching skin, responding to hallucinations may all suggest stimulant intoxication or induced psychosis; overactivity, intrusiveness suggest stimulants; catatonia or serenely responding to inner experiences imply hallucinogens; sleepy inactivity commonly found in opioid, cannabis and alcohol intoxication. Inappropriate giggling is common but not pathognomonic in cannabis intoxication.
>
> *Conversation:* Sedating substance intoxication generally slows the rate of speech and leads to the appearance that each word is being carefully chosen; stimulants accelerate speech, which can become loud, pressured, disjointed and difficult to follow.
>
> *Affect:* Mood alterations are features of all substances. Extreme irritability is more likely to be seen with stimulant intoxication, and less intensely as withdrawals set in. Anxiety is severe with alcohol withdrawals. Mild elevation or euphoria is common in cannabis and hallucinogen intoxication.
>
> *Perception:* Ask about auditory and visual hallucinations. Note whether the person appears to be responding to them. These are commonly seen in hallucinogens, but hallucinations are encountered in delirium from intoxication (e.g. cannabis, PCP), withdrawals (e.g. complicated alcohol or benzodiazepines) and in induced psychotic states.
>
> *Cognition:* Confusion, orientation and attentional impairment can indicate delirium, but inattention may signal sedative intoxication.
>
> *Insight:* Is the person aware that the symptoms they are experiencing are due to the substance they have taken, or have they lost this awareness, as may be seen in psychosis or delirium?

SYMPTOM CONTROL

Generally, the problems seen during acute situations by the paramedic such as intoxication or substance-induced disorders are managed symptomatically and the actual problem of substance using is addressed later. The paramedic, other health professionals and family members should aim to provide calm reassurance and reality orientation in a low-stimulus environment, regardless of where the person is helped. Some withdrawal states for alcohol require immediate treatment with medication, but generally other substances do not need urgent intervention (the exception being GHB withdrawal).

WHEN TO TRANSPORT?

While simple intoxication does not require a person to be transported, there are several situations in which the patient is best helped by transport to a treatment centre:

1. Risk (physical health or mental health) – for safety
2. High levels of distress – for patient relief
3. Symptoms of mental disorder that are not understood or are inconsistent with the expected effects of the substance – for diagnostic clarification and management
4. Severe alcohol withdrawals – confused or ataxic and withdrawing; withdrawing and has a history of withdrawals complicated by seizures or delirium – for treatment
5. Delirium due to substance withdrawals – for treatment.

In these situations, capacity may be very difficult to determine due to the substance use and may challenge the decision making by paramedics. Paramedics may need to activate early clinical, mental health and police support to provide care in the least confrontational and restrictive means possible. The support of the Operational Centre and local drug and alcohol treatment providers may also be of assistance.

LONG-TERM CARE OF PEOPLE WITH SUBSTANCE USE DISORDERS

Interventions depend on the severity of the disorder, particularly whether there is dependence or not.

ARE THEY 'ADDICTED' OR DEPENDENT?

- Consider whether withdrawal treatment is necessary as a first step.
- Motivation to change is needed; engage in treatment.
- Treatment options include a knowledgeable GP, drug and alcohol services, addiction specialist. Depending on the substance, this may include a combination of medication (e.g. anti-craving agents in alcohol dependence, or substitution with naltrexone/buprenorphine in opioid dependence) with psychosocial interventions.
- Consider 12-Step (e.g. Alcoholics Anonymous) or SMART groups if available.

ARE THEY NON-DEPENDENT?

They may respond to a brief intervention:

- Identify the problem.
- Recommend safe levels of use, including abstinence.
- Provide advice as to how this can be achieved.
- Follow up as appropriate, e.g. GP, drug and alcohol non-government organisation.

HAS THE SUBSTANCE CAUSED SYMPTOMS OF A MENTAL DISORDER?

Substance-induced mental disorders are temporary states, expected to resolve at the time or shortly after the substance is eliminated (certainly within a month) provided abstinence is maintained, but will return if use starts again. The time to recover varies according to the substance used based on its pharmacology. Reassurance and reality orientation in a safe, low-stimulus environment while waiting for the substance effects to subside may be all that is required in mildly psychotic patients. Medication (antipsychotics and/or benzodiazepines) is necessary if the patient has drug-induced psychotic symptoms and is distressed or agitated; and benzo-diazepines for those tormented by hallucinogen-induced psychotic states.

Depressive mood states and symptomatic anxiety are commonly seen in people with alcohol dependence because of alcohol's direct effects. Generally, the mood lifts and anxiety improves once withdrawal, if present, passes. It may take one to four weeks for the mood to lift once the person stops drinking. In the inter-vening time antidepressants will be of no use. Anxiety symptoms may be slower to improve, and are generally not very responsive to the antidepressant medica-tions normally prescribed for anxiety disorders. Long-term benzodiazepines should be avoided.

The critical determinants for the paramedic to decide where care is best pro-vided are risk and level of distress. In most cases, e.g. cannabis-induced delirium, management is possible out of hospital with an explanation as to what is happen-ing, the provision of comforting support and the reassurance that the person will begin to feel better quite soon. In some cases, notably chronic methamphetamine use leading to a severe substance-induced psychosis, it may require a brief initial psychiatric admission to provide a safe environment, antipsychotic medication and several weeks to recover. Antidepressants have no place in acute treatment settings for substance-induced depression.

WHAT TO DO ABOUT THE SUBSTANCE USE DISORDER

Paramedics have a unique opportunity to intervene when they encounter patients with chronic heavy substance use (suggestive of dependence), as well as those with milder use problems. Health crises often shape the person's resolve to act now to change their lives. Recovering from a substance use disorder requires time. The paramedic can use the opportunity to offer the person information as to where to start to address their problem. For most, contacting their state's alcohol and drug information phone line, or seeing their general practitioner is the starting point. Specialist drug and alcohol services inpatient facilities tend to focus on medical withdrawal management that may be required as the first step of treatment if the person is dependent. Drug and alcohol outpatient services tend to provide counselling, assisted withdrawals and opioid substitution treatments (for opioid dependence). They focus on those with severe use disorders. Most people with substance use disorders are managed in the community with their general practitioner and other services. Milder-severity substance use disorders do not require detoxification, and often respond to brief interventions.

The following is a list of substance use disorders with comments about the medication used in their management.

- *Alcohol dependence:* To treat withdrawal – benzodiazepines; to maintain abstinence – anti-craving agents (naltrexone or acamprosate) or disulfiram (an aversive agent).
- *Opioid dependence:* Withdrawal management – naloxone/buprenorphine or symptomatic medications; maintenance or substitution therapy – methadone or naloxone/buprenorphine. Maintenance therapy replaces the abused opioid with an alternative controlled prescribed opioid. This allows the person to undergo the necessary steps to recover from their dependence.
- *Benzodiazepine dependence:* Withdrawals managed by conversion to equivalent diazepam dosage and slow reduction. No maintenance therapy.
- *Cannabis, amphetamine-type stimulants and other illicits:* Withdrawals – symptomatic treatments using a variety of psychotropics to target specific symptoms; there are no agents of proven benefit for long-term treatment.

Psychosocial treatments for substance use disorders include cognitive behavioural therapies of various types and styles, therapeutic communities, groups (e.g. Alcoholic Anonymous, SMART recovery groups) that are delivered in private health, state/territory and non-government organisation settings. Motivational interviewing approaches recognise that confrontation is likely to ignite significant resistance to change.

RECOGNISING YOUR OWN EMOTIONAL RESPONSE

In most cases, unreasonable and threatening behaviour is the consequence of the effect of the substance. Repeated presentations for the same reason can prompt anger and cynicism. Often the person's presentation is entirely different once sober or once their mental health symptoms have resolved. This point in their life may be critical in helping them decide that it is time to stop taking the substance, or cease alcohol consumption, and to act. Remembering this, and that the problems of substance dependence are due to a chronic relapsing remitting condition, is helpful for the paramedic in controlling natural emotional responses to these situations. Many people do fully recover from their substance use disorders, but it may not be at this moment.

CONCLUSION

The paramedic is well equipped if they understand the effects that substances of abuse can have on the mental state and behaviour. The focus of the assessment is to decide which of the problems caused by substance use problems – intoxication, withdrawal or a substance-induced mental disorder – requires immediate action. Defining whether the problem is substance dependence or episodic abuse determines the correct course of action for aftercare.

LINKS AND RESOURCES

Phone information about treatment
- Alcohol and Drug Information Services – helpline available in each state.

Self-help for patients
- Alcoholics Anonymous (AA), Narcotics Anonymous (NA)
- SMART recovery groups

Self-help for families
- Available through Al-Anon and Alateen.
- Gordon, A., 2009. Comorbidity of Mental Disorders and Substance Use: A brief guide for the primary care clinician. Department of Health and Ageing, Canberra.
- Haber, P.L.N., Proude, E., Lopatko, O., 2009. Guidelines for the Treatment of Alcohol Problems. Australian Government Department of Health and Ageing, Canberra.
- http://www.alcohol.gov.au/internet/alcohol/publishing.nsf/Content/guidelines-treat-alc-09
- http://www.nationaldrugstrategy.gov.au/internet/drugstrategy/publishing.nsf/Content/FE16C454A782A8AFCA2575BE002044D0/$File/mono71.pdf

REFERENCES

Ali, R., Marsden, J., Srisurapanont, M., et al., 2010. Methamphetamine psychosis in Australia, Philippines, and Thailand: recommendations for acute care and clinical inpatient management. Addict. Disorder Treatment 9 (4), 143–149.

American Psychiatric Association (APA), 2013. Diagnostic and Statistical Manual of Mental Disorders, fifth ed. APA, Washington, DC. (DSM-5).

Australian Institute of Health and Welfare (AIHW), 2017a. National Drug Strategy Household Survey 2016: Detailed findings. AIHW, Canberra. Online. Available: https://www.aihw.gov.au/reports/illicit-use-of-drugs/2016-ndshs-detailed/contents/table-of-contents. 25 November 2019.

Australian Institute of Health and Welfare (AIHW), 2017b. Non-medical Use of Pharmaceuticals: Trends, harms, and treatment 2006–07 to 2015–16. AIHW, Canberra. Online. Available: https://www.aihw.gov.au/getmedia/d35a8ea3-e504-4cf2-8e72-d8e12f22d7ac/aihw-hse-195. pdf.aspx?inline=true. 25 November 2019.

Australian Institute of Health and Welfare (AIHW), 2018a. Impact of Alcohol and Illicit Drug use on the Burden of Disease and Injury in Australia: Australian Burden of Disease Study 2011. AIHW, Canberra. Online. Available: https://www.aihw.gov.au/reports/burden-of-disease/ impact-alcohol-illicit-drug-use-on-burden-disease/contents/table-of-contents.

Australian Institute of Health and Welfare (AIHW), 2018b. Mental Health Services in Brief 2018. Online. AIHW, Canberra. Available: https://www.aihw.gov.au/reports/mental-health-services/mental-health-services-in-australia-in-brief-2018/contents/table-of-contents. 25 November 2019.

Breet, E., Goldstone, D., Bantjes, J., 2018. Substance use and suicidal ideation and behaviour in low- and middle-income countries: a systematic review. BMC Public Health 18 (1), 549.

Cruickshank, C., Dyer, K., 2009. A review of the clinical pharmacology of methamphetamine. Addiction 104 (7), 1085–1099.

Greydanus, D., Merrick, J., 2016. Cannabis or marijuana: a review. J. Pain. Manage. 9 (4), 347–373.

Haber, P., Lintzeris, N., Proude, E., et al., 2009. Guidelines for the treatment of alcohol problems. Prepared for the Australian Government Department of Health and Ageing, Commonwealth of Australia, Canberra.

Hasin, D., O'Brien, C., Auriacombe, M., et al., 2013. DSM-5 criteria for substance use disorders: recommendations and rationale. Am. J. Psychiatry 170 (8), 834–851.

Kamal, R.M., van Noorden, M.S., Wannet, W., et al., 2017. Pharmacological treatment in gamma-hydroxybutyrate (GHB) and gamma-butyrolactone (GBL) dependence: detoxification and relapse prevention. CNS Drugs 31 (1), 51–64.

Koob, G., Volkow, N., 2016. Neurobiology of addiction: a neurocircuitry analysis. Lancet Psychiatry 3 (8), 760–773.

Kwako, L.E., Koob, G.F., 2017. Neuroclinical framework for the role of stress in addiction. Chronic Stress https://doi.org/10.1177/2470547017698140. 28 July 2018.

Kyzar, E., Nichols, C., Gainetdinov, R., et al., 2017. Psychedelic drugs in biomedicine. Trends Pharmacol. Sci. 38 (11), 992–1005.

Lankenau, S., Wagner, K., Bloom, J., et al., 2010. The first injection event: differences among heroin, methamphetamine, cocaine, and ketamine initiates. J. Drug Issues 40 (2), 241–262.

Lodge, D., Mercier, M., 2015. Ketamine and phencyclidine: the good, the bad and the unexpected. Br. J. Pharmacol. 172 (17), 4254–4276.

Lynagh, M., Sanson-Fisher, R., Shakeshaft, A., 2010. Alcohol-related harm: perceptions of ambulance officers and health promotion actions they do and would do. Health Promot. J. Austr. 21, 19–25.

Moszczynska, A., Callan, S., 2017. Molecular, behavioral, and physiological consequences of methamphetamine neurotoxicity: implications for treatment. J. Pharmacol. Exp. Ther. 362 (3), 474–488.

Sassano-Higgins, S., Baron, D., Juarez, G., et al., 2016. A review of ketamine abuse and diversion. Depress. Anxiety 33 (8), 718–727.

Sullivan, J., Sykora, K., Schneiderman, J., et al., 1989. Assessment of alcohol withdrawal: the revised clinical institute withdrawal assessment for alcohol scale (CIWA-Ar). Br. J. Addict. 84 (11), 1353–1357.

Tormoehlen, L., Tekulve, K., Nañagas, K., 2014. Hydrocarbon toxicity: a review. Clin. Toxicol. 52 (5), 479–489.

Volkow, N., Swanson, J., Evins, A., et al., 2016. Effects of cannabis use on human behavior, including cognition, motivation, and psychosis: a review. JAMA Psychiatry 73 (3), 292–297.

Yu, C., McClellan, J., 2016. Genetics of substance use disorders. Child Adolesc. Psychiatr. Clin. N. Am. 25 (3), 377–385.

Zammit, S., Allebeck, P., Andreasson, S., et al., 2002. Self reported cannabis use as a risk factor for schizophrenia in Swedish conscripts of 1969: historical cohort study. BMJ 325 (7374), 1199–1201.

Managing challenging behaviour and workplace violence

15

Scott Lamont and Scott Brunero

LEARNING OUTCOMES

By the end of this chapter, you should be able to:

- understand personal, patient, environmental and systemic risk factors associated with challenging behaviour and workplace violence in the pre-hospital setting
- understand the importance of maintaining therapeutic moments/interactions with patients presenting with challenging behaviour and violence
- identify specific strategies for managing challenging behaviour and violence
- become familiar with self-care concepts to maintain wellbeing when encountering challenging behaviour and violence.

INTRODUCTION

Challenging behaviour and workplace violence (WPV) in the health sector have multiple aetiologies and can pose a significant risk to all healthcare professionals. This risk is particularly prominent for paramedics when attending dynamic and unpredictable crisis situations with scarce information and resources. Despite the high likelihood of experiencing challenging behaviour and WPV, paramedics should not consider these as simply 'part of the job'.

The material in this chapter will assist you to prepare, recognise and respond effectively to challenging behaviour and WPV. The chapter will explore ways to promote and maintain healthy relationships with patients and others with whom you come into contact throughout your daily work, help you identify and develop strategies for managing challenging behaviour and WPV, and increase self-awareness regarding your own wellbeing.

CASE STUDY

Harry

You have been dispatched at a.m. 1.30 for a 25-year-old male who is running in and out of traffic on a busy road. The police do not have an available car to meet you at the scene. On arrival,

Harry is initially found sitting in the road with traffic having to drive around him. He is shirtless and bare footed. Upon seeing the ambulance he gets up and starts kicking out at cars before moving towards you raising his hands in the air and repeatedly yelling 'I AM JESUS'. Harry's friend, who is present, provides most of the answers to your questions while assisting you to calm Harry down.

Harry worked as a truck driver, but lost his licence this week after a repeated DUI (driving under the influence) charge. Six months ago he was admitted to a mental health intensive-care unit for an episode of drug-induced psychosis after having assaulted a stranger in the street. He does not presently take any regular medications or see anyone in community mental health.

After 10 minutes of listening to Harry and repeatedly reassuring him that you are there to help him, he is able to sit with his friend at the roadside and talk with you. He is observed to be hyper-ventilating, with large beads of sweat running off his forehead and with 4 mm dilated pupils. He has superficial abrasions to his hands, feet and forehead. He also complains of central chest pain. He remains distracted at times during the conversation, believing he has bugs crawling under his skin and continuing to talk to himself. With reassurance he allows you to take his vital signs and clean his wounds.

Vital signs
- Glasgow Coma Score: 15
- Oxygen saturations: 96%
- Respiratory rate: 26
- Heart rate: 120
- Blood pressure: 188/115
- Blood sugar level: 5.8 mmol
- Temperature: 37.9
- Wounds appear superficial and do not seem to require further treatment.

CRITICAL REFLECTION
- What potential safety issues can you identify from the above information? (Consider yourself, Harry and others.)
- How would you approach the immediate care of Harry? What are the priorities?
- What medical interventions would you consider?
- What role is Harry's friend fulfilling?
- What are the important aspects of communication in this case?

As Harry has become more engaged with you he admitts to injecting two points of 'ice' four hours ago, as he does every two days. He reports taking 15 x 50 mg Seroquel tablets two days ago, partly to slow down his thoughts but also with the thought of ending his life. He does not see any purpose in being alive.

In the past six months, he has experienced episodes of being awake for up to three days, during which time he describes feeling superhuman with powers to heal others. He admits to having approached strangers and placed his 'healing hands' on them. After his highs, he may sleep for two days and wake up feeling exhausted, depressed and experiencing stomach cramps.

CRITICAL REFLECTION
- What else would you like to know about Harry's background?
- What questions could you ask Harry to establish his current suicide risk?
- What legislative provisions might you want to consider at this time?
- What is your initial formulation/assessment of Harry (including mental state)?

Harry is reluctant to get into the ambulance to go to the emergency department (ED), but is able to comprehend that you are very concernevd about his heart rate and blood pressure, and that he requires further emergency medical attention. He remains agitated, alternating between being superficially cooperative and then confused, but agrees to lie down in the ambulance and take some medication to settle him before transfer to hospital.

CRITICAL REFLECTION

- What aspects of your engagement do you think helped facilitate Harry's agreement with you?
- What are your primary considerations before transferring Harry to hospital?
- What first-line medication would you consider administering to help Harry settle for the transfer?
- Given his fluctuating mental state, would you be happy to take Harry now in the ambulance, or would you wait until police arrive?

Harry is taken to the hospital as an involuntary patient.

ACTIVITY

- Complete a mental health certificate (or relevant legal order for your location) for Harry.
- Complete a clinical handover document for Harry to be given to ED staff.

DEFINING CHALLENGING BEHAVIOUR AND VIOLENCE

As a paramedic, you will encounter challenging behaviour in many of the interactions you have with patients. Challenging behaviour is an umbrella term which encompasses a range of behaviour which may include violence, sexual disinhibition, self-harm and manipulative, high-need or demanding behaviour (Brunero & Lamont, 2016).

WORKPLACE VIOLENCE (WPV) AND PARAMEDIC PRACTICE

The World Health Organization defines violence as 'the intentional use of physical force or power, threatened or actual, against oneself, another person, or against a group or community, which either results in or has a high likelihood of resulting in injury, death, psychological harm, maldevelopment, or deprivation' (World Health Organization, 2002, p. 4). A systematic review of WPV-related research in paramedic practice has highlighted the absence of a specific definition within this context (Maguire et al., 2018). However, the literature discusses consistent attributes of WPV related to paramedic practice, which we have developed as an operational definition for this chapter:

> *The experience of violence toward, and the witnessing of violence in paramedic practice encompasses; verbal assault, intimidation, physical assault, sexual harassment and sexual assault: the perpetrators of violence are predominantly patients, family members of patients and bystanders.*
>
> (Bigham et al., 2014; Boyle & McKenna, 2017; Maguire et al., 2018; Palmer, 2017; Ross et al., 2017)

PREVALENCE OF WORKPLACE VIOLENCE WITHIN PARAMEDIC PRACTICE

Internationally, violence towards paramedics has been reported as highly prevalent and a common risk factor within paramedic practice (Spencer & Johnson, 2016). In Australia, 12-month prevalence rates have been identified as high as 87.5% (Boyle et al., 2017), with international studies showing similarly high results, ranging from 75% to 90% over 12-month exposure (Bigham et al., 2014; Gabrovec, 2015; Maguire et al., 2018; Suserud et al., 2002).

A recent study published by Safe Work Australia (Maguire, 2018) examined 300 cases of serious claims of paramedic-injury-related assaults and WPV. In the study period reviewed, from 2001 to 2014, WPV-related cases increased from 5 to 40 per year, with a tripling of the number of cases of injury secondary to assault. There are also reports within the Australian literature that female paramedics are statistically significantly more likely to experience WPV than their male colleagues (Wongtongkam, 2017). Workplace violence is therefore a highly prevalent occupational risk hazard within paramedic practice, and needs to be understood within the context of its aetiology, before mitigating any associated deleterious effects.

CHALLENGING BEHAVIOUR

The following section discusses some concepts that are central to understanding and effectively responding to challenging behaviour.

REASONABLE AND UNREASONABLE BEHAVIOUR

Challenging behaviour may arise from a perceived need that is not being understood or met and where a person is unable to articulate their thoughts. When we perceive that someone is unreasonable, we may stop listening to them, start formulating judgments, and potentially become unreasonable ourselves. Consider challenging behaviour in the context of pain, loss, loneliness, stigma, bullying or trauma. It is important that you look beyond the external manifestation of what you perceive to be unreasonable, and consider what the reason for this 'unreasonable' behaviour may be.

THE LOSS OF POWER AND CONTROL

As a paramedic, you will experience a high degree of deference from patients and the general public due to your professional status and a person's need for care in times of crisis. This places you in a position of power, and patients in positions of vulnerability. You need to be aware of how you exercise this power, as it may negatively trigger reactions in people who are disempowered, marginalised or stigmatised. It is understandable to see how challenging behaviour can exist in this context.

DEFENSIVE BEHAVIOUR

Defensive behaviour is an instinctive trait which is activated when an individual perceives a threat. Defensive behaviour serves to protect individuals from discomfort or being viewed negatively by others. Of course, defensive behaviour can have a paradoxical effect which compromises an individual's engagement and social interaction with others, and thus presents challenging behaviour for paramedics.

Defensive behaviour is often interpreted as being uncaring or disrespectful, but it is important to try to see an individual's situation through their lens in a non-judgmental, empathic and professional manner. Achieving this will help you avoid negative 'labelling' and the challenges this brings when providing care to patients.

LABELLING

Mental illness often results in negative labelling and stigma such as 'dangerous' and 'risky', as well as 'frequent flyers' and 'absconders' (Brunero & Lamont, 2016). These labels sometimes influence how we perceive and interact with patients, and may also lead to individuals adopting such labels, or propagating behaviour associated with such labels. As a paramedic, you must be mindful of these attributes and the influence they may have on challenging behaviour. Negative labelling and stigma associated with mental illness can have immediate and long-term consequences for the way individuals access health services.

TRIGGERS OF CHALLENGING BEHAVIOUR AND WORKPLACE VIOLENCE

Challenging behaviour and WPV usually occur in the context of a multitude of factors, and an understanding of the context within which these behaviours occur is essential. For example, paramedics and patients often have different perceptions of why challenging behaviour and WPV are present; while paramedics may cite patient factors, patients may cite factors related to paramedics. The reality is that a range of socially determined factors, including patient, environmental, personal and cultural factors, act as precipitants to challenging behaviour and WPV (Brunero & Lamont, 2016).

THE ROLE OF THE PARAMEDIC

Challenging behaviour and WPV can often occur as a result of what we do, or in some circumstances do not do. We may not always be conscious of how we are being perceived by patients, or how our behaviours are influencing the behaviour of patients. Our knowledge, skills and attitudes and subsequent behaviour become an important aspect of preventing, mitigating and managing these behaviours.

Developing therapeutic relationships with patients is essential. This requires a commitment to engage purposefully with patients in a person-centred manner; developing an intimate knowledge of your patient as a person, showing respect and being courteous, actively listening to concerns, fears and frustrations, responding in an empathic manner, and communicating a genuine desire to help. Inattention to these issues may increase the likelihood of experiencing challenging behaviour and potential WPV (Stein-Parbury, 2014).

Therapeutic relationships can be compromised by a range of personal factors. For example, a paramedic's own mental health and personality style, current stressors in one's life, previous experience (or inexperience), tiredness and illness. Any of these factors can contribute to an interaction style that leads to a perception that paramedics are not interested or are simply ignoring the needs of patients. Further, paramedics who are impatient, controlling, authoritarian or coercive are less likely to have positive therapeutic moments, and thereby achieve desirable outcomes (McMain et al., 2015).

ENVIRONMENT

Being mindful of environmental risk factors is essential in understanding behaviours and potential mitigating risks. Upon call-out it is helpful to ascertain as much environmental information as possible. Is the location geographically isolated? Is it a high-crime area? In these situations, it may be prudent to park facing the way you intend to exit. Similarly, regarding any premises you may be required to enter, be aware of stairwells, lighting, working lifts and all possible exits from premises should a quick egress be required. Being close to the control panel and alarm within lifts is prudent, and awareness of other members of households who may be present, as well as of potentially aggressive animals, are aspects of 'situational risk awareness'. You may have to proceed with caution if you are aware of arguments or loud voices within premises, or indeed you observe firearms or other weapons.

SOCIO-ECONOMIC AND CULTURAL FACTORS

Potential risk factors associated with lower socio-economic status include unemployment, social marginalisation, decreased community participation, suboptimal housing and gang activities (Scott et al., 2014). Certain geographical areas will present more challenges during your work as a paramedic. Being mindful of this and preparing for any increased risks (see the section on safety and scene awareness for more information) will help reduce and manage some associated risks.

Culture has significant implications within the context of challenging behaviour and WPV (McCann et al., 2014). Within a local context, Indigenous Australians have had traumatic experiences of government control and coercion, and their perception of care may be influenced by this (Sambrano & Cox, 2013). As a paramedic, you need to be aware of any personal cultural biases and beliefs that may influence your communication or interaction with people.

CLINICAL PRESENTATIONS

Patients may display challenging behaviour and WPV in the context of drug and alcohol intoxication or withdrawal, psychosis, mood or personality disorder, situational crises and self-harm, neurocognitive disorders and other non-psychiatric conditions.

DRUGS AND ALCOHOL

Intoxicated patients may be challenging due to the disinhibiting effects of drugs and alcohol. Males who have a psychotic illness, combined with alcohol and illicit drug use, have an increased association with challenging and violent behaviour (Duke et al., 2018). Alcohol and other drugs have been linked to a range of challenging, violent and criminal behaviour, such as domestic violence, sexual assault, homicide, antisocial behaviour and property crime.

The increased abuse of stimulants has been associated with challenging or violent behaviour (McKenna, 2013), including hyper-sexuality and sexual assault (Coomber et al., 2016; Jessell et al., 2017). Preloading with alcohol has been a major factor associated with violence. Patients who mix drugs and alcohol also have an increased propensity for being perpetrators or victims of violence (McKetin et al., 2014; Tomlinson et al., 2016).

PSYCHOSIS

Psychosis is one of the most complex clinical presentations in the context of challenging behaviour. As a paramedic you will need to remember that the patient may be trying to interpret your actions in the context of their thoughts or perceptual disturbances. This means you need to be more mindful of how you communicate with someone who is experiencing psychotic symptoms. Communication needs to be considered and non-confrontational, and you may need to use the patient's name more than usual to keep them engaged and free from distraction (Brunero & Lamont, 2016). It is important to avoid challenging delusional ideas, but instead accept how these ideas are influencing the patients' emotions and behaviour. Patients who are paranoid are often frightened for their wellbeing, therefore reassurance regarding their safety and your intent to help is required. A statement such as: '*You look scared, what can I do to help?*' may be both validating of the patients' distress, and comforting because it communicates an offer of help.

MOOD DISORDER

Mood disorders can be a challenge for the paramedic. Patients experiencing depression may present as withdrawn and uncommunicative, have a loss of interest in activities, be irritable and lack motivation. Communication should be measured, empathic and reassuring. Patients experiencing mania may present with grandiosity, agitation or intrusiveness. Communication should be empathic and concise; you may be required to redirect the conversation frequently, and you will need to be more assertive with someone experiencing mania.

PERSONALITY DISORDER

Personality disorders are a pattern of behaviour, mood and social interaction that the patient and others find distressing. People with personality disorders have difficulty interacting with others, have a poor sense of self, and have difficulty trusting others. They respond poorly to 'rejection' from others, which may manifest in challenging behaviours, which are at times impulsive (Lowenstein et al., 2016). Offers from the paramedic may be dismissed even though clinically warranted, leaving the paramedic feeling angry and frustrated. Being aware of your own emotional reactions when interacting with a patient with a personality disorder may assist in de-escalating a situation (see the section of self-care in this chapter) (Colli & Ferri, 2015).

SITUATIONAL CRISIS

A situational crisis, defined as when circumstances overwhelm a person's internal and external resources, occurs with a precipitating event, and intensifies into emotions such as fear and intense anxiety. A crisis may arise as a result of bereavement, or problems with a relationship such as domestic violence. A patient may present with the following: hysteria, withdrawal, tearfulness, suicidal ideation, self-harm risk, panic symptoms or violence.

SELF-HARM

Deliberate self-harm can be confronting and challenging for paramedics. Deliberate self-harm often occurs in the context of situational crises, and patients may be so emotionally aroused that they exhibit hysterical or violent behaviour. A challenge for paramedics is in determining the suicide risk of an individual who has deliberately self-harmed. Most people who have self-harmed have no desire to die; rather, self-harm is a method of managing distressing thoughts or emotional dysregulation. Notwithstanding, paramedics must guard against complacency about self-harm, as each situation has its dynamic risks and idiosyncrasies (Lees et al., 2014).

NEUROCOGNITIVE DISORDERS AND OTHER NON-PSYCHIATRIC CONDITIONS

Patients with cognitive disorders can present with confusion, disorientation, wandering and potentially challenging behaviour. These behaviours are seen in patients with traumatic brain injury, dementia and delirium, and can pose a challenge to the paramedic. Other medical disorders which have been associated with challenging and violent behaviour (Fulde & Preisz, 2011; Rozel et al., 2017) include:

- hypoxia, hypercarbia – pneumonia, worsening chronic airway disease
- hypoglycaemia – diabetes, malnourished alcoholic
- cerebral insult – stroke, tumour, seizure, encephalitis, meningitis, trauma
- sepsis – systemic sepsis, urine infection in the elderly
- metabolic disturbance – hyponatraemia, thiamine deficiency, hypercalcaemia
- organ failure – hepatic or renal failure.

In summary, challenging behaviour and WPV often occurs as a complex integration of intrapersonal, interpersonal and environmental risk factors (Brunero & Lamont, 2016). Being mindful and attentive to these factors affords the best opportunity to understand and address these behaviours as well as your own response and communication.

RESPONDING TO CHALLENGING BEHAVIOUR AND WORKPLACE VIOLENCE

A wide range of personal, interpersonal and organisational skills are required when effectively responding to challenging behaviour, the choice being dependent on the situation and challenge presented to you.

SAFETY AND SCENE AWARENESS

The risk of adverse events is particularly high within the pre-hospital setting where paramedics attend situations that are dynamic and requiring quick assessment of safety, with limited information available and with limited resources. As a result, it is an expectation that paramedics become situationally aware of scene risks and safety, and are proficient at assessing risk. This will require you to look for hazards on approach, consider retreat options and exits, approach situations cautiously, stay close to your partner and avoid placing yourself or partner at risk (e.g. intervening in a challenging or violent incident), observe for potential weapons, and consider any additional resources required to safely assess and/or treat (South Australian Ambulance, 2017). Table 15.1 outlines some specific safety and risk mitigation factors you should consider before arrival, upon arrival, during assessment/treatment, and following return to base.

> ### ETHICAL DILEMMA
>
> You are dispatched to an address which is a known safety risk, where paramedics have previously been assaulted. The area is a high-crime area, occupied by gangs, with a high prevalence of drug- and alcohol-related assaults. The emergency call relates to a young male who is described by the caller as 'paranoid and crazy'. The male in question has been reportedly confronting members of the public and threatening them. It is also reported that he appears intoxicated and may be carrying a weapon. There is no immediately available police support, and on arrival at the scene you note there are large groups of youths in the surroundings, openly drinking alcohol. What do you do?

Table 15.1 Scene Safety and Risk Mitigation for Paramedic Call-outs

Prior to Call-out	Arrival at Call-out	Assessment/Treatment	Other Issues
• Recognise that risk is dynamic and that a 'low-risk' situation can change at any time. • Obtain as much information as possible about the patient and relevant others. • Obtain information about the location. For example: Is it in a high-crime area? Isolated? And/or have reduced accessibility to / availability of police? • Is the address listed as 'no go' or 'location of interest'? If so, consider police back-up.	• Park the ambulance facing the way you will be exiting, and avoid being blocked in. • Don't enter the premises if there are potentially aggressive animals which are not restrained. • Always check locking mechanisms at relevant entrances for quick egress if necessary. • Be aware of any arguments or other loud voices that may make a situation potentially unsafe.	• Be cautious when entering a person's home. • Leave immediately if you see any firearms (inform the police) or weapons. • Memorise all potential exits from premises or situations. • Ensure you position yourself between the person and exit (where possible). • Keep vehicle keys accessible for quick departure if necessary. • Only take what you need.	• Always report to base at regular intervals. • Ensure your workplace has a policy and response if you do not respond, e.g. activating a police response. • Always report 'near-misses' where risks did not eventuate. • Ensure you attend all workplace violence prevention / personal safety training offered by your service.

RECOGNISING AROUSAL

Challenging behaviour and WPV are often associated with or preceded by emotional arousal. Emotional arousal can be seen as a sign that something is wrong. Sometimes, despite our best attempts at providing professional and person-centred care, patients become frustrated, aroused and their behaviour escalates. While the behaviour may be directed at you as the paramedic, it is not directed at you as a person. This difference may appear subtle, but the implications are significant. Avoid personalising challenging behaviour; rather view it through the eyes of your professional role. This will help you to remain objective to these behaviours.

An integral part of paramedic work is the observation of a patients' demeanour, physical status and interactions with others. Some observations that may be suggestive of the increased potential for challenging behaviour and WPV, and thus requiring caution, include:

- flushed or red face
- hyperventilation
- increased muscle tone, such as clenched fists
- gritting teeth
- increased motor activity, such as pacing or shuffling
- ignoring requests
- prolonged eye contact or sudden lack of eye contact.

Think back to 'Harry', and his hyperventilation, increased perspiration, dilated pupils, reduced concentration and vital signs. Situational awareness and early intervention is paramount and may prevent escalation. Interventions may include attending to any related medical causes or using de-escalation communication techniques (see the section below).

SELF-AWARENESS AND PRINCIPLES FOR COMMUNICATING WITH CHALLENGING SITUATIONS

As a paramedic, you will need to respond to the potential for (or actual) behaviours in several ways. Firstly it is important to understand some general principles in interacting with someone who has the potential for, or is displaying, challenging or violent behaviour.

Verbal communication

Using an appropriate tone of voice, the rate at which we talk, the volume and pressure in our speech can influence how we engage patients. We are often unaware of when we have a high expressed tone that can negatively influence purposeful communication. You will need to fine-tune your tone of voice as the interaction with the patient occurs, testing and retesting your approach. Linking your words with actions can give a patient a sense that you are interested in and support therapeutic engagement. Alternatively, if you show incongruence between your words and actions, patients and others may interpret this as being untrustworthy and lacking authenticity.

Non-verbal communication

Your non-verbal communication is very important when engaging patients with the potential for challenging or violent behaviour. Through body language we constantly (sometimes unconsciously) send and receive non-verbal signals. The words you use to convey a message may be interpreted differently by the movements and gestures you make alongside them, which may create misunderstandings between you and the patient. Consider the following when engaging with someone who has the potential for challenging behaviour, and be mindful that your demeanour, movement and gestures may need to vary in differing situations:

- Pay attention to how you are sitting or standing, make sure that the expression on your face demonstrates warmth, acceptance or concern, and be aware of what you are doing with your hands.
- Personal space or distance can vary according to cultural and/or personal nuances.
- A relaxed, open posture with your hands visible can make you appear less threatening, and can also be protective during impulsive actions.
- It is helpful to have intermittent eye contact; thus avoiding prolonged staring, which may appear threatening, or avoidance, which may not be assertive enough when required.

Being flexible

Challenging behaviour and WPV require a flexible approach when engaging people. As a paramedic, the circumstances associated with your work will generally necessitate an assertive approach where you take control of situations. However, certain situations may require patience and caution, which may seem at odds with care requirements. Developing skills in redirecting and negotiating will also help when dealing with the potential for, or actual, challenging behaviour and WPV.

Active listening

Paramedics use active listening skills in most of their daily work with patients. Active listening is a skill that demonstrates through body language and verbal acknowledgement that you are interested in what is being conveyed. Active listening includes being congruent with words and actions, paraphrasing to ensure understanding, and the use of silence. Reflecting what the patient is saying while taking a position of not offering advice, or by expressing acceptance without agreeing, may help patients to acknowledge and talk about their emotions, as opposed to negatively acting on them.

Empathy and humility

Being empathetic or understanding the feelings of another gives someone a sense that you are acknowledging any concerns they may have and that you are trying to connect with them. An empathic demeanour is important when exposed to challenging behaviour and WPV. We can acknowledge and accept what someone is saying without necessarily agreeing with it. For example: *'I am sorry we took a long time to get here while you have been in pain.'* Empathy, apologies and humility are powerful ways of interacting with people and minimising challenging behaviour and WPV.

Assertive behaviour

Being assertive is a skill that requires careful consideration so as not to appear judgmental, punitive or aggressive. Assertiveness involves displaying high levels of empathy while setting limits on the behaviour presented to you. The following are examples of assertiveness statements which demonstrate setting limits in ways that are non-judgmental:

> *'You are threatening me, and I am finding it hard to help you.'*

> *'I am unable to communicate with you and help you when you are shouting at me.'*

Combining these statements with something like *'I appreciate you are trying'*, can also be helpful. It is important to avoid arguments, conflicting advice and convoluted explanations.

Provided that your demeanour is not aggressive and your response is consistent, this offers the best opportunity to manage challenging or violent behaviour in a non-threatening manner. Be mindful to acknowledge a satisfactory outcome and say *'thank you'*.

DE-ESCALATING CHALLENGING OR VIOLENT BEHAVIOUR

De-escalation as an intervention has been central to healthcare policy and professional guidelines aimed at managing challenging behaviour and WPV (Spencer & Johnson, 2016). Variously known as 'talking down', defusion or diffusion (Bowers, 2014), de-escalation is widely considered a first-line intervention when dealing with escalating behaviour (Price et al., 2015). General principles involve non-provocatively engaging someone using short-term psychosocial interventions that minimise restriction (Hallett & Dickens, 2017; Price et al., 2015) and enabling a mutually satisfactory outcome for both parties.

Themes, principles, and attributes of de-escalation

A multitude of techniques (Price & Baker, 2012), domains (Richmond et al., 2012), themes (Hallett & Dickens, 2017; Price & Baker, 2012), and validated scale items (Mavandadi et al., 2016; Nau et al., 2009) have been identified within the international literature suggesting the principal components of de-escalation. However, a recent concept analysis of de-escalation in healthcare settings, which included 79 studies, has attempted to resolve concerns over clarity by proposing the following theoretical definition:

a collective term for a range of interwoven staff-delivered components comprising communication, self-regulation, assessment, actions, and safety maintenance which aims to extinguish or reduce patient aggression/agitation irrespective of its cause, and improve staff–patient relationships while eliminating or minimising coercion or restriction.

(Hallett & Dickens, 2017, p. 16)

This definition arguably provides the most comprehensive understanding of de-escalation as a concept, and provides an opportunity to explore theory–practice translational aspects of de-escalation. Table 15.2 details various themes, principles, attributes and suggestions for verbal engagement and management in de-escalation situations (Hallett & Dickens, 2017; Lamont & Brunero, 2018).

Successful de-escalation, therefore, comprises a complex set and interaction of skills and behaviours, which can be helpful in addressing challenging behaviour and WPV exposure, and may prevent the need for more restrictive practices such as sedation and restraint (Hallett & Dickens, 2017).

RESTRICTIVE PRACTICES AND CHALLENGING BEHAVIOUR

Restrictive practice is a term which generally involves limiting an individual's movement, and in the paramedic context can refer to physical, mechanical and/or chemical restraint. Restrictive practices should be used only as a last resort to prevent harm to self or others.

Physical and mechanical restraint

There may be occasions where your attempts to de-escalate have been unsuccessful, and consequently a decision is made to physically intervene to prevent the risks associated with challenging or violent behaviour. It should be emphasised that the physical and mechanical restraint of patients is an intervention of last resort, and should only be carried out with the appropriate training. You should always consider whether any alternative strategies are available, and whether these have been exhausted. Also, ask yourself what would happen if you did nothing. This question may be asked in the context of alleged assault when considering whether reasonable force should be applied, either in a patient's best interests or as a basis for self-defence. Restraint carries with it significant risks of injury to patients, and in some cases even death (Boumans et al., 2014). Box 15.1 sets out some guiding principles to follow when restraining a patient.

Pharmacological restraint (chemical restraint)

Pharmacological interventions may also be required for patients whose behaviour puts them or others at immediate risk of serious harm, where de-escalation interventions have been unsuccessful, or behaviour is impulsive or unpredictable. The following are general principles that should be applied when using pharmacological

Text continued on p. 373

Table 15.2 De-escalation, Themes, Principles, Attributes and Interventions

Themes and Principles	How You Could Do This	What You Could Say
Communication		
Engage early in de-escalation	One person only should engage, in a calm and measured way, as it can be confusing and counter-productive when more than one person is speaking. Use the person's name (and yours), and use tactful language and a sensitive use of humour (only if you feel it safe to do so).	'Hello John, my name is Jane and this is Simon. That looks painful: can I take a look at it?'
Non-provocative engagement	Display a calm demeanour and appropriate tone of voice, and engage assertively (not emotively or confrontationally). Eye contact should be intermittent to avoid staring. Awareness of one's own body language and adoption of an open, non-threatening posture with arms visible (not folded or behind the back). Use of humour can help, but only when appropriate.	Avoid saying the following: 'You need to calm down', 'Don't speak to me like that' or 'You're upsetting other people'.
Determine needs/ wishes	Violent behaviour is a primitive form of communicating that something is wrong, or a need is not being met. Look beyond the external manifestation of this to ask how you can be of help.	'I understand that you are frustrated, let's sit down and discuss that' or 'We're here to help you, how best can we do that?'
Listen actively	Convey through body language and verbal acknowledgment that you are interested, and repeat back (paraphrasing) that you understand. Be congruent in actions and words. Use of silence can allow a person time to clarify their thoughts.	'You said that you want ...?' or 'Am I correct in saying ...?'
Display empathy	Demonstrate empathy in verbal and non-verbal communication. Listen and offer understanding (not sympathy), while acknowledging the person's feelings/situation.	'That would frustrate me, too' or 'I can appreciate how this is affecting you'.
Be clear and concise	A person's ability to concentrate is compromised when in an emotionally aroused state. Avoid jargon or medical terminology. Speak clearly and slowly – information may have to be repeated several times.	'Let's sit down and discuss your pain' or 'We're concerned about your health and your safety'.
Agree or accept	Concentrate on opportunities for agreement. Validate concerns where relevant and accept that concerns are distressing for the person (even if you may not agree with them).	'I'm sorry this has happened to you, it's unacceptable' or 'I would feel angry too if I had to wait this long'.
Offer choices and optimism	Offering choice, where relevant, is empowering and can enable a sense of internal control, while providing an acceptable 'out' from challenging behaviour. Also offer things perceived as acts of kindness, where relevant, such as food/drink, pain relief, etc. Be honest and don't make promises that can't be kept, or compromise others.	'Can I get you some water and medication for your pain? Then we can discuss this' or 'I'm sorry, but I'm unable to do that ... what I can do is help you with ...'.

Continued ...

Table 15.2 De-escalation, Themes, Principles, Attributes and Interventions *continued*

Themes and Principles	How You Could Do This	What You Could Say
Self-regulation		
Remain calm	Appearing fearful may make someone feel unsafe or may escalate behaviour in the context of manipulation. Maintain emotional regulation, self-control and confidence. Concentrate on your breathing; count to three before engaging; and having positive inner dialogues that you can successfully negotiate and de-escalate can contribute to effective self-control plans.	Say to yourself: *I'm confident I can connect with (name) and successfully de-escalate the situation'* or *'This will resolve with everyone safe'.*
Non-judgmental approach	Separate your feelings about the person and the problem. Avoid making judgments about the person and don't personalise any challenging behaviour.	*'I don't think that of you at all'* or *'I'm sorry you think that of me'* or *'I didn't mean to give you the wrong impression'.*
Self-reflection	Personal reflection following an incident allows you to consider and make sense of what went well or not so well. This enables consistency or modification of engagement/intervention strategies.	Ask your colleague: *'How did I do?'* or *'Could I have done anything different?'*
Assessment		
Is it safe/ When to intervene	Assess the risks associated with any intervention. Early intervention is always recommended for escalating behaviour, but patience and caution, if safe, may be more prudent when assessing benefit–harm ratio. Ask yourself what would happen if you did nothing, or waited for support.	*'Can we take a minute, then I'll attend to that?'* or *'I need you to put that down before I can treat that'* or *'Do you mind if we wait for my colleague, as he has something that can help with your pain?'*
Here and now	Assess the person's emotional state or the immediate situation in relation to safety for all. Other aspects of assessment and intervention can wait.	*'You look distressed (or angry), can you talk to me about it?'*
Escalating aggression	Observe for and recognise known early-warning signs of violence; for example, pacing, clenched fists, kicking objects, loud voice, staring, tense facial expressions / posturing, ignoring requests.	*'I need you to sit down so I can attend to your …'.*

Actions

Positional imitation	Stand if the person is standing (personal safety); sit if they are sitting, as this reflects a sense of equity required for successful de-escalation.	'Do you mind if I sit down?' or 'Do you mind if I join you?'
Reduce stimuli / Creating a safe space	Decrease environmental stimulus and encourage private interaction free from any potential triggers or antagonists. Attempt to remove the person, or others, from situation, thus creating a safe space for engagement and intervention.	'Can we move over here and talk in private?' or 'Can we sit in the ambulance, so we can attend to …?'
Distraction	Redirect the person's attention from escalating behaviour. Bringing in a different person to interact with the individual may change the dynamic of unsuccessful de-escalation.	'Is there anyone you'd like me to call to let them know you're safe or where you are going?' or 'This is my colleague Jane, do you mind if she attends to you while I get you something for the pain?'
Limit-setting	Be clear about what you would like to happen and that you want to help, in a non-confrontational and respectful way. A discussion of behavioural expectations may help, if safe to do so. Acknowledge if you are feeling uncomfortable, as humility is a very powerful tool!	'When you are shouting I find it hard to understand how I can help you' or 'I can't attend to your needs while you're threatening me'.
Therapeutic treatment	Identifying and alleviating causes of escalating behaviour; for example, pain, confusion, etc., can quickly inform de-escalation strategies and required treatments.	'Can I give you something to help with the pain?' or 'Can I give you some medication to help take your mind off it?'

Continued …

Table 15.2 De-escalation, Themes, Principles, Attributes and Interventions *continued*

Themes and Principles	How You Could Do This	What You Could Say
Maintaining safety		
Situational awareness	Situational awareness is being aware of what is happening around you in terms of where you are, whether anyone or anything around you is a threat, and what supports may be available. It is essential to remain vigilant. Awareness of the environment in terms of isolation, quick egress and exit routes, and the removal or moderation of potential weapons, dangers and triggers is paramount.	'Can we talk somewhere else?' or 'Do you mind if I sit here?' or 'Can you put the syringe down and I'll attend to that?'
Situational support	Communication with colleagues is essential. Identify availability of back-up should it be needed, while being mindful that excessive show of force can escalate a person's behaviour.	'No one's in trouble, the police are here for everyone's safety' or 'I need to contact control to let them know we'll be longer than expected'.
Approach with caution	Approach in a measured way, careful to avoid sudden movements. Avoid being too close to someone fearful or confused, as this may appear threatening, while maintaining a distance which protects from a potential punch or kick until you feel it safe for close proximity.	'Can we take a look at that injury?' or 'Someone phoned as they are concerned about your safety'.
Respect personal space	Acknowledge that more personal space than usual may be required, while being mindful not to appear fearful or disinterested.	'Do you mind if I have a look at that?' or 'I won't come any closer, I just want to chat'.
Debrief all involved	Debriefing with persons displaying challenging behaviour helps maintain therapeutic aspects of the relationship. It is important that a person does not feel isolated following resolution, irrespective of how this has been achieved. Debriefing with colleagues ensures that psychological first aid can be administered. Bystanders may also require debriefing if witnessing potentially traumatic events. Debriefing allows learning from situations that may prove useful in future crises.	'I'm sorry we did that, I know you didn't want to, we did this because …' (Patient) or 'That must have been very difficult to witness, are you OK? Can I contact someone to take you home?' (Bystander) or 'How do you think that went? Should we do anything different next time?' (Colleague).

BOX 15.1   PRINCIPLES FOR SAFE RESTRAINT

1. Restraint should only be used as a last resort when other less coercive interventions are unsuccessful or inappropriate.
2. Any restriction to a patient's liberty and interference with their rights, dignity and self-respect is kept to a minimum and should cease as soon as the patient has regained self-control.
3. All actions undertaken by a paramedic are to be justifiable and proportional to the patient's behaviour, and use the least amount of force necessary.
4. Paramedics must ensure the safety, comfort and humane treatment of patients in restraint.
5. Communication should be maintained with the patient at all times, with all opportunities taken to de-escalate the situation.
6. The patient's physical condition should be continuously monitored, with any deterioration, in particular to the airway, noted and managed promptly.
7. Face-up restraint (supine) is to be used where it is safe to do so. Face-down restraint (prone) is only to be used if it is the safest way to protect the patient and paramedic.
8. Post-restraint debrief of patient, paramedic and any relevant others is to be undertaken in all situations.

BOX 15.2   PRINCIPLES FOR PHARMACOLOGICAL SEDATION

1. Pharmacological management should be used only when verbal de-escalation is unsuccessful.
2. Oral medications are preferable to parenteral medications when there is no imminent risk to self, the patient or others.
3. The desired clinical end point is the relief of distress/agitation.
4. The choice of medication should be guided by local service clinical guidelines.
5. Use lower doses and caution in patients who are frail or medically compromised.
6. Appropriate monitoring of the patient's vital signs is required whenever parenteral sedation is utilised.

---

agents for sedation (see Box 15.2). You should follow relevant state clinical guidelines for the administration of these agents.

SELF-CARE AND CHALLENGING BEHAVIOUR

There is increasing evidence of the stress burden associated with emergency services practice. Exposure to trauma, challenging behaviour and WPV are correlates of this burden within paramedic practice. While most people will cope well with the daily demands of practice; there are times when our ability to cope is compromised by internal or external factors. Research within the paramedic context has identified that social support is a significant positive predictor of wellbeing, and post-traumatic growth (positive psychological change following a highly stressful event) significantly and negatively predicts post-traumatic stress disorder. The same research found that self-efficacy significantly and positively predicts wellbeing, while shift work significantly and negatively predicts post-traumatic stress disorder (Shakespeare-Finch & Lurie-Beck, 2014).

It is therefore essential, when exposed to highly stressful and potentially traumatising situations, that maintaining one's health becomes paramount. To engage therapeutically and professionally with challenging behaviour, you must be able to recognise your own needs and develop personal and professional plans to support your own emotional and psychological wellbeing. As the saying goes: 'Who cares for carers?' Being self-aware and able to evaluate one's actions and behaviour will help you engage therapeutically with patients. Some individuals naturally engage in reflective thinking to enhance self-awareness, while others may require some formal structure or support to engage in this practice.

RECOGNISING YOUR OWN EMOTIONS

When someone is displaying challenging or violent behaviour, you will need to be able to make sense of and manage your own emotions and behaviour (Dahl et al., 2012). The natural response we have is known as the 'fight–flight response'. This is evoked when people are threatening, angry and/or violent, resulting in an immediate response to defend yourself (Roberts & Grubb, 2014). Paramedics should be aware that the fight–flight response is normal and you should expect it to occur. Some of the physical signs that you may experience include:

- increased pulse rate and blood pressure
- shallow, rapid respirations
- muscular tension; dry mouth; and excessive perspiration.

You may, in turn, experience the following:

- irritability
- anxiety or panic
- ruminating or worrying thoughts
- mood changes
- poor concentration and memory lapses.

MAXIMISING SELF-CONTROL

To assist you in managing your response to challenging or violent behaviour, a self-control plan can be helpful in preparing your response. For example, concentrating on your breathing or counting to five before you engage someone may help you respond in a calm and measured way. Inner dialogues are also posited as a strategy for successfully approaching challenging situations. For example, if we approach a situation with a negative perception that things are not going to go well, this will likely influence our behaviour and the resulting outcome. Be aware of what you are telling yourself or thinking to yourself. Thinking the worst or catastrophic thinking can lead you to behave in a negative way. Conversely, having an inner dialogue that enables you to negotiate a successful resolution to a challenging situation will likely help you to utilise skills and resources in doing so. Creating an individual 'self-control plan' can help you counteract the 'fight–flight response'.

CRITICAL REFLECTION

- What might be your emotional responses when someone is shouting, intimidating or demanding your attention?
- What physical reactions are you having?
- What thoughts are going through your mind?

The following workload practices can also help in maintaining psychological and emotional wellbeing: working collaboratively where the workload is shared and delegated appropriately; being honest and transparent about your limitations (we all have bad days), but also maintaining professional conduct; and engaging in more formal, structured processes of reflective practice and clinical/peer supervision. Clinical/peer supervision is a practice endorsed across all professional groups, with a focus on personal and professional development in the context of safe, efficient healthcare (Brunero & Lamont, 2012).

Ambulance services also have a range of services aimed at providing mental health support and wellbeing for staff. These may include employee assistance programs and specialist psychological services, peer support and grievance support officers, and chaplaincy services. You should identify what is available locally within your service.

CARING FOR OTHERS

During paramedic work, there may be more than 'one patient' at a scene requiring attention, support and care. Consider family members, witnesses and bystanders to traumatic events (as can be seen in Table 15.2), those experiencing grief or loss, or those who may have intervened in a violent incident (Bloch et al., 2018), any of whom may require psychological first aid or debriefing. They are often 'first responders' who unselfishly (at times) intervene in highly challenging, stressful and potentially traumatic situations.

Consider also the victims of intimate partner violence (or in some cases child victims or witnesses to this) who may be present during the call-out to a perpetrator of this. Intimate partner violence is highly prevalent in Australia, and paramedics frequently encounter this (Sawyer et al., 2018). Such incidences require a careful and sensitive approach to identify relevant needs and safety issues. Police involvement may be required, which presents a challenge in itself and potential moral conflict. It is therefore important that you familiarise yourself with relevant geographical legislation, policy and guidance relating to mandatory reporting in the context of perceived or actual violence. Recent research within Australia has seen the development of a comprehensive, consensus-based guideline, which is aimed at paramedic identification and referral of people affected by intimate partner violence (Sawyer et al., 2018).

You may even be required to care for a colleague who has had a stressful or traumatic response to a call-out, or perhaps be required to navigate a challenging situation or disagreement with a colleague.

ETHICAL DILEMMA

There may be times when there is discord between you and your colleague(s) on how best to manage a challenging situation. Consider a scenario similar to 'Harry' where you believe it is safe to transfer him as a voluntary patient with oral sedation during transportation, while your colleague believes that this is not safe, and it is best to transfer using mental health legislation and intramuscular (IM) sedation. How do you approach/resolve this?

In principle, a supportive working relationship with colleagues based on trust, mutuality, respect and openness can contribute significantly to your own and their wellbeing, as can regular debriefing and peer supervision. Simply asking *'Are you OK?'*, finding time to reflect and discuss challenging call-outs, validating and acknowledging their positive professional impact in situations, and complimenting their skills and qualities during challenging situations will enhance working relationships with colleagues. When caring for others, identification of professional and community-based psychosocial services and supports should be an integral part of paramedic care delivery.

CONCLUSION

Providing care and treatment to patients exhibiting challenging behaviour and WPV is a significant demand for paramedic practice. These behaviours have deleterious effects on patients, paramedics and others. This chapter has some theoretical aspects relevant to understanding challenging behaviour and WPV, which must be considered within any framework of mitigating and managing such behaviours. The chapter has also presented some general principles, techniques and interventions that are applicable to all challenging behaviour including WPV.

As can be seen in the case study with 'Harry', you will encounter complex call-outs with competing medical and mental healthcare issues. Sensitive engagement, assessment and empathic communication were required to build a rapport with Harry. This allowed the paramedic to ultimately gain some agreement and cooperation with care goals and transfer to hospital to attend to his physical, mental health and psychosocial needs. Despite his recent suicidal behaviours, Harry had some protective factors and social supports, which are essential to identify and engage, in relation to immediate safety and future care planning. As your skills in managing challenging situations improve, and self-care and support become routine parts of practice, you are likely to perceive fewer situations as challenging. Consequently you are more likely to manage them effectively, and be less emotionally and psychologically affected by them.

REFERENCES

Bigham, B., Jensen, J., Tavares, W., et al., 2014. Paramedic self-reported exposure to violence in the Emergency Medical Services (EMS) workplace: a mixed-methods cross-sectional survey. Prehosp. Emerg. Care 18 (4), 489–494.

Bloch, C., Liebst, L., Poder, P., et al., 2018. Caring collectives and other forms of bystander helping behavior in violent situations. Curr. Sociol. 66 (7), 1049–1069.

Boumans, C., Egger, J., Souren, P., et al., 2014. Reduction in the use of seclusion by the methodical work approach. Int. J. Ment. Health Nurs. 23 (2), 161–170.

Bowers, L., 2014. A model of de-escalation. Ment. Health Pract. 17 (9), 36.

Boyle, M., McKenna, L., 2017. Paramedic student exposure to workplace violence during clinical placements – a cross-sectional study. Nurse Educ. Pract. 22, 93–97.

Brunero, S., Lamont, S., 2012. The process, logistics and challenges of implementing clinical supervision in a generalist tertiary referral hospital. Scand. J. Caring Sci. 26 (1), 186–193.

Brunero, S., Lamont, S., 2016. Challenges, risks and responses. In: Evans, K., Nizette, D., O'Brien, A. (Eds.), Psychiatric and Mental Health Nursing, fourth ed. Elsevier, Sydney.

Colli, A., Ferri, M., 2015. Patient personality and therapist countertransference. Curr. Opin. Psychiatry 28 (1), 46–56.

Coomber, K., Pennay, A., Droste, N., et al., 2016. Observable characteristics associated with alcohol intoxication within licensed entertainment venues in Australia. Int. J. Drug Policy 36, 8–14.

Dahl, H.S., Røssberg, J., Bøgwald, K., et al., 2012. Countertransference feelings in one year of individual therapy: an evaluation of the factor structure in the Feeling Word Checklist-58. Psychother. Res. 22 (1), 12–25.

Duke, A., Smith, K., Oberleitner, L., et al., 2018. Alcohol, drugs, and violence: a meta-meta-analysis. Psychol. Violence 8 (2), 238.

Fulde, G., Preisz, P., 2011. Managing aggressive and violent patients. Aust. Prescr. 34 (4), 166–168.

Gabrovec, B., 2015. The prevalence of violence directed at paramedic services personnel. Obzornik Zdravstvene Nege 49 (4), 284–294.

Hallett, N., Dickens, G., 2017. De-escalation of aggressive behaviour in healthcare settings: concept analysis. Int. J. Nurs. Stud. 75, 10–20.

Jessell, L., Mateu-Gelabert, P., Guarino, H., et al., 2017. Sexual violence in the context of drug use among young adult opioid users in New York City. J. Interpers. Violence 32, 2929–2954.

Lamont, S., Brunero, S., 2018. The effect of a workplace violence training program for generalist nurses in the acute hospital setting: a quasi-experimental study. Nurse Educ. Today 68, 45–52.

Lees, D., Procter, N., Fassett, D., 2014. Therapeutic engagement between consumers in suicidal crisis and mental health nurses. Int. J. Ment. Health Nurs. 23 (4), 306–315.

Lowenstein, J., Purvis, C., Rose, K., 2016. A systematic review on the relationship between antisocial, borderline and narcissistic personality disorder diagnostic traits and risk of violence to others in a clinical and forensic sample. Borderline Personal. Disord. Emot. Dysregul. 3, 14.

Maguire, B., 2018. Violence against ambulance personnel: a retrospective cohort study of national data from Safe Work Australia. Public Health Res. Pract. 28 (1), e28011805–e28011805.

Maguire, B., O'Meara, P., O'Neill, B., et al., 2018. Violence against emergency medical services personnel: a systematic review of the literature. Am. J. Ind. Med. 61 (2), 167–180.

Mavandadi, V., Bieling, P., Madsen, V., 2016. Effective ingredients of verbal de-escalation: validating an English modified version of the 'De-Escalating Aggressive Behaviour Scale'. J. Psychiatr. Ment. Health Nurs. 23 (6–7), 357–368.

McCann, T., Baird, J., Muir-Cochrane, E., 2014. Attitudes of clinical staff toward the causes and management of aggression in acute old age psychiatry inpatient units. BMC Psychiatry 14, 80.

McKenna, S., 2013. 'We're supposed to be asleep?' Vigilance, paranoia, and the alert methamphetamine user. Anthropol. Conscious. 24 (2), 172–190.

McKetin, R., Lubman, D., Najman, J., et al., 2014. Does methamphetamine use increase violent behaviour? Evidence from a prospective longitudinal study. Addiction 109 (5), 798–806.

McMain, S., Boritz, T., Leybman, M., 2015. Common strategies for cultivating a positive therapy relationship in the treatment of borderline personality disorder. J. Psychother. Integr. 25 (1), 20.

Nau, J., Halfens, R., Needham, I., et al., 2009. The de-escalating aggressive behaviour scale: development and psychometric testing. J. Adv. Nurs. 65 (9), 1956–1964.

Palmer, S., 2017. Intoxication and violence during ambulance call-outs. J. Paramed. Pract. 9, 483–485.

Price, O., Baker, J., 2012. Key components of de-escalation techniques: a thematic synthesis. Int. J. Ment. Health Nurs. 21 (4), 310–319.

Price, O., Baker, J., Bee, P., et al., 2015. Learning and performance outcomes of mental health staff training in de-escalation techniques for the management of violence and aggression. Br. J. Psychiatry 206 (6), 447–455.

Richmond, J., Berlin, J., Fishkind, A., et al., 2012. Verbal de-escalation of the agitated patient: consensus statement of the American Association for Emergency Psychiatry Project BETA De-escalation Workgroup. West. J. Emerg. Med. 13 (1), 17.

Roberts, R., Grubb, P., 2014. The consequences of nursing stress and need for integrated solutions. Rehabil. Nurs. 39 (2), 62–69.

Ross, L., Adams, T., Beovich, B., 2017. Methamphetamine use and emergency services in Australia: a scoping review. J. Paramed. Pract. 9 (6), 244–257.

Rozel, J., Jain, A., Mulvey, E., et al., 2017. Psychiatric assessment of violence. In: Sturmey, P. (Ed.), The Wiley Handbook of Violence and Aggression. John Wiley & Sons, West Sussex.

Sambrano, R., Cox, L., 2013. 'I sang Amazing Grace for about 3 hours that day': understanding Indigenous Australians' experience of seclusion. Int. J. Ment. Health Nurs. 22 (6), 522–531.

Sawyer, S., Coles, J., Williams, A., et al., 2018. Paramedics as a new resource for women experiencing intimate partner violence. J. Interpers. Violence https://doi.org/10.1177/0886260518769363.

Scott, K., Al-Hamzawi, A., Andrade, L.H., et al., 2014. Associations between subjective social status and DSM-IV mental disorders: results from the World Mental Health surveys. JAMA Psychiatry 71 (12), 1400–1408.

Shakespeare-Finch, J., Lurie-Beck, J., 2014. A meta-analytic clarification of the relationship between posttraumatic growth and symptoms of posttraumatic distress disorder. J. Anxiety Disord. 28 (2), 223–229.

South Australian Ambulance, 2017. Clinical Practice Guideline, Intensive Care Paramedic Challenging Behaviours. SA Health, Government of South Australia, Adelaide.

Spencer, S., Johnson, P., 2016. De-escalation Techniques for Managing Aggression. Cochrane Library. John Wiley & Sons, West Sussex.

Stein-Parbury, J., 2014. Patient and Person: Interpersonal skills in nursing. Elsevier Health Sciences, Sydney.

Suserud, B., Blomquist, M., Johansson, I., 2002. Experiences of threats and violence in the Swedish ambulance service. Accid. Emerg. Nurs. 10 (3), 127–135.

Tomlinson, M., Brown, M., Hoaken, P., 2016. Recreational drug use and human aggressive behavior: a comprehensive review since 2003. Aggress. Violent Behav. 27, 9–29.

Wongtongkam, N., 2017. An exploration of violence against paramedics, burnout and post-traumatic symptoms in two Australian ambulance services. Int. J. Emerg. Serv. 6 (2), 134–146.

World Health Organization (WHO), 2002. World Report on Violence and Health: Summary. WHO, Geneva.

Understanding personality and changes in personality

16

Francesca Valmorbida McSteen and Paul Cammell

LEARNING OUTCOMES

By the end of this chapter, you will be able to:

- understand the concept of personality, its multifactorial development, and models with which to describe it
- describe personality disorder, be aware of theories of aetiology, and be familiar with common classification systems
- appreciate the basics of generalised personality assessment and how this informs physical and psychiatric assessment and management, as well as be able to tailor this to a pre-hospital setting
- appreciate the impact of personality pathology on the person, their general health and function, those around them and our healthcare systems
- be aware of general treatment goals, principles of management and approaches for people with personality disorders
- be comfortable in assessing and working with a person presenting in crisis, employing a collaborative and holistic approach.

INTRODUCTION: WHAT IS PERSONALITY?

Of the many areas of mental health, the idea of personality is perhaps one that seems most accessible to a non-clinical audience. In everyday conversation we refer to the word and associated descriptors often. Statements such as 'she's a great personality' or 'he's narcissistic' are common. Most of us have an inherent understanding that the differences we notice in each other, the unique qualities and characteristics, constitute personality. However, while the concept is largely accepted, the area is fraught with ambiguity, and defining exactly what personality is remains difficult.

In a clinical context, personality can both predispose to psychiatric and medical conditions, as well as influence their presentation. As a clinician, an empathic understanding of those we treat relies on an appreciation of the varied ways in which people experience and respond to the world around them. A person's personality will affect their attitude towards clinicians and treatment options, and will, to some extent, dictate which therapeutic approaches will be most successful.

This chapter largely focuses on disorders of personality; that is, when aspects of personality cause problems for an individual and those with whom they interact. However, in order to think about disordered personality, we must first understand what is 'normal'.

MODELS OF PERSONALITY

Models of personality can be broadly divided into three types: trait, categorical and structural (Poole & Higgo, 2006).

TRAIT MODELS

Trait models attempt to identify certain characteristics or behaviours that are present in individuals to different extents. Each trait is expressed on a spectrum, with some people possessing it strongly, and others, more weakly. For example, a 'normal' level of self-confidence would be in the middle, with extremes, either severe self-doubt or inflated confidence, labelled as abnormal. Theorists have identified and measured different traits, including extraversion–introversion, neuroticism, psychoticism, openness to experience, conscientiousness and agreeableness (Taylor & Vaidya, 2009). The International Classification of Diseases (ICD-11) employs a trait model in its classification of personality disorders (World Health Organization [WHO], 2018).

CATEGORICAL MODELS

A categorical model of personality aims to define 'types' of personalities, clusters of characteristics that often occur together, rather than the expression of specific traits. This model draws on Kraepelinian theory that classifies mental disorders based on patterns of symptoms, clearly differentiating illness from normality. While this model struggles to describe the full diversity of personality (Poole & Higgo, 2006), the clarity of definition is useful in research, and provides a language for clinical diagnosis. One of the most widely used systems of classification of mental illness, the *Diagnostic and Statistical Manual of Mental Disorders (DSM-5)*, uses a categorical model of personality classification, describing 10 distinct personality disorders, grouped into three clusters.

STRUCTURAL MODELS

Structural models rely on a theoretical basis of human development, subsequent structure of personality and behaviour. Both psychoanalytic and cognitive behavioural theories approach personality in this way. Sigmund Freud (1856–1939) described a dynamic unconscious that developed through early childhood experiences and was made up of thoughts, feelings and desires. He argued that human behaviour was the consequence of interactions between three competing parts of the mind: the unconscious, primitive id that desires immediate gratification, the reasonable and pragmatic ego, and the conscious and moralistic superego. In contrast, cognitive theory suggests that one's behaviour is a result of learning through prior experience that forms automatic processes and implicit memory. While these approaches have been criticised due to a lack of empirical evidence, they have been highly influential in our understanding of personality, in particular in how it develops.

PERSONALITY DEVELOPMENT

Given the ambiguity in defining personality, it is not surprising that understanding its development is complicated. As such, personality development is likely multifactorial, including biological, psychological and environmental influences.

GENETIC

Studies of sets of twins have suggested that personality traits are inherited, particularly extraversion and neuroticism (McGuffin & Thapar, 1992). Personality characteristics and disorders are associated with multiple genes, which have a collective, rather than individual, effect (Harrison et al., 2018).

BIOLOGICAL

Current research is investigating areas such as hormones, enzymes and neurotransmitters that have bearing on certain personality traits.

EARLY CHILDHOOD

Newborns exhibit early differences and seem to be born with varying characteristics; some settle more easily, some feed with fewer problems; others seem less disturbed by new or changing environments. These early traits continue into later childhood but are modifiable, becoming more or less prominent, depending on environmental influences.

While these early qualities are the beginning of the infant's personality development, they also shape the parental attitude and response. The innate temperament of the child not only influences the child's development from within, but also has a direct effect on the environment in which they are developing, including on the parent. The parent and child essentially shape each other's behaviour.

It is generally accepted that our experiences throughout childhood, adolescence and even early adulthood shape us into the adults we eventually become. Multiple theories exist to explain how this occurs, some of which will be outlined below. While research in this area is difficult due to multiple variables and lifetime-spanning follow-up periods (Harrison et al., 2018), studies such as the Dunedin cohort study, which began in the 1970s and continues today, have found evidence that links early childhood experiences to later adult outcomes (Reuben et al., 2016).

PSYCHODYNAMIC THEORY

Freud argued that personality develops in stages characterised by internal psychological conflict. Unresolved conflicts leave the child 'fixated' at that stage, creating personality and interpersonal difficulties later in life. While Freud's theories have received significant criticism due to lack of scientific evidence and a seeming gender bias, they are still widely referenced in psychiatry and popular culture, and form the basis for much of personality theory.

One of the most influential theories of personality development is attachment theory, which was described by John Bowlby in 1969. He stressed the importance of a close and reliable relationship with early caregivers in terms of social, emotional and cognitive development. He contrasted this 'secure-attachment' with 'insecure' types, either 'ambivalent' or 'anxious', that led to problems in relationship formation (Harrison et al., 2018). Subsequent researchers added a 'disorganised' type, reflecting a history of impaired attachment experiences and leading to difficulties with self-regulation, personality and relationship style (Liotti, 2004).

DISORDERS OF PERSONALITY AND THEIR CLASSIFICATION

While our personality defines us as individuals and is responsible for our strengths, it also leaves vulnerabilities, predisposition to emotional or relationship difficulties, and even mental health problems. In this context, even personalities we would consider 'abnormal' are not necessarily disordered. Some people viewed as odd or eccentric may be able to function relatively well despite their difference. Others, however, struggle with social interactions and function, causing distress to themselves and those around them.

Just as there are different models in understanding personality and its development, there are different models of defining and classifying personality disorder. Disorders are diagnosed when a person's experience and way of interacting with the world lies outside the norm and causes significant distress and dysfunction. The two most commonly used classification systems that define personality disorders are the ICD-11 and *DSM-5*. The former is informed by a trait or dimensional model, the latter employs a categorical model while acknowledging the general international move towards a dimensional approach in the 'emerging methods and models' section (American Psychiatric Association [APA], 2013).

As the *DSM-5* is the most widely used in Australia, it will form the basis for further reference for the rest of this chapter. It describes personality disorder as 'an enduring pattern of behaviour and inner experience that deviates significantly from the individual's cultural standards, is pervasive and inflexible, has an onset in adolescence or early adulthood, is stable over time and leads to distress or impairment' (APA, 2013).

Ten discrete disorders are described, organised into three clusters grouped by similarities. Cluster A includes disorders with odd, aloof features, Cluster B includes dramatic, impulsive and erratic features, while Cluster C includes anxious

---

BOX 16.1   DSM-5 PERSONALITY CLUSTERS

Cluster A
- Schizotypal
- Schizoid
- Paranoid

Cluster B
- Narcissistic
- Borderline
- Antisocial
- Histrionic

Cluster C
- Obsessive-compulsive
- Dependent
- Avoidant

Source: APA, 2013

and fearful features. Each disorder has a specific set of criteria, and an exclusion for difficulties that occur due to another cause, such as another psychiatric illness.

EPIDEMIOLOGY OF PERSONALITY DISORDERS

Personality disorders are common. Rates differ, however, depending on the classification system used and the country in which the research is conducted. A review from 2016 found that studies from the UK, Norway and Australia showed a prevalence ranging between 4.4% and 13.4%, while data from the USA showed a prevalence range between 9% and 21.5% (Quirk et al., 2016). Within the mental health system, around 50% of patients will have a personality disorder, often comorbid with another psychiatric disorder (Sadock et al., 2015).

Those with personality disorders have a higher incidence of health problems, and higher utilisation of the healthcare system, and are therefore prevalent in primary care populations (Huprich, 2018). Personality traits, perceptions of self and the quality of interpersonal relationships all influence healthcare outcomes (Huprich, 2018).

In the emergency department (ED), patients with frequent, high-intensity usage are more likely to have a personality disorder (Beck et al., 2016), while such a diagnosis also increases the attendance of people with substance use disorders (Huynh et al., 2016). Factors associated with ED presentation in individuals with personality disorders include female gender, youth and the involvement of police. These patients are likely to have a prolonged stay but eventually be discharged home (Penfold et al., 2016).

Given the high presentation of people with personality disorders to the ED, it is likely that there will be a correspondingly high prevalence of personality pathology in the population of patients cared for by paramedics. There is, however, little research in this area.

ASSESSMENT OF PERSONALITY DIFFICULTIES AND DISORDER

In any clinical setting, assessment of personality, even in the absence of a disorder, is important as it allows us to understand and predict what may be stressful for our patients and how they may react to or engage with clinical staff and proposed treatments. Paramedics are often the first health professionals involved in the care of people who have self-harmed or attempted suicide, many of whom have personality pathology.

While a person's behaviour usually reflects their underlying personality style, care must be taken in a clinical context as this does not necessarily hold true. As clinicians, particularly in an emergency setting, we interact with people during the most challenging situations of their lives. The behaviour we observe reflects how that person functions under extreme stress, which may be significantly different from their usual behavioural and communication style. In a pre-hospital assessment it is important to be aware of potentially confounding factors that could affect behaviour, including the role of intoxication or withdrawal, or a comorbid disorder such as depression, mania or psychosis. While a person is intoxicated or suffering an affective illness, the assessment of personality is so impeded that it is nearly impossible.

A full assessment of personality includes gathering information from other sources; this is called collateral history. With the luxury of time, history can be gathered from old reports from school, the general practitioner, colleagues or employers (with consent). In a time-limited setting, valuable information can be gathered from friends and family who may be present. People who know the patient well can advise whether or not the presentation differs from usual behaviour. Information can also be sought regarding previous episodes, interactions with clinical staff and previous hospitalisations. Gathering information from multiple sources allows the development of a rounded view of the patient and recognition of patterns of behaviour.

TYPES OF PERSONALITY DISORDERS
CLUSTER A PERSONALITY DISORDERS

Cluster A incorporates the odd, eccentric and suspicious. These disorders share some features with psychotic disorders and are more common in relatives of those with schizophrenia (Sadock et al., 2015).

Studies show a prevalence of around 1.6% (Newton-Howes, 2015); however, given that these are often socially isolated people who rarely seek treatment, this is likely to be an under-representation. It is often the family, rather than the individual, who become concerned at unusual behaviour, diminishing social circles or difficulties in the workplace.

**BOX 16.2 CLINICAL FEATURES OF PARANOID
PERSONALITY DISORDER**

- Mistrustful
- Suspicious
- Extremely sensitive
- Unforgiving
- Jealous and doubtful of partner
- Irritable
- Litigious

Attendance at emergency departments is usually in the context of comorbidity. In extreme cases, the disorder itself may precipitate presentation if it resembles another diagnosis such as psychosis, or if disregard for social norms has led to poor self-care or hoarding which have become a safety concern (Newton-Howes, 2015).

Paranoid personality disorder (PPD)

- Prevalence of roughly 2–4% (Sadock et al., 2015)
- Some go on to be diagnosed with a delusional disorder or schizophrenia

Clinical features

PPD is characterised by an irrational mistrust, often suspecting others of attempting to harm, exploit or deceive them, and perceiving innocent comments as attacking or demeaning. Social interactions are difficult and result in few friendships. People with PPD are unforgiving, tend to bear grudges and are usually quick to anger.

In relationships, people with PPD are usually jealous and question their partner's fidelity without justification. They tend to observe hierarchy, devaluing those they perceive to be inadequate or imperfect.

People with PPD tend to be tense and alert, their interaction style formal, confrontational and lacking in emotional depth. They mostly lack humour, externalise their emotions and put forward highly logical or obsessional arguments, believing strongly in their own correctness and objectivity. These people are often baffled by a suggestion to see a psychiatrist despite the significant impact on social functioning (Grant et al., 2004).

Differential diagnosis

The main differentials that should be considered are of a paranoid psychosis or a delusional disorder. Psychosis is normally discernible due to the lack of hallucinations, formal thought disorder and other symptoms of psychosis in PPD. Paranoid beliefs in PPD can be so intense that they border on delusional ideas, resembling a delusional disorder. Usually in PPD, with sufficient exploration these beliefs can be categorised as overvalued ideas and the persecutory assumptions as 'sensitive ideas of reference' (Harrison et al., 2018). However, in some cases there may not be a clear distinction.

> ### BOX 16.3 CLINICAL FEATURES OF SCHIZOID PERSONALITY DISORDER
>
> - Detached from social relationships
> - Cold and unemotional
> - No desire for friendships
> - Little interest in sexual relationships
> - Introspective
> - Prefer solitary pursuits

Schizoid personality disorder (SdPD)

- Prevalence of roughly 5% (Sadock et al., 2015)
- A small minority go on to develop schizophrenia (Harrison et al., 2018)

People with SdPD have a pervasive detachment from social relationships as well as a cold, aloof and introspective style. They neither desire nor enjoy personal closeness and have little, if any, interest in sexual relationships. They can seem indifferent to praise or criticism, and struggle to express their emotions. In social situations they are uncomfortable, at times employing unusual patterns of speech.

These people prefer spending time alone, and often end up in careers with minimal contact with other humans. They can seem to take pleasure in few things, but may have excessive interest in a particular area such as mathematics or metaphysical constructs (Sadock et al., 2015). People with SdPD are quite introspective and have rich fantasy worlds. Sometimes, their attachment to animals is more successful than with other people.

Differential diagnosis

SdPD shares some features with autism spectrum disorder; however, differences include no difficulties with communication or the use of language, and lack of stereotyped behaviours and developmental difficulties.

Schizotypal personality disorder (SPD)

- Prevalence of roughly 3% (Sadock et al., 2015)
- Significant link with schizophrenia, with neurobiological similarities (Newton-Howes, 2015) and a higher frequency among relatives of those with schizophrenia (Harrison et al., 2018)
- Research suggests that 10% eventually commit suicide (Sadock et al., 2015)

People with SPD tend to be those individuals whom we perceive as very odd or eccentric, sometimes encountered as a clairvoyant or one who claims to have magical powers. They have pervasive patterns of social and interpersonal deficits, difficulty with close relationships, and cognitive and perceptual distortions.

Social interactions are often difficult due to an excessive anxiety that stems from paranoid tendencies rather than negative self-judgment. Their style of interaction is awkward, with inappropriate emotional responses, and a vague, circumstantial,

---

**BOX 16.4   CLINICAL FEATURES OF SCHIZOTYPAL
PERSONALITY DISORDER**

- Eccentric
- Magical thinking
- Social anxiety
- Suspiciousness
- Vague, metaphorical speech
- Desire but struggle to attain friendships
- Odd appearance

---

over-elaborate style. Unsurprisingly, those with SPD struggle to make friends. In contrast to those with SdPD, they desire friends, but often feel out of place and lonely. Their appearance alone can be peculiar, failing to follow social norms and often exhibiting odd mannerisms.

Schizotypal people often have magical thinking and beliefs that are at odds to those around them. Common themes are superstition, clairvoyance, the supernatural, magical powers, telepathy or having a sixth sense. They can describe ideas of reference (not to the point of delusions) as well as strange perceptual experiences such as bodily illusions.

Differential diagnosis

Like PPD, SPD is differentiated from schizophrenia by an absence of frank psychotic symptoms.

CLUSTER B PERSONALITY DISORDERS

Cluster B disorders are the more dramatic and flamboyant. They are also those that are seen most frequently in clinical practice, often coming to attention in acute and emergency situations. While most personality disorders become apparent in the context of treating a comorbidity, Cluster B disorders are themselves the focus of treatment.

These disorders seem to have a genetic basis. Research has linked 'gross physical neglect' as well as physical and sexual abuse in childhood with all Cluster B disorders (Johnson et al., 1999).

Histrionic personality disorder (HPD)

- Prevalence of roughly 1–3% (Sadock et al., 2015)
- Associated with somatisation (the manifestation of psychological distress through bodily symptoms) and alcohol use disorders (Sadock et al., 2015)
- Diagnosed more frequently in women than in men
- Symptoms become less prominent with age (Sadock et al., 2015)

HPD is characterised by drama, extroversion and excessive emotionality. While uncomfortable when not the centre of attention, there is often insecurity about

---

BOX 16.5   CLINICAL FEATURES OF HISTRIONIC PERSONALITY DISORDER

- Dramatic
- Extroverted
- Attention-seeking
- Inappropriately seductive
- Difficulty maintaining attachments
- Easily bored
- Insecure
- Shallow and labile affect
- Impressionistic speech
- Self-deceptive
- Suggestible

---

individual value, physical appearance or attractiveness. There is a tendency towards suggestibility, as well as deception both of themselves and others.

Interactions can be intense and theatrical, with impressionistic, colourful and superficial speech. They demonstrate rapidly shifting and shallow emotions, but have difficulty understanding and expressing inner feelings and motivations. Demonstrative acts such as suicidal gestures or self-harm are not uncommon.

Both men and women with HPD seek intimacy and can be inappropriately seductive or provocative, often believing relationships to be more intimate than they truly are. Ultimately, relationships tend to be superficial and they struggle to maintain meaningful attachments.

Differential diagnosis

HPD share some features with borderline personality disorder, and the two disorders can and often do co-occur.

Borderline personality disorder (BPD)

- Prevalence of around 1–4% (Sadock et al., 2015)
- Diagnosed more frequently in women; however, recent studies suggest a more even gender distribution (Harrison et al., 2018)
- Associated with major depressive disorder (MDD) and alcohol use disorders

BPD, also known as emotionally unstable personality disorder, is probably the most widely known of the personality disorders. These people tend to be high users of emergency and psychiatric services, often presenting in dramatic situations with high levels of expressed emotion, suicidal ideation, suicide attempts and self-harming behaviours.

Aetiology

Why people develop BDP is not completely understood despite significant research. Current understanding involves genetic, biological and environmental factors.

BOX 16.6   CLINICAL FEATURES OF BORDERLINE PERSONALITY DISORDER

- Intense, unstable interpersonal relationships
- Fear of abandonment
- Alternation between idealised and devalued views of others
- Emotional instability
- Intense anger
- Unstable sense of self
- Emptiness
- Dissociation
- Impulsive
- Risky behaviours
- Self-harm
- Suicidal ideation
- Brief psychotic symptoms

There is a significant genetic link with studies of twins showing heritability, and first-degree relatives being 10 times more likely to also have BPD or a similar personality pathology (Harrison et al., 2018).

A current focus of research is identifying genes that help regulate emotions and impulses. Another is functional brain imaging (fMRI), which has shown changes in the connections between different brain networks. Epigenetic research has demonstrated that environmental factors can impact on gene expression (Pier et al., 2016).

Culturally, lack of stable familial relationships seems to increase one's risk of having BPD. Psychoanalytic theory describes contributing problems with development and attachment. Early life trauma is significantly linked with the development of BPD, with high rates of reported physical abuse, sexual abuse or neglect during childhood (National Health and Medical Research Council [NHMRC], 2012).

Clinical features

People with BPD struggle with relationships, often feel insecure, have a poor sense of self and struggle to contain their emotions and impulses.

Interpersonal relationships alternate between idealisation and devaluation, considering others as all good or all bad. Intimate relationships tend to be intense and unstable due to a constant fear of rejection and abandonment, and frantic efforts to avoid this. Persistent demands for closeness and love can often paradoxically drain partners (Harrison et al., 2018). Fear of loneliness can lead to vulnerability, possibly accepting strangers as friends or entering into intimate relationships quickly (Sadock et al., 2015).

A core feature is severe mood swings and difficulty containing emotions. Someone with BPD can sink into the depths of despair, but can recover to a positive state in a matter of hours or days. Their experience of anger can be extreme and uncontrollable, anxiety can be debilitating and excitement overwhelming, and the person is often unaware from where each emotion stems.

People with BPD usually struggle with a sense of self and stable identity. Feelings of emptiness and detachment are common. Despite the severe mood swings, they can often feel detached from their emotional experience and situation. In severe cases, people can dissociate, detaching from emotional and physical surroundings.

Impulsivity is another key feature, with those with BPD often engaging in risky activities. Spending excessively, sexual promiscuity, substance use and erratic driving are not uncommon. Substance use can also serve the purpose of numbing the extreme emotional experiences.

Acts of self-harm, suicidal statements or suicidal acts are a common and very visible feature of BPD. These behaviours can be a coping mechanism to relieve tension, a method to gain care and support or an expression of anger.

At times, those with BPD experience stress-related psychotic-like symptoms such as paranoid ideas or auditory or visual hallucinations. As opposed to the psychotic symptoms associated with schizophrenia, these tend to be short lived, are often dramatic, emotionally laden and thematically related to real stressors. They tend not to be accompanied by the usual distraction evident in schizophrenia, and differ also in the lack of associated thought disorder.

The severity of the disorder varies significantly. Some people are able to function well, maintaining employment and relationships, and only experiencing symptoms in times of stress. Others find that their function is impacted more severely. Some have repeated crises, often involving self-harm and impulsive aggression (National Institute for Health and Care Excellence [NICE], 2009).

Course and prognosis

BPD is often not formally diagnosed before adulthood; however, symptoms are often clearly evident in adolescence. The course is variable. While many people recover over time with treatment, some may continue to experience social and interpersonal difficulties (NICE, 2009).

MDD is frequently comorbid in those with BDP (Sadock et al., 2015), as well as other personality disorders (NICE, 2009), post-traumatic stress disorder (PTSD), and anxiety and eating disorders. BPD is associated with substantial impairment in social, psychological, occupational functioning and quality of life, with sufferers at an increased risk of completed suicide (NICE, 2009).

Antisocial personality disorder (ASPD)

- General prevalence of around 0.2–3% and more common in lower socio-economic and urban areas (Sadock et al., 2015)
- Prevalence of just under 50% in a prison population (NICE, 2009)
- Three times more common in men than in women (NICE, 2009)
- Five times more common among first-degree relative of men with the disorder (Sadock et al., 2015)

Some differences exist in the definition of ASPD. The *DSM-5* requires that a person meet the criteria for conduct disorder as a child or teen to receive a diagnosis of

---

BOX 16.7   CLINICAL FEATURES OF ANTI-SOCIAL PERSONALITY DISORDER

- Disregard for others
- Frequent criminal activity
- Manipulative
- Impulsivity
- Irresponsible
- Aggressive and irritable
- Violent
- Shallow and short-lived relationships
- Can be charming and ingratiating
- Lack of remorse and empathy
- Failure to learn from previous experiences

ASPD as an adult. The ICD does not have this requirement, and uses the term 'dissocial'.

Aetiology

Adoption studies have suggested a genetic link, with children of parents with ASPD more likely to have the disorder even when separated at birth (Harrison et al., 2018). Biological factors are being studied with monoamine oxidase A (MAOA) predisposing to adult antisocial behaviour in men, particularly those who have experienced early adversity (Byrd & Manuck, 2014).

There are a number of developmental theories for ASPD. Bowlby, in 1944, suggested that early separation from mothers could lead to antisocial behaviour and difficulty forming relationships (Harrison et al., 2018). Violent and inconsistent parenting has been shown to predispose to antisocial behaviour (Pollock, 1990), while backgrounds of fractured families with frequent parental conflict are common in those with ASPD (NICE, 2009). Children in these contexts are often removed from families, leading in turn to delinquency, substance misuse and truancy, which later predisposes to unstable accommodation and limited education and employment (NICE, 2009).

ASPD is characterised by a consistent disregard for and violation of the rights of others (APA, 2013), with high rates of impulsivity, aggression and manipulation. People with ASPD generally fail to respect legal and social boundaries, often purposefully deceiving or manipulating others either for gain or pleasure.

People with ASPD rarely consider consequences, taking large risks with their own and others' safety. Inconsistency and irresponsibility make it difficult to sustain employment or relationships.

Interactional styles can oscillate between demanding and manipulative, utilising suicide threats and somatic complaints, to charming, ingratiating and seductive. They can appear composed, despite high levels of irritability, aggression and hostility. Relationships tend to be shallow and short lived, often ending when the other person is no longer perceived as useful. These people can be controlling and degrading to spouses and family members, with domestic violence and infidelity not uncommon.

There is a striking lack of remorse and empathy for others, often rationalising damaging behaviour or denying responsibility. In traumatic situations, people can appear numbed, showing little if any anxiety or distress. These people have a marked inability to learn from negative experiences and consequence.

Course and prognosis

ASPD is often comorbid with depression, anxiety and substance misuse (NICE, 2009). The course of the disorder is variable. Some people's behaviour and relationships seem to improve with age, while others continue to have severe difficulties throughout their lives.

A note on the 'psychopath'

The label 'psychopath' is heavily stigmatising, engenders fear, implies badness, danger and treatment resistance, and is used frequently in both popular culture and everyday language. Psychopaths are described as chillingly callous and lacking empathy, with an ability to credibly demonstrate remorse without experiencing it. While the concept crosses over with the terms 'dissocial' or 'antisocial', current psychiatric practice considers it as a personality trait rather than a disorder, and uses it rarely. The term is found predominantly in forensic psychology (Harrison et al., 2018).

Narcissistic personality disorder (NPD)

- Prevalence ranges from 1–6% (APA, 2013)

People with NPD demonstrate a pattern of grandiosity, need for admiration and lack of empathy for others (APA, 2013). They have an inflated sense of self-importance and uniqueness, and show boastful, arrogant and pretentious qualities. Entitlement is common, with unreasonable expectations of superior service and unquestioning

---

BOX 16.8   CLINICAL FEATURES OF NARCISSISTIC PERSONALITY DISORDER

- Grandiosity
- Need for admiration
- Lack of empathy
- Inflated sense of self-importance
- Disdaining and condescending
- Entitlement
- Fantasises about success and power
- Exploitative
- Envious of others
- Fragile self-esteem
- Highly sensitive

compliance. They will often gravitate towards those with perceived high status or power, but show disdain and condescension to others.

These people lack empathy for others and can be exploitative; relationships are consequently difficult. They either partner with others who are dependent, of whom they eventually bore, or end up enraging partners and eventually rejecting them (Sadock et al., 2015).

Narcissists tend to fantasise about success, power, brilliance, beauty, intellectual prowess or ideal love (APA, 2013). They tend to be envious of the possessions and achievements of others, and believe others to be envious of them. Underneath, there is often a fragile self-esteem. Criticism or failure are not well tolerated, is frequently met with anger, and can precipitate a fall into crisis and depression through narcissistic injury.

Course and prognosis

The features of NPD are chronic, and its treatment difficult, as it involves frequent challenges to the person's narcissistic core. Ageing for these people can be difficult and they have a predisposition to midlife crises as they attempt to cling to youthful qualities (Sadock et al., 2015). Narcissistic patients are at a higher risk of suicide and depressive disorders compared with that of the general population.

CLUSTER C PERSONALITY DISORDERS

These disorders share the common trait of anxiety. While potentially disabling for the sufferer, they can have minimal negative impact on those around them. Patients are less commonly seen in clinical contexts, only coming to attention when very severe, or if presenting with another illness (Poole & Higgo, 2006).

Avoidant personality disorder (APD)

- Prevalence roughly 2–3% (Sadock et al., 2015)
- Limited research regarding aetiology

BOX 16.9   CLINICAL FEATURES OF AVOIDANT PERSONALITY DISORDER

- Social inhibition
- Feelings of inadequacy
- Hypersensitive to criticism
- Avoid interpersonal situations
- Timid and anxious
- Lack confidence
- Believe themselves to be inferior and unappealing
- Socially inept
- Fearful of relationships but crave human contact
- Avoid new situations

People with APD experience social inhibition, feelings of inadequacy, hypersensitivity to disapproval (APA, 2013) and may be described colloquially as having an 'inferiority complex' (Sadock et al., 2015).

They tend to avoid interpersonal contact, particularly in new situations, for fear of criticism, embarrassment or failure, with significant impact on their social and occupational functioning. They are often shy, lack confidence and are self-deprecating, with core beliefs that they are unappealing, inferior or unlikeable. Hampered by these fears, which worsen with perceived disapproval, they come across as socially inept.

People with APD are fearful of relationships unless they are certain of being liked. Social contacts are often limited to family and intimate relationships are uncommon, hindered by fears of rejection. Despite this, they crave companionship but need incredible reassurances of acceptance.

Differential diagnosis

While similar to schizoid PD, those with APD differ in that they desire social connections, often reporting loneliness. They differ from those with dependent PD as they have less fear of abandonment (Sadock et al., 2015).

Treatment

Treatment is difficult. There has been some evidence of success using cognitive behavioural therapy (CBT) in a group format (with peers) within a forensic setting (Duggan et al., 2007). Other approaches include social skills training and addiction services.

Obsessive-compulsive personality disorder (OCPD)

- Prevalence of 2–8% (APA, 2013)
- More common in men than in women, and in first-degree relatives of people with the disorder (Sadock et al., 2015)
- Limited evidence regarding aetiology

BOX 16.10   CLINICAL FEATURES OF OBSESSIVE-COMPULSIVE PERSONALITY DISORDER

- Emotional constriction
- Perfectionism
- Inflexibility
- Preoccupied with details and rules
- Inefficient
- Stiff, rigid interpersonal style
- Lack of humour, spontaneity or imagination
- Authoritarian
- Moralistic
- Judgmental
- Avoidance of change
- Hoarding

OCPD is characterised by emotional constriction, preoccupation with orderliness, perfectionism and excessive mental control at the expense of flexibility and efficiency (APA, 2013). Those with OCPD adhere rigidly to rules and cannot tolerate deviations. Excessive focus on detail and order can mean that the point of an activity can be lost. High levels of perfectionism can decrease efficiency and lead to indecisiveness as they struggle to meet their own unrealistically high standards.

Interpersonal skills are often limited, with a stiff, formal and over-inclusive style that lacks spontaneity and humour. Their inability to compromise or tolerate different attitudes can be alienating, often holding strict and inflexible views in ethical, moral and political domains. Consequently, they can often be judgmental and struggle to adapt to new situations. Those with OCPD often devote the majority of their time and energy to work, meaning that relationships suffer and they often have few friends but manage to have stable employment and partners.

There is a tendency towards hoarding with OCPD, with an unwillingness to discard objects. Similarly, with money, there is a propensity to save unreasonably in case of an emergency.

Differential diagnosis

Confusion can arise due to the similarity of name between OCPD and obsessive-compulsive disorder (OCD). In the latter, recurrent obsessions and compulsions are present, and, if noted in someone with OCPD, a diagnosis of OCD should be considered.

Course and prognosis

The course of OCPD is variable and unpredictable. Some diagnosed with this personality disorder go on to develop schizophrenia, OCD or MDD. As yet, it is difficult to predict who these people will be. On the other hand, a significant proportion of people improve over time, becoming less rigid and obsessional with age.

Treatment

Unlike many of the other personality disorders, those with OCPD are often aware of their suffering and are motivated to seek treatment. A behavioural approach is usually favoured, aiming to teach the patient to avoid situations that may increase difficulties as well as improving their coping mechanisms. There is no substantial evidence for the use of medications, even those known to be helpful in OCD.

Dependent personality disorder (DPD)

- Prevalence of around 0.6% (APA, 2013)
- More common in women than in men

Persons with DPD have a strong need to be taken care of that leads to submissive and clinging behaviour and fears of separation (APA, 2013). They struggle to make even simple decisions without advice and reassurance, and find it very difficult to take responsibility for multiple areas of their life.

> **BOX 16.11   CLINICAL FEATURES OF DEPENDENT PERSONALITY DISORDER**
>
> - Submissive
> - Fear separation
> - Struggle to make decisions
> - Need excessive reassurance
> - Give up responsibility
> - Hesitant to make demands
> - Compliant and subordinate
> - Low self-confidence
> - Vulnerable to abuse

People with DPD struggle to disagree or make demands, as they fear disapproval. They will go to abnormal lengths to obtain approval and support, meaning they are unduly compliant, devalue their own needs, and are willing to withstand extreme discomfort if it guarantees support. Due to low self-confidence, people with DPD struggle to start tasks and can appear amotivated.

These people struggle to be alone, as they fear that they are unable to look after themselves. They tend to end up with partners who are more energetic and driven and are willing to support them. This means that they can often remain in a relationship that is abusive for long periods of time to avoid a separation. Similarly, when a relationship does end, a replacement relationship is sought urgently. Often, these people only come to attention when a partner leaves or dies.

Differential diagnosis

Dependent traits are common in both histrionic and borderline personality disorder; however, those with DPD usually have longer and more consistent relationships, and tend to be less manipulative (Sadock et al., 2015).

Course and prognosis

People with DPD can have significant amounts of social and occupational impairment. Relationships are limited to those who can tolerate dependency, making them vulnerable to exploitation and abusive situations (Sadock et al., 2015).

GENERAL PRINCIPLES OF MANAGEMENT

Given the difficulties of engaging this population in treatment, it is not surprising that there is minimal firm evidence for the treatment of many personality disorders (Bateman et al., 2015). Much of the research looks at BPD given its prominence in clinical settings, and at ASPD, focusing on the associated criminality. Psychosocial interventions are usually a focus of treatment rather than medications, which are used only for symptoms or comorbidities.

Management generally focuses on helping the person to improve their function (Harrison et al., 2018). Exacerbating factors, such as substance abuse, social difficulties and other psychiatric illnesses, should be treated and minimised.

Mainstays of treatment are a trusting therapeutic relationship, collaboration, and encouragement of patient autonomy (Harrison et al., 2018). Given the complexity of managing those with personality disorders, most regions have developed working groups and guidelines for a multidisciplinary and multiservice approach.

The Project Air Strategy (2005), an organisation that offers research, education and treatment guidelines for personality disorders, highlights a need for:

- collaboration between patients, individual clinicians and multidisciplinary teams, and integration of services (hospitals, community teams, police, ambulance and social services) to ensure consistency
- an individualised treatment model that is shared and understood by the patient, clinicians and carers
- consistent policies around admission and referral pathways
- support and supervision of individual clinicians.

Managing people with personality disorders can be challenging and requires significant skill and self-awareness. Clinical supervision is always recommended to allow self-reflection and debriefing.

MEDICATIONS

Despite the minimal evidence for the use of medications in personality disorders, psychotropic prescription, often polypharmacy, is widespread among this patient population. Often it is focused on symptom control (e.g. emotional lability) and comorbid mood, anxiety and psychotic disorders.

PSYCHOTHERAPIES

Generally, referral to an area mental health or personality disorder service that offers a theoretical approach, motivated therapists and supervision will be of benefit regardless of the specific modality used. Group therapies can sometimes be helpful in addressing dependency and teaching social skills (Harrison et al., 2018). Most personality irregularities can be worked on in standard outpatient psychotherapy (Sadock et al., 2015).

For all personality disorders, if the patient is willing and motivated to engage in treatment, psychotherapeutic approaches are the mainstay. A number of structured therapies have been developed, all of which are commonly used and evidence based. These include, among others, dialectical behaviour therapy (DBT), mentalisation-based treatment, CBT for personality disorders, transference-focused psychotherapy and cognitive analytical therapy (Newton-Howes, 2015). The most robust evidence is for DBT.

MANAGEMENT OF BPD

Psychotherapy has long been the mainstay of treatment for BPD, with the use of medication, as already discussed, firmly taking a back foot. There is extensive research in this area, with numerous different approaches emerging over time. The strongest evidence is for the use of structured psychotherapies with experienced clinicians (NHMRC, 2012).

Goals of treatment are negotiated between the clinician and the patient; however, they usually focus on improving function by gaining better control over emotional states, engaging in healthier relationships, and reducing impulsivity and self-harm behaviours by developing coping strategies as well as ultimately finding a sense of direction and purpose.

Forms of psychotherapy include psychoanalytic, psychodynamic, cognitive-behavioural and short-term integrative therapies such as DBT, Mentalisation-based treatment and transference-focused psychotherapy. Common characteristics of psychotherapeutic approaches for BPD include manualised therapies, encouraging patient autonomy, an attempt to link emotions to their context and behaviour, a responsive, validating and educational stance, and supervision of the therapist themselves (Harrison et al., 2018).

A general principle amongst all of these psychotherapeutic approaches is the emphasis on establishing rapport, adopting a collaborative approach to decision making, including the discussion of how to handle risky behaviours such as self-harm and suicidality. There is an underlying assumption that it is desirable for the individual to take as much responsibility and control of their situation, including crises, as they can. This will be explored in a case history below.

Hospitalisation

There is extensive evidence to suggest that prolonged hospitalisation for people with BPD is not helpful and can often worsen symptoms, reinforce maladaptive behaviours and be of no long-term benefit. The NHMRC states that people with BPD should be admitted to hospital for only short, time-limited periods, when in crisis and at risk of significant harm, with specific goals agreed upon prior to admission (2012).

People with BPD are frequent presenters at emergency departments (Shaikh et al., 2017). The paramedic is often the first contact with the health service, and can set the tone and impression for future interactions. Mental health treatment should occur concurrently to physical treatment, when self-injurious behaviour has occurred (NHMRC, 2012). De-escalation of agitated patients can be attempted first by enquiring about concerns, sources of frustration and distress, then offering reassurance and firmly and calmly setting boundaries regarding appropriate behaviour. If agitation is severe, medications can be used to relieve distress (Shaikh et al., 2017).

In the case study below, examples will be given of how paramedics can engage a client with these issues, assessing risk, adopting a problem-solving approach, and exploring crisis-based and self-management techniques to assist the client.

PERSONALITY COURSE ACROSS THE LIFETIME

Most definitions of personality disorder describe patterns of difficulties that are chronic and enduring. There is, however, growing evidence to suggest that while personality traits might be stable over the course of one's life, the level to which these impact on function and behaviour is not (Newton-Howes, 2015).

Externalising, self-destructive traits seem to lessen in intensity with age, while rigid, introspective traits may become more prominent (Newton-Howes, 2015). This can affect observed prevalence across age groups, with Cluster B disorders becoming less visible as these people age, and vice versa for Clusters A and C (Newton-Howes, 2015).

Patients with BPD tend to have varied outcomes. Research in 2006 suggested that 88% achieved remission across a 10-year period, those with substance abuse faring worse (Harrison et al., 2018). Those with BPD are at increased risk of many health conditions, including cardiovascular disease, diabetes, chronic fatigue, fibromyalgia, chronic pain and obesity. They tend to be more neglectful in terms of preventative healthcare and, despite consulting greater numbers of practitioners, often fail to complete recommended investigations or treatment (Bertsch & Herpetz, 2018; Sansone & Sansone, 2015). These patients are also known to have higher rates of completed suicide.

Generally, those with personality disorders have poorer health outcomes than the general population (Bertsch & Herpetz, 2018), and have a life expectancy that is 17.7 years lower than the general population's (Fok et al., 2012).

ORGANIC PERSONALITY CHANGE

There are a number of physical health conditions that can lead to sustained personality and behaviour change. As these changes may be the first evidence of disease, they are worth being aware of, to avoid mis-diagnosis. The particulars depend on aetiology; however, the medical condition needs to have been active prior to the noted changes.

The following areas of disease are more likely to affect personality:

* neurodegenerative disorders including frontotemporal dementias, Huntington's disease or other dementing illnesses
* structural damage, particularly to the temporal or frontal lobes, caused by head trauma or a lesion such as a carcinoma
* epilepsy
* heavy metal poisoning
* infections such as syphilis or HIV.

CASE STUDY

Emma

You have been dispatched to a suburban house at 12.25 a.m. to attend a 23-year-old woman who is bleeding from what is reported to be a self-inflicted laceration to her arm. She is conscious but distressed and saying that she wants to die. There are no other known injuries. When you arrive at the house, a young man greets you. He explains that he came home to find his girlfriend in the bathroom, crying and bleeding from multiple cuts on her forearm. He is shaking, shocked and overwhelmed by the situation, but is not angry or hostile. He confirms that there is no one else at home.

As you walk through the house you notice that it is reasonably neat and tidy. There is a wine bottle on the kitchen table. When you get to the bathroom, you can see a young woman sitting on the floor, with a number of lacerations on her left wrist. There is a broken glass on the ground. Emma is turned away from you, sobbing. From the doorway you introduce yourself and your partner and state that you are here to help, but get no response. You assess the room. The broken glass is not within arm's reach of Emma. There is a small amount of blood on the floor. In the bathroom cabinet you can see multiple objects, including some medications.

CRITICAL REFLECTION – INITIAL IMPRESSIONS AND SCENE ASSESSMENT

Stop, look, listen

- You have already started your scene assessment, but what else do you want to know from Emma's partner before you walk into the room?
- Conduct a safety assessment of the scene and develop an immediate safety plan with your partner before you engage Emma.
- Consider the makeup of the paramedic team. How would it make a difference if the two paramedics were:
  - both male?
  - both female?
- Are there any gender, religious or cultural factors that need to be considered?
  If any of these situations are potentially a problem, how would you mitigate against it?

What would you consider initially?

- The report is suggestive of an act of self-harm; however, it is important to keep an open mind to other possible causes of Emma's injuries.
- An appraisal of dangers to yourself and your partner from the environment or anyone who may be at the scene.
- Recognition that the patient is distressed, likely making the interview more challenging and potentially posing a risk to herself and others.
- You would need to consider the possibility of intoxication or other psychiatric illness that could affect her mental state.
- It will likely be necessary to gather information from other sources. A person's home environment can give multiple clues to the situation, especially when the patient is unable or unwilling to communicate. These should be documented to inform clinicians who may be involved later.
- In this example, the organised and tidy house suggests that, while things are dramatic currently, previously this was a settled household. It makes the likelihood of a prolonged and severe psychiatric illness, such as a psychotic or affective illness, slightly less likely.
- The wine bottle should remind us about the possibility of alcohol use, which must be factored into the assessment.

You and your partner enter the room. You remove the broken glass and place it out of the way. You approach Emma and repeat your name. There is still no response. As you ask for permission to look at her wrist, she begins to yell at you to *'Go away!'* … *'I just want to die!'* She appears angry and distressed, her knees pulled up to her chest, pushing herself away from you into the corner. You can now see that the lacerations to her forearm appear to have stopped bleeding. Her face has a good level of colour and she is speaking in complete sentences.

Primary assessment and de-escalation
- The first priority is to assess safety. Any objects that could potentially be used as weapons need to be removed, and you should be alert to the possibility of there being further such objects that are not immediately obvious.
- This woman's distress, her defensive body language and statements telling others to go away suggest that she feels cornered and will need space. Impulsive behaviour that could potentially be dangerous for both herself and those around her is more likely in this context.
- Respecting her space and adopting a non-confrontational manner can be helpful. Sitting side-on to the patient, with some distance between you, allowing her a free pathway to the exit, would be appropriate.
- You should adopt a calm, warm, non-judgmental and patient manner, repeating that you are there to help, but allowing the patient time before progressing to further questions.
- Validating the woman's feelings by stating that she appears to be very upset and scared can be helpful. It is important to remember that, while for clinical staff this is not an unusual situation, for the patient and her partner this is likely to be one of the most difficult periods in their lives.
- The woman's physical state should be assessed as soon as possible. The minimal amount of blood, the fact that she is not actively bleeding and her appearance are reassuring.

After some time sitting in silence, the young woman appears to relax a little. She has stopped crying and is looking around the room. You ask her if she will allow you to look at her arm, and she agrees. Your assessment confirms that the lacerations are superficial and will be able to heal without sutures. Her other physical examination and vital signs are normal. You now attempt to ask her what happened. She states, *'I've just had enough … no one can help me … I don't want to be alive anymore.'* She tells you that she had had an argument with her boyfriend earlier in the evening and that he had left the house. She had felt incredibly distressed and was unable to reach him by phone. She had had a few glasses of wine before going into the bathroom with the intention of cutting her arm *'to make it all go away'*.

Secondary assessment
Now that Emma has calmed, it is possible to attempt a more comprehensive assessment. Unlike a full assessment of personality described earlier in this chapter (the principles of which do still apply), the situation above calls for the assessment of a crisis situation. The aim will be to understand the woman's current dilemma as well as, as much as time permits, the contextual and historical factors that will inform management decisions.

This assessment should include the following:

- An attempt to understand the events leading up to the current situation. For example, details of the argument, associated thoughts and feelings and actions taken. The young woman should be encouraged to recount the evening's events chronologically.
- An understanding of the person's previous history. Patients will often be aware of a diagnosis of a personality disorder, and Emma may therefore be able to let you know about diagnosis, similar previous situations and any current or past treatment. Sometimes patients will be able to describe their usual ways of coping or distraction techniques that they utilise, which can be helpful in determining a management plan.
- Examination of the current mental state, screening for features suggestive of other psychiatric illnesses.

- Appraisal of the contribution of intoxication. Many patients in crisis will be intoxicated. Often the intoxication will have some direct responsibility for the self-harm or suicidality, or intoxication may be a result of this crisis from an attempted overdose (Ryan et al., 2015). In this example, Emma has reported drinking alcohol. It is worth assessing her level of intoxication, as there is limited utility in attempting an assessment and the creation of a management plan with someone who is acutely intoxicated. In this case, it would be better to allow her to sober up, either at home or in an emergency department, prior to making a further plan. The possibility of intoxication from overdose is also worth assessing and enquiring about. The woman has made suicidal statements, and medications have been noted in the bathroom. People in crisis do not always offer all of the relevant information immediately, and it is not unknown for an overdose to be concealed if not asked about directly while the focus is on something such as deliberate self-harm.
- Gathering of collateral history. Emma's partner will likely be able to provide valuable information about her history, corroborate her story and give some indication as to whether this behaviour deviates significantly from previous experiences. At times, assessments may be of a first-time crisis situation, but at others, patients may have self-harmed or been suicidal numerous times previously. In the latter case, previous successful management approaches can inform the current situation.

In a crisis situation such as this, a risk assessment and any risk-mitigation plan needs to involve a collaborative approach with the client.

CRITICAL REFLECTION – RISK ASSESSMENT

Commence a risk assessment for Emma
- What other information do you need to know?
- From who and where will you get this information?
- Document protective factors as well.

Now complete a risk mitigation plan for Emma
- Taking the risk factors that you have already identified, what can you do as a paramedic to mitigate against these risks? Who else, and what other resources, can you use to assist?

CRITICAL REFLECTION – COMMUNICATION

Consider the ways in which you would use communication (both verbal and non-verbal) as a therapeutic tool, both to engage and calm Emma, and also to decrease any identified risk factors.

A collaborative approach to management

Once the primary and secondary assessments have been completed, a decision will need to be made about whether to transport this young woman to an emergency department or whether management can continue in the community. Most current guidelines for the management of personality disorders advocate for a collaborative approach that is guided chiefly by the person's views and wishes. Additionally, there is recognition that inpatient admissions have limited utility, and are therefore recommended only as a last resort and for brief periods of time. Obviously, any concerns over physical health will need to be addressed first, and may necessitate transport to an emergency department, irrespective of the mental health assessment.

The following should be considered in devising a management plan:

- The person's opinions on how best to help themselves. In the scenario above, the young woman should be encouraged to express what she would like to do next and what she would find most helpful.

- Opinions of significant others and their ability to provide support and care. If a person is to remain at home with others after a crisis presentation, it will be necessary that the other people are comfortable and agree with this plan. If the patient and their family or friends have differing opinions on this, open discussion should be encouraged with an attempt to facilitate compromise.
- Possible interventions – Once the antecedents of the crisis have been discussed, it can be useful to attempt to identify any issues that may be open to intervention (Ryan et al., 2015). These may include practical interventions regarding housing or finances, problem solving or attempts at conflict resolution with partners or family.

Sometimes a person will request a plan that seems unrealistic, unsafe or at odds with what you would expect them to usually do (Ryan et al., 2015). In these cases, the person's capacity for decision making needs to be assessed. Capacity can be impaired by intoxication, cognitive difficulties, the presence of major mental illness or temporarily by intense levels of distress. If there is suspicion of any of the above, the person would likely need transport to an emergency department to facilitate further investigation and assessment. While the use of an appropriate legal order may need to be considered, it is important to note that simply making an impulsive decision does not mean that the person lacks capacity (Ryan et al., 2015).

If a decision is made for transport to an emergency department, it is important that both the patient and their support people are aware that this is for the purpose of an assessment and will not necessarily result in an admission. It is worth considering any further potential risks prior to transport, including a search of the patient and belongings for any items that could be used for further self-harm either enroute or once in the emergency department. On arrival at an emergency department a comprehensive handover should be given, highlighting aspects of the presentation, examination and history, as well as the patient's role in development of the agreed plan. If a decision is made to remain with community management, the patient should be referred on to an appropriate mental health service. Both the patient and their family/supports should be provided with avenues to seek further support, treatment and advice on what to do if the situation were to deteriorate.

CONCLUSION

This chapter has described normal and abnormal personality, emphasising the lack of clear delineation between the two, and examining the biological, environmental and psychological factors that shape both normal and abnormal development.

The heavy presence of people with personality disorders in pre-hospital and emergency department environments is well documented. Being called to see suicidal patients, those who have attempted or are threatening self-harm, or those who are aggressive, demanding and manipulative is not uncommon. Given this, it is important that paramedics have a thorough understanding of personality, its pathologies and assessment, and how this can be factored into pre-hospital care.

The forensic system, area mental health services, primary care, pre-hospital and emergency settings are all impacted by personality pathology, while those with a personality disorder have poorer health outcomes, higher mortality rates and significant social, occupational and intra/interpersonal dysfunction.

Communication difficulties during assessments are often related to personality. The environment, usual patterns of communication and behaviour, and the collateral history offered by family, friends and partners, are all integral to the assessment.

Treatments include predominantly psychotherapies, with caution advised regarding psychotropic medication or prolonged admissions. A collaborative, validating and non-judgmental approach is recommended, balancing the need to respect autonomous decision making with an attempt to provide care in a safe and containing way.

LINKS AND RESOURCES

For clinicians:

- nice.org.uk – management guidelines for various personality disorders that were reviewed in 2015
- nhmrc.gov.au – Australian clinical practice guidelines
- spectrumbpd.com.au – personality disorder service for Victoria

For patients and their families

- Headspace.org.au – Self-referral service for young people aged 12–25. The website provides educational information on all forms of mental health problems, but with good coverage of personality disorders, geared at young people. Videos provide a 'lived experience' perspective.
- Projectairstrategy.org – Personality disorder information with fact sheets, personal stories and treatment guidelines.

REFERENCES

American Psychiatric Association (APA), 2013. Diagnostic and Statistical Manual of Mental Disorders, fifth ed. American Psychiatric Association, Washington, DC. (DSM-5).

Bateman, A., Gunderson, J., Mulder, R., 2015. Treatment of personality disorders. Lancet 385 (9969), 735–743.

Beck, A., Sanchez-Walker, E., Evans, L., et al., 2016. Characteristics of people who rapidly and frequently reattend the emergency department for mental health needs. Eur. J. Emerg. Med. 23 (5), 351–355.

Bertsch, K., Herpetz, S., 2018. Personality disorders, functioning and health. Psychopathology 51 (2), 69–70.

Byrd, A.L., Manuck, S.B., 2014. MAOA, childhood maltreatment, and antisocial behaviour: meta-analysis or a gene-environment interaction. Biol. Psychiatry 75 (1), 9–17.

Duggan, C., Adams, C., McCarthy, L., et al., 2007. Systematic review of the effectiveness of pharmacological and psychological strategies for the management of people with personality disorder. NHS National R&D Program in Forensic Mental Health.

Fok, M., Hayes, R., Chang, C., et al., 2012. Life expectancy at birth and all-cause mortality among people with personality disorder. J. Psychosom. Res. 73 (2), 104–107.

Grant, B., Haisin, D., Stinson, F., et al., 2004. Prevalence, correlates, and disability of personality disorders in the United States: results from the national epidemiologic survey on alcohol and related conditions. J. Clin. Psychiatry 65 (7), 948–958.

Harrison, P., Cowen, P., Burns, T., et al., 2018. Shorter Oxford Textbook of Psychiatry, seventh ed. Oxford University Press, Oxford.

Huprich, S., 2018. Personality pathology in primary care: ongoing needs for detection and Intervention. J. Clin. Psychol. Med. Settings 25 (1).

Huynh, C., Ferland, F., Blanchette-Martin, N., et al., 2016. Factors influencing the frequency of emergency department utilization by individual with substance use disorders. Psychiatr. Q. 87 (4), 713–728.

Johnson, J., Cohen, P., Smailes, E., et al., 1999. Childhood maltreatment increases risk for personality disorders during early adulthood. Arch. Gen. Psychiatry 56 (7), 600–606.

Liotti, G., 2004. Trauma, dissociation, and disorganized attachment: three strands of a single braid. Psychotherapy: Theory Res. Pract. Train. 41 (4), 472–489.

McGuffin, P., Thapar, A., 1992. The genetics of personality disorder. Br. J. Psychiatry 160, 12–23.

National Health and Medical Research Council (NHMRC), 2012. Clinical Practice Guidelines for the Management of Borderline Personality Disorder. National Health and Medical Research Council, Melbourne.

National Institute for Health and Care Excellence (NICE), 2009. Borderline Personality Disorder: Recognition and Management, Clinical Guideline. National Institute for Health and Care Excellence, London.

Newton-Howes, G., 2015. Personality Disorder: Oxford psychiatry library. Oxford University Press, Oxford.

Penfold, S., Groll, D., Mauer-Vakil, D., et al., 2016. A retrospective analysis of personality disorder presentations in a Canadian university-affiliated hospital's emergency department. Br. J. Psych. Open 2 (6), 394–399.

Pier, K., Marin, L., Wilsnack, J., et al., 2016. The neurobiology of borderline personality disorder. Psychiatric Times 33 (3).

Pollock, V., 1990. Childhood antecedents of antisocial behavior; parental alcoholism and physical abusiveness. Am. J. Psychiatry 147 (10), 1290–1293.

Poole, R., Higgo, R., 2006. Psychiatric Interviewing and Assessment. Cambridge University Press, Cambridge.

Project Air Strategy for Personality Disorders, 2015. Treatment Guidelines for Personality Disorders, second ed. University of Wollongong, Illawarra Health and Medical Research Institute, Wollongong.

Quirk, S., Berk, M., Chanen, A., et al., 2016. Population prevalence of personality disorder and associations with physical health and comorbidities and health care service utilization: a review. Personal. Disord. 7 (2), 136–146.

Reuben, A., Moffitt, T., Caspi, A., et al., 2016. 'Lest we forget': comparing retrospective and prospective assessments of adverse childhood experiences in the prediction of adult health. J. Child Psychol. Psychiatry 57 (10), 1103–1112.

Ryan, C., Large, M., Gribble, R., et al., 2015. Assessing and managing suicidal patients in the emergency department. Australas. Psychiatry 23 (5), 513–516.

Sadock, B., Sadock, V., Ruiz, P., 2015. Kaplan & Sadock's Synopsys of Psychiatry, eleventh ed. electronic book. Wolters Kluwer, Philadelphia.

Sansone, R., Sansone, L., 2015. Borderline personality disorder in the medical setting: suggestive behaviours, syndromes, and diagnoses. Innov. Clin. Neurosci. 12 (7–8), 39–44.

Shaikh, U., Qamar, I., Jafry, F., et al., 2017. Patients with Borderline personality disorder in emergency departments. Front. Psychiatry 8, 136.

Taylor, M., Vaidya, N., 2009. Descriptive Psychopathology: The signs and symptoms of behavioural disorders. Cambridge University Press, Cambridge.

World Health Organization (WHO), 2018. The ICD-11 for Mortality and Morbidity Statistics, Mental, Behavioral or Neurodevelopmental Disorders: Personality disorders and related traits. WHO, Geneva.

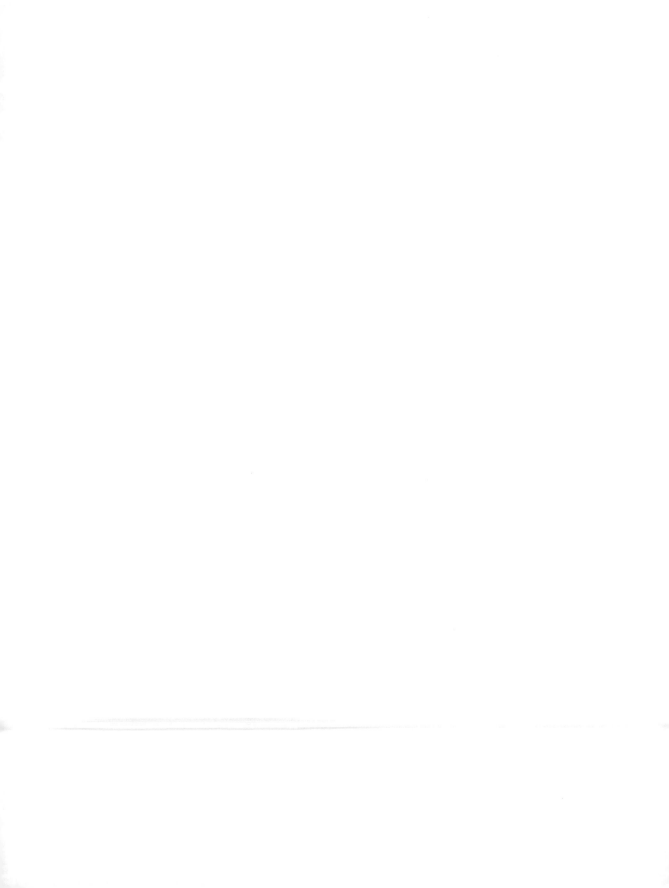

Common psychological interventions

17

**Anthony Venning, Madeleine Herd, Sharon Brown,
Fiona Glover, Lian Hill and Paula Redpath**

LEARNING OBJECTIVES

By the end of this chapter, you should be able to:

- have a broad understanding of common therapeutic approaches and strategies
- identify which therapies and strategies target different presentations
- understand that the use of transdiagnostic strategies to empower patients may reduce the reliance on paramedics.

INTRODUCTION

A paramedic is defined as a health professional who provides rapid response emergency medical assessment, treatment and care in an out-of-hospital setting. It has been reported that in Australia paramedics attend more than 1.3 million call-outs each year (Productivity Commission, 2018), of which 20% are for mental-health-related presentations (e.g. anxiety, depression and/or psychosis) with the most common being anxiety related (Beyond Blue, 2019). A paramedic's role in supporting people experiencing mental health issues requires complex abilities around negotiation, communication and advanced knowledge to make critical decisions (Paramedics Australasia [PA], 2016). In line with this, a recent study by Beyond Blue (2019) indicated that paramedics desired more training to support patients in ways other than transporting them to the emergency department (ED), but two out of three felt unprepared to use communication skills in place of transport to the ED (Beyond Blue, 2019). While the authors acknowledge that paramedics face substantial barriers to supporting people with mental health issues in alternative ways (e.g. organisational norms, legislative responsibilities, time constraints), this chapter seeks to provide paramedics with information to help engage, empower and build capacity in patients with mental health issues, and ultimately make better decisions around their care.

COMMON PSYCHOLOGICAL APPROACHES

While several different approaches and therapeutic techniques are discussed below, it is important to note that the authors do not suggest that paramedics need to be experts in or proficient with these approaches and strategies, as this is impractical given the barriers faced and constraints of a call-out. Rather, it is suggested that if a paramedic has an understanding of the types of therapies a patient with mental health issues may have been exposed to, and the common therapeutic strategies within these, this may then inform the way they engage with a patient to direct their approach, de-escalate situations, and ultimately empower patients through the interaction. While not an exhaustive list, outlined below are 12 **therapeutic approaches** (information only) followed by eight **transdiagnostic strategies** (practical tools that can be used to engage with patients).

COGNITIVE BEHAVIOURAL APPROACHES TO THERAPY

Cognitive behavioural approaches refer to a range of therapies that are the most widely employed, scrutinised and validated forms of psychotherapy (Hayes & Hofmann, 2017; Venning et al., 2016). First-generation approaches focus on the modification of behaviour, second-generation approaches *combine* changing behaviour with changing cognitions, and third-generation approaches focus on changing an individual's relation to thoughts and emotions rather than their content (Hayes & Hofmann, 2017; Venning et al., 2016).

First-generation behavioural approaches

Behaviour therapy is based on the theory that behaviour is learnt and, accordingly, can be changed (Australian Psychological Society [APS], 2018). When depressed, a person disengages with life and reduces the amount of meaningful and routine activities they engage with, which can then lead to a cycle of low mood, hopelessness and helplessness. **Behavioural activation (BA)** is an effective therapy to break a person's low mood cycle and provide a scaffold for them to make the specific and gradual changes needed to overcome depression (Venning et al., 2017b). The premise of BA is that by scheduling routine pleasurable and necessary activities, a person can 'act' themselves out of depression by progressively increasing activities that promote a sense of purpose and achievement, which in turn reduces the amount of negative and limiting thoughts they have. By supporting someone to do *more* of the things that they are doing less of (e.g. walking and socialising) and *less* of the things that they are doing more of (e.g. sedentary behaviour, isolating themselves, and consuming a poor diet), self-efficacy is restored and regular engagement with meaningful activity is activated.

If an individual experiences a high level of anxiety, they can feel so overwhelmed that avoiding or escaping certain situations is seen as the only way to manage the intense feelings. The temporary relief created by the avoidance then serves as a reinforcer for unhelpful behaviour and develops into a long-term pattern of avoidance. While this may work in the short term, in the long term it has a serious impact on a person's life by preventing them from undertaking tasks of daily living (Venning et al., 2017a; Wells, 2013). The aim of **exposure therapy (ET)** within a habituation model is to support an individual to learn that anxiety-provoking situations can be approached in a gradual way to help them overcome fear. Individuals would generally rank *graded* tasks from moderately anxiety provoking to highly anxiety provoking. Once the tasks have been agreed upon, individuals are encouraged to *focus* on the physical and cognitive processes that take place during the task, and support is then provided to ensure that the individual remains in the situation for a *prolonged* period until anxiety reduces. In order to consolidate new learning, individuals undertake the same task in a *repeated* manner until anxiety is no longer provoked.

Second-generation cognitive approaches

When people face challenges in life and experience psychological distress, significant changes can occur in the way they interpret themselves, the world and future events. For example, in the case of disorders such as anxiety and depression, it is common for individuals to become introspective and perceive challenges and difficulties as unmanageable, the past as regretful and the future as overwhelming (Beck, 2011). **Cognitive therapy (CT)** is based on Beck's theory that unpleasant emotions and maladaptive behaviours are the result of the maladaptive interpretation of events and the meaning derived from these interpretations (APS, 2018). Therefore, CT contains strategies that bring about behaviour change by supporting people to identify maladaptive thoughts, explore evidence for and against, and then generate alternative ways of thinking by engaging in behavioural experiments (BE) between therapy sessions. BEs are planned activities to test and establish the validity of an individual's current beliefs about themselves, others and the world, and generate new information to challenge unhelpful thinking patterns and develop more adaptive ways of experiencing life (Papworth et al., 2014).

Cognitive behaviour therapy (CBT) is a psychotherapy with a wide application that concentrates on how an individual's thoughts, behaviours and emotions are connected. CBT is a combination of behaviour therapy and CT, which focuses on the '*here and now*', and is based on the premise that cognitions influence feelings and behaviours, and that subsequent feeling and behaviours can then influence cognitions (APS, 2018). Typical elements of CBT include: (a) a brief, collaborative but therapist-led approach; (b) Socratic questioning (open-ended inquiry); (c) the definition and prioritisation of goals; (d) techniques to identify and modify cognitive distortions; (e) behavioural strategies to modify symptoms directly (e.g. exposure, behavioural activation, problem-solving and stress-management techniques); (f) relapse prevention; and (g) ongoing homework and evaluation (Venning et al., 2016; Wells, 2013).

Cognitive behaviour therapy for psychosis (CBTp) is a therapeutic approach adapted from CT to reduce the distress associated with symptoms of psychosis and to improve functioning. CBTp can be delivered in a brief or a full format (e.g. over six months), with a focus on three elements over and above traditional CBT (Brabban et al., 2016). These are: (1) the development of a shared formulation to inform the understanding and how psychotic symptoms are maintained; (2) the normalisation of the psychotic experience to address the stigma associated with the illness; and (3) the acceptance of psychotic symptoms rather than alter the occurrence of the symptoms (Brabban et al., 2016).

Interpersonal therapy (IPT) is a time-limited therapy that aims to relieve symptoms of distress and improve interpersonal functioning in individuals who are depressed and/or suffering problems with relationships or significant life changes. The underlying assumption of IPT is that an individual's mental health problems and interpersonal problems are interrelated (APS, 2018). Therefore, IPT focuses on helping individuals to understand the relationship between interpersonal circumstances and mental health problems. IPT aims to improve a person's social support network, communication, and interpersonal skills to better manage interpersonal distress (APS, 2018; Stuart & Robertson, 2003). IPT consists of five phases including: (1) assessment (a standard clinical interview); (2) initial sessions (socialising an individual to IPT); (3) middle sessions (where the major problem is addressed); (4) termination sessions (to review progress); and (5) maintenance sessions (to prevent relapse) (Robertson et al., 2008). IPT requires therapists to have adequate micro-counselling and psychotherapy skills, and to adopt specific techniques such as non-directive and directive exploration, clarification, encouragement of affect, communication analysis, role play, problem solving and a therapeutic relationship (Stuart & Robertson, 2003).

Third-generation approaches

Unlike second-generation CBT, which focuses on changing what a person thinks about, third-generation CBT focuses on changing the context in which a person's thoughts and emotions are *experienced* (O'Brien et al., 2008). To illustrate this, Baer and Huss (2008) provide an indication of how second- or third-generation therapy would approach an individual's sad mood. A second-generation approach would focus on changing an individual's emotional state, by identifying the thought that triggered the low mood and the distortion behind it, and then examining the evidence for and against the distortion, before developing and testing a more rational and balanced thought. In contrast, a third-generation approach would encourage the individual to observe the feeling of sadness and adopt an attitude of openness, curiosity and compassion to the thought in order to diminish its behavioural impact. Ultimately a third-generation approach aims to redirect the energy that otherwise would have been expended on identifying and changing the maladaptive thoughts towards the pursuit of valued goals (Venning et al., 2011).

Acceptance and commitment therapy (ACT) is a mindfulness-based behavioural therapy that seeks to help people to willingly experience all thoughts and feelings without attempting to avoid, escape or stop them, and which uses cognitive de-fusion (e.g. giving up control over thoughts and feelings) and value-directed behaviour. The therapy was created in 1986 by Steve Hayes as one of the first 'third-generation' therapies, and has a large body of empirical data to support its efficacy across a broad spectrum of presentations, such as chronic pain, anxiety and depression (A-Tjak et al., 2015; Harris, 2006; Tighe et al., 2018). The goal of ACT is not to reduce unwanted experiences – labelled as 'symptoms' – as the ongoing process of attempting to reduce these symptoms is often considered responsible for the development of clinical disorders in the first place. Furthermore, ACT avoids utilising the word 'symptom' due to its connotations of something 'pathological', and teaches individuals to perceive these experiences as harmless and to 'create a rich and meaningful life, while accepting the pain that inevitably goes with it' (Harris, 2006). ACT differs from other third-generation approaches in that it has been demonstrated to be effective with a wide range of clinical conditions (e.g. depression, OCD, workplace stress, the stress of terminal cancer, chronic pain, anxiety, PTSD, anorexia, heroin abuse, marijuana abuse and even schizophrenia), with various populations, and can be applied either briefly or long term. Two main processes are crucial in ACT interventions: (1) developing acceptance of unwanted experiences that are out of personal control; and (2) commitment and action towards a valued life (Hayes et al., 1999).

Mindfulness-based cognitive therapy (MBCT) is a theory-driven therapeutic approach developed to prevent the relapse and recurrence of major depression. MBCT emphasises mindfulness meditation as the primary therapeutic approach (APS, 2018), and in doing so encourages individuals to see emotions and cognitions as merely 'mental events' – as opposed to aspects of the self or accurate reflections of reality. In MBCT, individuals are encouraged to intentionally, and non-judgmentally, focus their attention on present experiences rather than focusing on the past or the future (Teasdale et al., 2000), and change their relationships to their thoughts rather than challenge them (APS, 2018). MBCT is an integration of aspects of CBT for depression (Beck et al., 1979) with components of the mindfulness-based stress-reduction program developed by Kabat-Zinn (1990).

Dialectical behaviour therapy (DBT) is a multimodal therapeutic approach originally developed for suicidal women, and subsequently refined for the treatment of borderline personality disorder (BPD); however, it has developed over time to include treatment for comorbid disorders across a range of clinical settings and ages (Salsman & Linehan, 2006). DBT is built on the principles of CBT, dialectical philosophy and mindfulness, and focuses on helping individuals find a balance between acceptance and change and finding a life worth living (Feigenbaum, 2008; Salsman & Linehan, 2006; Toms et al., 2019). The DBT model is based on an assumption of a pervasive skills deficit (e.g. an individual with BPD would be seen to lack interpersonal and self-regulation skills) and is applied with the aim of facilitating the learning of new skills, embedding them and applying them across various personal and environmental contexts in an individual's life.

Family and systemic therapy (FT) is a brief therapy that aims to explore and resolve conflict within the family unit. The emphasis of the therapy is not on any particular individual within the family, but rather on the family structure as a whole by examining the interacting dynamics of family members and situations. The goal of FT is to help family members develop problem-solving skills and achieve the family's goals, and ultimately modify any problematic or dysfunctional behaviours. FT adopts a CBT approach and emphasises the central role of cognitions (Friedberg, 2006).

PSYCHODYNAMIC APPROACHES TO THERAPY

Psychodynamic therapy is a transference-based therapeutic approach that can either be brief (six to eight sessions) or long term (unlimited sessions), and helps people work through internal conflict (APS, 2018). While psychodynamic approaches have been traditionally used to treat depression and other serious psychological disorders, they have also been effectively applied to treat problems such as addiction, social anxiety and eating disorders (Gaskin, 2012; Shedler, 2010). Specific techniques used in psychodynamic approaches can include: (a) exploring clients' attempts to avoid topics or engage in activities that obstruct therapeutic progress; (b) identifying patterns in actions, thoughts, feelings, experiences and relationships; (c) emphasising past experiences; and (d) exploring dreams, wishes or fantasies (Blagys & Hilsenroth, 2000). Within the psychodynamic approaches is **psychoanalytic therapy (PT)**. PT positions psychological problems as stemming from the unconscious mind, and aims to help people understand how these are related (McWilliams, 2004). Unlike CBT, the focus in PT is on *past* experiences and emotions, with the assumption that people hold painful and distressing feelings, memories and experiences in the unconscious by using defence mechanisms such as denial, repression and rationalisation.

Mentalisation-based treatment (MBT) is a therapeutic approach designed to treat people with borderline personality disorder (BPD) by helping people to separate their own thoughts and feeling from those around them (Bateman & Fonagy, 2010). Individuals with BPD are sensitive to interpersonal interactions, so MBT focuses on creating a well-managed attachment relationship between an individual and therapist to stabilise their emotional expression, allow them to consider internal representations, and reinstate lost mentalisation (Bateman & Fonagy, 2010; Daubney & Bateman, 2015). Mentalising is the insightful understanding of what another is feeling and why; mentalising is the process by which we make sense of others and ourselves in terms of subjective states and mental processes (Bateman & Fonagy, 2010). Typically lasting 12 to 18 months, MBT focuses on helping individuals to maintain mentalising within interpersonal contexts, to set goals to improve life functioning, and reduce self-destructive processes and behaviours that interfere with therapy (Daubney & Bateman, 2015).

COMMON TRANSDIAGONOSTIC THERAPEUTIC STRATEGIES

While a general understanding of the 12 psychotherapies presented above is important to provide context for a paramedic during a call-out, we expect that an understanding of those specific techniques that are core to each therapy may be more practically useful than understanding the general theory of the psychotherapies themselves. To that end, we provide eight transdiagnostic strategies below that are common to all of the above therapies that a paramedic could incorporate into their communication with individuals experiencing a mental health emergency. We expect that paramedics are most likely already utilising many of these strategies to de-escalate situations with patients, and thus we have ordered the strategies beginning with those we suggest are more pragmatic in an emergency situation, followed by those which a paramedic may wish to incorporate in their skill set for specific situations.

Micro-skills

Micro-skills are subtle verbal and non-verbal actions paramedics may use when interacting with patients to help develop rapport and elicit information. Common micro-skills include: (a) phrases to show active listening (e.g. 'mmm', 'okay', 'aha' or 'yes'); (b) paraphrasing content to help move an assessment forwards and provide greater clarity; (c) summarising to organise content; (d) reframing information to offer new meaning; and (e) reflecting feelings to empathise with the patient and help them explore their feelings further.

Normalising

Paramedics can use 'normalising' to help patients realise that their distressing thoughts and erratic behaviours may just be the body's normal response (e.g. 'fight/flight/freeze') to whatever challenge they are facing. By helping a patient to normalise their experience, a paramedic conveys a level of understanding about the way patients think, feel and behave in certain situations without judgment, and that their reactions have a rationale which, when relayed to people, offers some relief.

Grounding

Grounding is a technique that paramedics can use to de-escalate patients who are overwhelmed by what may be happening to them, by encouraging them to 'slow down', ground themselves and reorientate focus back to the present moment. This technique involves encouraging the patient to *disengage* with the *past* and *future* (which is where their thoughts may be taking them) and *re-engage* with the *present*. If a patient's thoughts are appearing as scattered, then encouraging them to focus their attention on tangible things, such as 'what they hear' / 'what they see' / 'what they smell', while engaging in and recognising their controlled breathing, may allow them to interrupt their unhelpful thoughts, feelings and behaviours to ultimately engage better.

Controlled breathing

When a person is anxious or stressed, they tend to breathe rapidly and erratically, think their thoughts and behaviours are abnormal, and feel overwhelmed, making it difficult to think clearly. An increased breathing rate is an important aspect of our stress response when we feel threatened – to get more oxygen in the blood and prepare us to either 'fight', 'flee' or 'freeze'. However, when we are not actually under threat, only a *perceived* threat, this type of breathing leads to people making reactive rather than mindful decisions (i.e. well 'thought-out'), as incoming information is directed away from the pre-frontal cortex (i.e. where we make rational and 'thought-out' decisions). Controlled breathing (CB) is a technique paramedics can use with patients who are exhibiting symptoms of anxiety or panic and are not thinking clearly – to assist them to effectively 'switch-off' the 'fight or flight' response, pay attention to their body until their symptoms reduce, and send incoming information back towards the pre-frontal context. CB, which pays deliberate attention to drawing air *in*to and expelling air *out* of the body, is an umbrella term that includes a number of systematic breathing techniques that can be easily used (e.g. counting breaths, inhaling and exhaling for a certain amount of time, or deep abdominal breathing). When breathing is deliberately regulated over time, the brain is primed to focus, think first and counteract the nervous system's 'fight', 'flight' or 'freeze' response.

Socratic questioning

Socratic questioning is a questioning technique that paramedics may employ to guide people's thoughts from the 'concrete' (or what they perceive as absolute) to the 'possible', in order for them to generate a stronger problem-solving ability (e.g. developing alternative responses to negative automatic thoughts) (Beck, 1995). Put another way, using a Socratic rather than didactic style, individuals are guided to develop new perspectives and foster critical thinking (Neenan, 2009). Typical types of questions include clarification questions ('what do you mean by … ?'), probing questions ('what would happen if … ?'), exploratory questions ('can you tell me more about … ?'), and questions about the question ('why is … important?').

Automatic negative thoughts (ANTs)

If individuals are not coping, it is common to experience thinking traps from time to time, and this is more likely when individuals are under stress. Individuals are also more vulnerable to thinking traps when they are not taking good care of themselves, such as not eating or sleeping, or if they are not successfully managing a medical or psychological condition. Thinking traps – defined as exaggerated or unhelpful thoughts people have about themselves, others, their future, or the world around them – can predispose people to interpret situations in a way that fits their perspective (i.e. thinking traps) as opposed to changing their perspective to fit the situation. Therefore, when individuals are trapped in this cycle of thinking, their ability to problem solve is limited (refer to Table 17.1 for a list of common thinking traps). With an understanding of these common thinking traps, a paramedic may be able to assist a patient who is 'stuck' by helping them become more aware of their distorted thinking, which in turn may help to highlight an alternative way of interpreting the situation. Questions that help to identify a patient's ANTs may

Table 17.1 Common Thinking Traps

We all tend to think in extremes, and when stressful events happen we think that way even more. Here are some common thinking traps.

1	**All-or-nothing thinking:** You see things in black-and-white categories. If your performance falls short of perfect, you see yourself as a total failure.
2	**Over-generalisation:** You see a single negative event as a never-ending pattern of defeat.
3	**Mental filter:** You pick out a single negative detail and dwell on it exclusively so that your vision of all reality becomes darkened, like the drop of ink that discolours the entire cup of water.
4	**Disqualifying the positive:** You reject positive experiences by insisting they 'don't count' for some reason.
5	**Jumping to conclusions:** You make a negative interpretation even though there are no definite facts that convincingly support your conclusion.
6	**Mind reading:** You arbitrarily conclude that someone is reacting negatively to you and don't bother to confirm it.
7	**The Fortune Teller error:** You anticipate that things will turn out badly and feel convinced that your prediction is an already-established fact.
8	**Magnification (catastrophising) or minimisation:** You exaggerate the importance of things (such as your mistakes or someone else's achievement), or you inappropriately shrink things until they appear tiny (your own desirable qualities or the other person's imperfections).
9	**Emotional reasoning:** You assume that your negative emotions reflect the way things really are: 'I feel it, therefore it must be true.'
10	**Personalisation:** You see yourself as the cause of some negative external event, even though you were not primarily responsible.

help to shift their thinking and provide a way of communicating that is purposeful and educative.

Motivational interviewing

Motivational interviewing (MI) is a directive, client-centred communication approach that enhances an individual's reasons to change by exploring and helping them to resolve ambivalence (Miller & Rollnick, 2013). Originally, MI was used in addiction settings with individuals who were not maintaining recommended routines. More recently, MI is used broadly in a variety of clinical and corporate settings to support people in how to manage life-changing conditions that impact on their health (e.g. asthma, heart problems or diabetes). The main principles behind MI are: (a) express empathy through reflective listening; (b) develop a discrepancy between an individual's goals or values and current behaviour; (c) work *with* rather than oppose resistance (i.e. rolling with resistance); and (d) support self-efficacy and optimism (Miller & Rollnick, 2013). Put another way, MI helps people to find and keep their motivation so they can change the behaviour that is preventing the healing process. This technique could be utilised by paramedics to de-escalate situations, re-focus patients back to managing difficult/life-changing conditions, and foster collaborative shared decision making about the next step in a patient's care.

Problem solving

People are often overwhelmed with the many problems they face (real or perceived). However, sometimes the presenting worry may be unrealistic and/or an unlikely prediction of the future, which one has little control over. Therefore, although it appears 'real' to the individual, the problem is not necessarily one that requires a solution. Alternatively, some problems can be real with potential solutions, for which a problem-solving strategy may be useful. If it is a 'real' problem, problem solving (PS) is a constructive thought process focused on how one can effectively deal with problems. The three steps to PS are: (1) identifying what the problem is; (2) thinking of possible ways to deal with the problem; and then (3) examining the pros and cons for each of these. Some questions paramedics may use include: (a) 'Is it a real and likely problem?'; (b) 'Is the problem something that is happening now?'; and (c) 'Is the problem something they have some control over?' For example, the price of fresh food is something an individual has no control over (unsolvable), but the type and quantity of foods purchased to attain a healthy/balanced diet is very much in their control (solvable). Once a current and actual problem is identified, or an element of that problem, a paramedic may be able to help a patient engage in one or more of the six steps of problem solving: (1) *state the problem* as clearly as possible (be objective about the behaviour, situation, timing and circumstances that make it a problem); (2) *generate possible solutions* (be creative and list all the possible solutions, regardless of their quality – then eliminate the unreasonable or impractical solutions, and list the remaining ones in order of preference); (3) *evaluate alternatives* (evaluate the top few in terms of their advantages and disadvantages); (4) *decide on a plan* (i.e. *who* will take action, *when*, and *how*); (5) *implement the plan*; and (6) *evaluate the outcome*.

UNDERSTANDING HOW THE APPROACHES FIT TOGETHER

As already stated, it is not suggested that paramedics develop expertise in the therapeutic approaches listed or be proficient with common strategies employed, as this is impractical given the time and constraints of a call-out. However, with the aim of facilitating a shared decision-making process between patients and paramedics, the 'Strategy Compass' (SC) (Fig. 17.1) provides a quick reference as to what therapeutic approaches target, and what common strategies are used. The SC may help paramedics to understand which type of therapy and/or strategies patients have been engaged in and to determine what approach to take to engage the patient. The central component of the SC lists some common patient presentations that a paramedic may encounter at a call-out (e.g. depression, mania, anxiety, interpersonal conflict, etc.). The next outside layer provides a paramedic with a quick reference

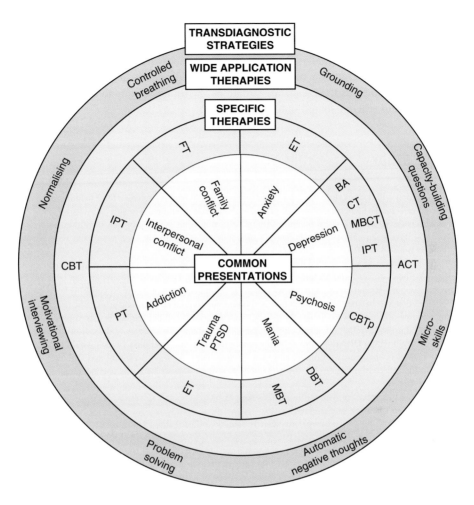

CBT = Cognitive behaviour therapy
FT = Family and systemic therapy
BA = Behavioural activation
ET = Exposure therapy
DBT = Dialectical behaviour therapy
CT = Cognitive therapy

ACT = Acceptance and commitment therapy
IPT = Interpersonal therapy
PT = Psychoanalytic therapy
MBT = Mentalisation-based treatment
CBTp = Cognitive behaviour therapy for psychosis
MBCT = Mindfulness-based cognitive therapy

FIGURE 17.1

Strategy Compass demonstrating specific, wide and transdiagnostic strategies that can be used when working with patients presenting with mental health issues.

as to what types of therapies are commonly applied to treat these issues, whereas the next layer outlines those therapies that have a wider application to most issues (e.g. CBT and ACT). Finally, the outermost layer indicates those transdiagnostic strategies that are common to most therapeutic approaches and which could be utilised by paramedics to de-escalate situations, facilitate communication and build rapport to help reach a shared outcome.

CASE STUDY
Anita

This section will now explore the use of the common mental health strategies for a mental-health-related call-out. Evidence suggests that one of the most common mental health call-outs for paramedics is anxiety related (Beyond Blue, 2019). Following is an example of one such interaction.

You have been called to the home of Anita (female, 32 years of age), who lives with her partner Bob.

Bob answers the door, stating there is something wrong with his partner Anita. Anita is looking scared. She is dressed in tracksuit pants and a T-shirt, and her hair is in a ponytail. She is teary, restless, confused and talking quickly as you enter the house. As you begin to speak to her, you observe that she has her arms folded and is rubbing her shoulders, head and neck. She proceeds to sit down and hold her knees tightly (i.e. in a ball position), and her partner insists you help. It should be noted here that all approaches adopted by paramedics to patients in the out-of-hospital setting begin with a DRABC check (Danger [operational safety], Response [which would include how patient is engaging with others and their environment], Airway, Breathing and Circulation) to consider all possible causes for the presentation. While not described, this is conducted by the paramedics.

Paramedic: Anita, can you tell me what's happening?

Bob: Can't you see, she's scared!

Anita: I can't breathe properly, my heart is beating so fast. I don't know what's happening to me.

Paramedic: OK, that must be really scary and we are here to help. Can you tell us if there is anything else happening at the moment? (**Socratic questioning and active listening**)

Anita: My fingers are tingling. I feel dizzy. You've got to do something. I just don't feel right.

Paramedic: We are going to check you out. What are you most worried about right now? (**Socratic questioning**)

Anita: I can't breathe properly: when I try to take a deep breath my chest hurts and makes me feel dizzier. I can't control this! It's getting worse!

Paramedic: So you feel dizzy and can't breathe? (**paraphrasing**)

Anita: Yes!

Paramedic: And you said you can't control it?

Anita: I don't know what's wrong! I feel like I'm going to die.

Bob: You need to help her!

Paramedic: That must be really scary, Anita. (**reflection of feeling**) Let's see if we can work out what is happening for you right now.

Anita: It's horrible, I just want it to stop.

Paramedic: These feelings and thoughts can be scary. When did they start?

Anita: It came on a few hours ago and it's getting worse! I'm freaking out! That's why I called 000.

Bob: We didn't know what to do … can you do something other than ask questions!

Paramedic: Well I'm glad you did call and that we are here to help. Bob, I know you're scared. You want the best for Anita, right? (**beginning of motivational interviewing**)

Bob: Yes, she's the most important person in my life!

Paramedic: OK. So that's why it's important for you to let me do a few tests to see what might be going on for Anita. It can seem like we aren't doing anything, but we are.

Bob: OK.

Paramedic checks Anita's vital signs. In Anita's case paramedics would consider all potential causes for her panicked state, such as cardiac and respiratory illness. If safe to do so, you would include a 12-lead electrocardiogram, vital sign observations, and history taking for any past experiences that may indicate a cardiac or respiratory cause, as well as the possibility of an anxiety disorder. In Anita's case, all look unremarkable.

Paramedic: All right, Anita, we've checked your vital signs and everything looks OK with your heart.

Anita: But something's going on to make me feel like this! I've called heaps of people and they all told me to call an ambulance.

Paramedic: OK. What is happening to you is very real and you are worried. Let's just give something a go before we do anything else. So, stay where you are and focus on the sound of my voice. Concentrate on what you can hear right now. You don't need to respond. Bring your attention to what you can see in the room and pick an object to focus on. Describe the shape … the colour … . Now move to another object and describe the shape and colour – *pause* – Now bring your focus to your breath. Begin to breathe in more deeply and slowly through your nose *(repeat a few times)*. Now breathe in and hold for 2, 3 – *pause* – out and hold for 2, 3 – each time lengthening the breath by one count - *pause*. OK. (**grounding / controlled breathing**)

Paramedic: So tell me what is happening for you now?

Anita: Things seem to be settling down a bit, but I still don't know what is going on.

Paramedic: Well, we have had an initial look at the way your heart and lungs are functioning and the results are good; there might be alternative explanations for what is going on. While we were doing those tests earlier Bob was saying to my partner that you have been pretty stressed lately, and that you've told Bob that things feel 'out of control', is that right? … [Anita nods] … Stress can lead to things happening in your body that can feel different, and as a result you might think that something is not right. These physical sensations and distressing thoughts are very consistent with panic, and these are actually very common when we are feeling stressed, as our body reacts and goes into fight/flight/freeze which is a normal response when we think we are in danger. When I came in you were rubbing your neck and shoulders: sometimes this is something people do to relieve the tension when they feel stressed. (**normalising**)

Anita: So you're saying I'm not going to have a heart attack?

Paramedic: At this point your heart looks OK and anxiety attacks can feel terrible.

(*What follows is a discussion on anxiety* – refer to Chapter 9 for a full discussion.)

Paramedic: Now you know a bit more about anxiety, let's talk about what you can do to manage this if it comes up again. (**beginning to problem solve**)

Anita: I'll just call an ambulance again. I have no other options?

Paramedic: Of course, calling us again is an option; another might be that you try to sit down, focus on your body and wait until the symptoms reduce.

Anita: You mean to realise that this might just be anxiety and not that something bad might happen? That I am not having a heart attack?

Paramedic: Absolutely, so what do we now know about anxiety, it comes in … ?

Anita: Waves. If I can keep myself grounded and regulate my breathing, my feeling of anxiousness will eventually pass.

Paramedic: Yes. Remember when I first arrived you said you can't control what was happening?

Anita: Yes.

Paramedic: While you can't stop yourself from feeling anxious, you can try some techniques. And if you feel it has taken a hold then sitting down and letting your body calm down all on its own will work. You just told me some ways that help – keeping yourself grounded and regulating your breathing and reminding yourself that this is not likely to be a heart attack but anxiety. (**challenging ANTs**). There are some other things you can do too. You could talk to your GP about how you have been feeling stressed and out of control. They might be able to offer you some support and refer you to someone who can give you more strategies to help manage the anxiety. What we do know is that anxiety can be treated, particularly if it's picked up early.

CONCLUSION

With paramedics asking to be better equipped to distinguish between mental health presentations and types of therapeutic techniques used (Roberts & Henderson, 2009), the current chapter set out to answer this call by providing information to scaffold a paramedic's interactions with a client via an understanding of common therapeutic approaches and strategies. Aided by the 'Strategy Compass' and eight transdiagnostic strategies, we envisage that paramedics may feel better equipped when faced with a mental health crisis on a call-out by recognising and positioning the key terminology and core processes common to a psychotherapy a client may be undertaking. This understanding and familiarity may then provide an additional opportunity for communication to develop, rapport to be established, and a shared and beneficial outcome reached between paramedic and patient.

REFERENCES

A-Tjak, J.G., Davis, M.L., Morina, N., et al., 2015. A meta-analysis of the efficacy of acceptance and commitment therapy for clinically relevant mental and physical health problems. Psychother. Psychosom. 84 (1), 30–36.

Australian Psychological Society (APS), 2018. Evidence-based psychological interventions in the treatment of mental disorders: a review of the literature, fourth ed. Online. Available: https://www.psychology.org.au/getmedia/23c6a11b-2600-4e19-9a1d-6ff9c2f26fae/Evidence-based-psych-interventions.pdf. (12 October 2018).

Baer, R., Huss, D., 2008. Mindfulness-and acceptance-based therapy. In: Lebow, J.L. (Ed.), Twenty-first Century Psychotherapies. Wiley, Hoboken, pp. 123–166.

Bateman, A., Fonagy, P., 2010. Mentalization based treatment for borderline personality disorder. World Psychiatry 9 (1), 11–15.

Beck, A.T., Rush, A., Shaw, B., et al., 1979. Cognitive Therapy of Depression. The Guilford Press, New York.

Beck, J., 1995. Cognitive Therapy: Basics and beyond. The Guilford Press, New York.

Beck, J., 2011. Cognitive Therapy: Basics and beyond, second ed. The Guildford Press, New York.

Beyond Blue 2019 Beyond the Emergency: Turning point. Online. Available: https://www.beyondblue.org.au/docs/default-source/default-document-library/beyond-the-emergency-report.pdf. (24 July 2019).

Blagys, M.D., Hilsenroth, M.J., 2000. Distinctive features of short-term psychodynamic-interpersonal psychotherapy: a review of the comparative psychotherapy process literature. Clin. Psychol. Sci. Pract. 7 (2), 167–188.

Brabban, A., Byrne, R., Longden, E., et al., 2016. The importance of human relationships, ethics and recovery-orientated values in the delivery of CBT for people with psychosis. Psychosis 9 (2), 1–10.

Daubney, M., Bateman, A., 2015. Mentalization-based therapy (MBT): an overview. Australas. Psychiatry 23 (2), 132–135.

Feigenbaum, J., 2008. Dialectical behaviour therapy. Psychiatry 7 (3), 112–116.

Friedberg, R., 2006. A cognitive-behavioural approach to family therapy. J. Contemp. Psychother. 36, 159–165.

Gaskin, C., 2012. The Effectiveness of Psychodynamic Psychotherapy: A systematic review of recent international and Australian research. Psychotherapy and Counselling Federation of Australia, Melbourne.

Harris, R., 2006. Embracing your demons: an overview of acceptance and commitment therapy. Psychother. Aust. 12 (4), 2–8.

Hayes, S., Hofmann, S., 2017. The third wave of cognitive behavioural therapy and the rise of process-based care. World Psychiatry 16 (3), 245–246.

Hayes, S.C., Strosahl, K.D., Wilson, K.G., 1999. Acceptance and Commitment Therapy: An experiential approach to behaviour change. The Guilford Press, New York.

Kabat-Zinn, J., 1990. Full Catastrophe Living: Using the wisdom of your body and mind to face stress, pain, and illness. Dell Publishing, New York.

McWilliams, N., 2004. Psychoanalytic Psychotherapy: A practitioner's guide. The Guilford Press, New York.

Miller, W., Rollnick, S., 2013. Motivational Interviewing: Helping people change, third ed. The Guilford Press, New York.

Neenan, M., 2009. Using Socratic questioning in coaching. J. Rational-Emotive Cognit. Behav. Ther. 27 (4), 249–264.

O'Brien, K.O., Larson, C.M., Murrell, A.R., 2008. Third-wave behaviour therapies for children and adolescents: progress, challenges and future directions. In: Greco, L.A., Hayes, S.C. (Eds.), Acceptance and Mindfulness Treatments for Children and Adolescents: A practitioner's guide. New Harbinger Publishers, Oakland, pp. 15–35.

Papworth, M., Marrian, T., Martin, B., et al., 2014. Low Intensity Cognitive Behaviour Therapy: A practitioner's guide. Sage, London.

Paramedics Australasia (PA) 2016 Paramedic role descriptors: paramedic, report, pp. 1–22. Online. Available: https://paramedics.org/wp-content/uploads/2016/09/PRD_211212_WEBONLY.pdf. (5 May 2018).

Productivity Commission (PC) 2018 Ambulance services – report on government services 2018, PC, Canberra. Online. Available: https://www.pc.gov.au/research/ongoing/report-on-government-services/2018/health/ambulance-services. (24 July 2019).

Roberts, L., Henderson, J., 2009. Paramedic perceptions of their role, education, training and working relationships when attending cases of mental illness. J. Emerg. Prim. Health Care 7 (3), 1–16.

Robertson, M., Rushton, P., Wurm, C., 2008. Interpersonal psychotherapy: an overview. Psychother. Aust. 14 (3), 46–54.

Salsman, N., Linehan, M., 2006. Dialectical-behavioural therapy for borderline personality disorder. Prim. Psychiatry 13 (5), 51–58.

Shedler, J., 2010. The efficacy of psychodynamic psychotherapy. Am. Psychol. 65 (2), 98–109.

Stuart, S.A., Robertson, M., 2003. Interpersonal Psychotherapy: A clinician's guide. Taylor & Francis Group, London.

Teasdale, J.D., Segal, Z.V., Williams, J.M.G., et al., 2000. Prevention of relapse/recurrence in major depression by mindfulness-based cognitive therapy. J. Consult. Clin. Psychol. 68 (4), 615–623.

Tighe, J., Nicholas, J., Shand, F., et al., 2018. Efficacy of acceptance and commitment therapy in reducing suicidal ideation and deliberate self-harm: systematic review. JMIR Ment. Health 5 (2), 1–11.

Toms, G., Williams, L., Rycroft-Malone, J., et al., 2019. The development and theoretical application of an implementation framework for dialectical behaviour therapy: a critical literature review. Borderline Personal. Disord. Emot. Dysregul. 6 (2), 1–16.

Venning, A., Eliott, J., Kettler, L., et al., 2011. Cognitive behavioural therapy. In: Levesque, R.J. (Ed.), Encyclopaedia of Adolescence. Springer, New York, pp. 439–447.

Venning, A., Kettler, L., Redpath, P., et al., 2016. Cognitive behavioural therapy. In: Levesque, R.J. (Ed.), Encyclopaedia of Adolescence, second ed. Springer, New York, pp. 439–447.

Venning, A., Redpath, P., Orlowski, S., 2017a. One Step at a Time: Graded exposure. Flinders Human Behaviour and Health Research Unit. Flinders University, Adelaide.

Venning, A., Redpath, P., Orlowski, S., 2017b. Move Yourself Out of Depression: Behavioural activation. Flinders Human Behaviour and Health Research Unit. Flinders University, Adelaide.

Wells, A., 2013. Cognitive Therapy of Anxiety Disorders: A practice manual and conceptual guide. John Wiley & Sons, Chichester.

Psychopharmacology

18

Richard Summers

LEARNING OBJECTIVES

By the end of this chapter you should be able to:

- understand the range of pharmacotherapies and their application to mental health issues
- understand the pharmacology of the pharmacotherapies and apply this to clinical practice
- determine the potential complications of pharmacotherapies used in mental health and how to manage or avoid such issues
- determine the implications of psychopharmacotherapies to practice in the pre-clinical setting.

INTRODUCTION

In this chapter we discuss the major categories of the drugs used in mental health. We will discuss the specific mental health conditions, and outline the classes of drugs used and their therapeutic applications. For each condition we will overview the various neurochemical hypotheses and drug categories, how they work and how they apply to the actions of the therapies used. This background information will assist in understanding their application to clinical practice and their implications with respect to patient presentations. In addition, we will explore the potential adverse effects along with some of the important toxicities that may present in the clinical setting.

Drugs used in mental health have significant potential to interact with other medications, foodstuffs and substances of abuse or misuse, and therefore it is important to put these into context to appropriately manage patients and their responses to medical intervention. A comprehensive patient history and having knowledge about the medications used will assist you in interpreting the clinical significance of the patient presentation.

ANXIETY DISORDERS – BENZODIAZEPINES AND ANXIOLYTICS

Anxiety is characterised by excessive worry and brings about defensive behaviour associated with fear. This anticipatory reaction can become maladaptive and impair an individual's ability to function, impacting significantly on their quality of life.

There is evidence suggesting an overlap exists between depression and generalised anxiety disorder (GAD) (Olfson et al., 2017). Similarity of symptoms, risk factors, patterns of psychiatric comorbidity and the fact that they can often co-exist, strengthens this association. They can also co-exist with other conditions such as pain syndromes, hyperactivity disorders and bipolar disorders.

The amygdala, pre-frontal cortex and the hypothalamic-pituitary-adrenal (HPA) axis are associated with anxiety, and are responsible for the emotional and motor responses (Pagliaccio et al., 2015).

While elevated cortisol levels in the short term assist in the evasion of an imminent threat, on a chronic basis this can have detrimental consequences contributing to chronic disease states such as cardiovascular disease, type 2 diabetes and stroke (Rosmond & Björntorp, 2000). Additional autonomic and cardiovascular responses associated with fear, such as change in heart rate and elevated blood pressure, can be responsible for comorbidity issues, such as hypertension, atherosclerosis, myocardial infarction, and sudden death.

Anxiety triggered by memories of past traumatic events involves and is modulated by a number of neurotransmitters – serotonin, gamma-aminobutyric acid (GABA), dopamine, noradrenaline (norepinephrine), glutamate, and the voltage gated ion channels (Stahl, 2013). It has also been shown that a correction of the cortisol levels in post-traumatic stress disorder (PTSD) improved anxiety symptoms (De Kloet et al., 2005).

As symptoms of anxiety and depressive disorders overlap (Olfson et al., 2017), antidepressants can also show efficacy with anxiety symptoms by increasing the levels of serotonin, a major neurotransmitter associated with fear and worry. A Cochrane review found no difference in the efficacy between antidepressants and benzodiazepine use in panic disorders (Bighelli, 2018).

BENZODIAZEPINES

Benzodiazepines (BDZ) (see Table 18.1) are a class of drugs that act selectively on gamma-aminobutyric acid A (GABA$_A$) receptors to potentiate the actions of GABA, the principal inhibitory neurotransmitter found in the brain. They bind to subunits of the GABA receptor, enhancing its affinity for the neurotransmitter. When GABA binds to the receptor it opens the chloride ion channel and increases the influx of chloride ions into the neuron, which hyperpolarises the cell membrane and decreases the excitability of the cell (Sigel & Ernst, 2018).

All benzodiazepines potentiate the inhibitory effects of GABA in various regions of the brain (spinal cord, hippocampus, cerebellar and cerebral cortices), and vary in terms of their individual clinical application and in their duration of action. Benzodiazepines should only be used short term or intermittently due to their abuse potential (euphoria and sedation), tolerance and dependence. They should be avoided in patients with respiratory depression, hepatic impairment, sleep apnoea or myasthenia gravis (Rossi, 2019).

Table 18.1 Benzodiazepines

BZD	Indication	Duration	Onset
Alprazolam	Anxiety, panic disorder	Short (half-life 6 to 12 hours)	Rapid (<1 hour after oral administration)
Clonazepam	Epilepsy (refractory to other therapy, absence, myoclonus, infantile spasms), status epilepticus	Long (half-life >24 hours)	Rapid (<1 hour after oral administration) Peak 2 to 3 hours
Diazepam	Anxiety, agitation, acute alcohol withdrawal, muscle spasm, surgical premedication, conscious sedation, status epilepticus	Long (half-life >24 hours)	Rapid (<1 hour after oral administration)
Flunitrazepam	Insomnia	Long (half-life >24 hours)	Rapid (<1 hour after oral administration)
Lorazepam	Anxiety, insomnia (short term associated with anxiety), surgical premedication, anticipatory nausea and vomiting associated with cytotoxic chemotherapy	Moderate (half-life 12 to 24 hours)	Readily absorbed after oral administration Peak 2 hours
Midazolam	Conscious sedation, induction of anaesthesia, sedation during ventilation, premedication, status epilepticus	Very short (half-life <6 hours)	Rapid (<10 minutes after buccal/intranasal administration)
Nitrazepam	Insomnia, infantile spasms	Long (half-life >24 hours)	Readily absorbed after oral administration Peak 0.5 to 2 hours
Oxazepam	Anxiety	Short (half-life 6 to 12 hours)	Readily absorbed after oral administration Peak 2 to 3 hours
Temazepam	Short-term treatment of insomnia	Short (half-life 6 to 12 hours)	Rapid (<1 hour after oral administration)

Adapted and modified from Rossi, 2019

Therapeutic indications include the following:

- insomnia
- generalised anxiety disorders
- Epilepsy
- anticipatory nausea and vomiting associated with cancer chemotherapy
- agitation
- acute alcohol withdrawal
- conscious sedation.

Benzodiazepines that have rapid onset are highly lipid-soluble, facilitating their ability to cross the blood–brain barrier to elicit a response. Patients with renal impairment have an increased sensitivity to the effects of benzodiazepines, and elderly patients are particularly sensitive to over-sedation contributing to an increased falls risk (Brett & Murnion, 2015), memory impairment and ataxia. This is particularly concerning, as benzodiazepine use is more prevalent as age increases, yet estimates suggest only a third of benzodiazepine use in the elderly is appropriate (Airagnes et al., 2016).

In the management of anxiety disorders, benzodiazepines are only used for a short term in an acute phase, for 2 to 4 weeks (Reinhold & Rickels, 2015). They have a rapid onset of effect; however, the risk for dependence is high, and adverse effects, rebound anxiety and withdrawal symptoms are problematic (Brett & Murnion, 2015).

Adverse effects

- Drowsiness
- Confusion
- Aggression (paradoxical reaction)
- Memory impairment
- Loss of muscle coordination
- Muscle weakness
- Dependence and tolerance.

Dependence and tolerance

With all benzodiazepines, tolerance can develop and is seen as a need for dose escalation to produce the desired response. While the mechanism is not yet fully understood, there may be multiple processes that alter the GABA receptors which can lead to development of tolerance (Gravielle, 2016).

It is also known that sudden withdrawal of benzodiazepines with a short half-life (e.g. temazepam and alprazolam) will have more pronounced, earlier onset and increased severity of withdrawal symptoms (Milhorn, 2018). Other factors include high dose, extended duration, abrupt cessation, drug abuse history or underlying panic disorder. In addition, rebound anxiety is more commonly associated with the sudden cessation of benzodiazepines with short half-lives (Riss et al., 2008).

Dependence is a significant issue with benzodiazepine use, and suddenly stopping after weeks or months of therapy can result in elevated rebound symptoms of anxiety, along with dizziness, headache, insomnia, irritability, restlessness, sweating, tremor, seizures, palpitations, hypertension and delusions. Rebound insomnia on withdrawal may perpetuate usage, so withdrawal should be gradual – changing to long-acting agents and then reducing doses slowly, which may take up to 10 weeks (Brett & Murnion, 2015).

Dependence can involve both physical and psychological withdrawal symptoms, and is based on dosage, duration and potency of therapy (Milhorn, 2018). Long-term use can also lead to psychological over-reliance, with a reluctance to cease through irrational fear or anticipatory anxiety and the therapeutic dependence category (Milhorn, 2018).

Toxicity

Benzodiazepines are involved in up to one-third of intentional self-poisonings (Murray et al., 2015). With supportive care for central nervous system (CNS) depression, the prognosis is favourable (Buckley et al., 1995). Benzodiazepines and hypnotics are involved in 14% of self-poisoning presentations to emergency departments in England (Geulayov et al., 2018) and diazepam was associated with 45.5% of the calls to Australian poisons information centres relating to sedative poisoning exposures (Huynh et al., 2018).

Following a benzodiazepine overdose, the onset of symptoms are generally seen within 1 to 2 hours. The initial presentation is ataxia, lethargy, slurring of speech, sedation and reduced reaction times. Significant coma is rarely seen, but airway obstruction can be complicated by apnoea (Murray et al., 2015).

In general, benzodiazepine overdose on its own usually manifests as mild to moderate sedation requiring supportive care; however, with significant overdoses bradycardia, hypotension and hypothermia can occur, and the altered mental status significantly increases pulmonary aspiration risk (Milhorn, 2018). It is also important to screen for ingestion of other substances and undertake an electrocardiogram (ECG) and check blood glucose level (Murray et al., 2015). Other substances can enhance CNS depression, and concurrent benzodiazepine use with opioids or alcohol has been associated with an increased risk of death from drug overdose (Park et al., 2015). Overdoses involving benzodiazepines as a single-drug class death involved alcohol in 72.1% of cases from Drug Abuse Warning Network data in the United States (Jones et al., 2014).

Resuscitation, monitoring and supportive care are priorities. Management may include flumazenil, a competitive benzodiazepine antagonist. Flumazenil is used in anaesthetics for the reversal of benzodiazepine effects, but can be used as a diagnostic aid in suspected toxicity and as a therapeutic option to reverse the effects (Penninga et al., 2016). While severe consequences with overdoses of benzodiazepines on their own are rare, the risk of convulsions and death increases in cases where there are multiple substances involved (Milhorn, 2018). These may contribute to seizures in their own right or the reversal of seizure control with administration of flumazenil (Rossi, 2019).

ANXIETY DISORDERS – ALTERNATIVE THERAPIES

Selective serotonin reuptake inhibitors (SSRIs) and serotonin noradrenaline (norepinephrine) reuptake inhibitors (SNRIs) have demonstrated in many randomised controlled trials significant beneficial responses (Reinhold & Rickels, 2015), and are regarded as the most effective first-line pharmacotherapies in GAD (Fowler, 2019) – see Table 18.2. Usage needs to be balanced against the potential for class adverse effects, such as weight gain, sedation, agitation and sexual dysfunction.

SNRIs, venlafaxine and duloxetine, have shown efficacy in a number of studies (Reinhold & Rickels, 2015). The choice of venlafaxine for long-term treatment

Table 18.2 Pharmacotherapy for General Anxiety Disorder

Pharmacotherapy for GAD	First-line	Second-line	Alternative
Selective serotonin reuptake inhibitors (SSRIs)	X		
Serotonin noradrenaline (norepinephrine) reuptake inhibitors (SNRIs)	X		
Benzodiazepine			Only short term
Tricyclic antidepressant (TCA)		X	
Buspirone			X
Gabapentin			X

Adapted from Fowler, 2019

in anxiety may be considered even in the absence of depression; however, cautious consideration to its potential for toxicity in overdose is warranted (Fowler, 2019).

Tricyclic antidepressants have demonstrated efficacy in anxiety syndromes, but are considered second-line agents because they are associated with many side effects and, as they have substantial lethality in overdose, caution is particularly warranted with use in patients with comorbidities of depression or those with suicidal ideation (Fowler, 2019).

ANTIDEPRESSANTS

The aims of treatment focus on alleviating depressive symptoms, reducing the risk of recurrence or relapse, and improving the quality of life. Strategies in the management of depression include psychotherapy, pharmacotherapy and electroconvulsive therapy (Fowler, 2019).

NEUROCHEMICAL BASIS FOR DEPRESSION

While the exact cause of depression is unknown, an accepted hypothesis relates to an abnormality in the central nervous system (CNS) monoaminergic neurotransmission. Many antidepressant drugs exert their effects by increasing catecholamines at their receptor sites, and depression is associated with reduced levels of catecholamines, particularly noradrenaline (norepinephrine), but also other amines at the adrenergic receptor sites in the brain. This is known as the catecholamine or the monoamine hypothesis (Schildkraut, 1965).

This hypothesis needs to be interpreted with reference to how the levels of catecholamines are modulated within the CNS. Noradrenaline (norepinephrine) can regulate serotonin (5 hydroxytryptamine or 5HT) neurons enhancing (by α_1 receptors) or dampening (by α_2 autoreceptors) 5HT release. Within the brain there are overlapping areas influencing noradrenaline (norepinephrine), dopamine and serotonin neurotransmitter systems, which can influence not only their own release and function but also the release of other monoamines (Stahl, 2013).

While dysfunction of these monoamines in varying brain circuits imparts some explanation for depression, there are several other influencing factors. Stressful life events may affect brain circuits and increase a depressive episode risk (Risch et al., 2009) and chronic stress has been linked to treatment resistance (Liu et al., 2017). Gene variants to serotonin transporter (SERT) systems may influence vulnerability and neuroplasticity – the adaptability of the neuronal system to external stimuli and how it will respond in the future through structurally reorganising connections and function (Kennedy et al., 2016; Liu et al., 2017).

Brain structural changes affecting emotional regulation may be associated with severity of depression (Zhang et al., 2016). Emotional changes of decreased positive affect (decreased pleasure, loss of joy) are possibly associated with dopamine dysfunction, and increased negative affect (guilt, fear, irritability, aggression, loneliness) associated with serotonin, whereas noradrenaline (norepinephrine) dysfunction may have an involvement in both. The use of drug therapy that enhances the function of serotonin and noradrenaline (norepinephrine) may improve depressed mood and symptoms linked to the negative affect, whereas dopamine and noradrenaline (norepinephrine) enhancement impacts on those symptoms associated with positive affect (Stahl, 2013).

Another mechanism proposed for antidepressants is decreasing presynaptic glutamate release, as increased glutamate levels have been consistently shown in depressed patients (Küçükibrahimoğlu et al., 2009; Sanacora, Treccani & Popoli, 2012). Ketamine, an inhibitor at N-methyl-D-aspartate (NMDA) glutamate receptors, produces an immediate antidepressant effect in unipolar or bipolar depression. It is also known that glutamate synapses can undergo structural or functional change in response to external or environmental stimuli such as emotional processing, memory and learning. The dampening effect of antidepressants on glutamate release induced by stress may also explain their anxiolytic action (Sanacora et al., 2012).

There are many different classes of antidepressants that principally act to enhance monoamine levels in the brain. One way they do this is to block the transport systems for one or more of the monoamines – serotonin, dopamine or noradrenaline (norepinephrine). This is considered a classic mechanism of action for antidepressants. First-line agents include SSRIs, SNRIs, bupropion, mirtazapine and vortioxetine, whereas agomelatine, moclobemide, selegiline and tricyclic antidepressants (TCAs) are considered second-line, and monoamine oxidase inhibitors and reboxetine third-line (Fowler, 2019; Kennedy et al., 2016).

SELECTIVE SEROTONIN REUPTAKE INHIBITORS (SSRIs)

This class of antidepressants includes citalopram, escitalopram, fluoxetine, fluvoxamine, paroxetine and sertraline.

These antidepressants all selectively inhibit the presynaptic reuptake of 5HT by inhibiting SERT. This aims to enhance or concentrate more of the neurotransmitter to be in the synapse that downregulates the receptors. By blocking the pump responsible for the reuptake of serotonin there is an increased availability, and consequently it blocks the negative feedback mechanism leading to downregulation of the neurotransmitter, resulting in a dampening effect.

This class of antidepressants is indicated for a variety of conditions, including major depression, PTSD, bulimia nervosa, premenstrual dysphoric disorder, social phobia, and anxiety disorders such as obsessive-compulsive disorders and panic disorder (Rossi, 2019).

Tolerability and adverse effects

Newer-generation antidepressants have been implicated in causing the following side effects:

- bleeding
- weight gain
- sexual dysfunction
- cardiovascular side effects
- dry mouth
- gastrointestinal adverse effects
- hepatotoxicity
- suicidality
- overdose safety
- hyponatraemia
- seizures
- sleep, sweating.

Concerns about antidepressants and their association with suicidality in adolescents and young adults have resulted in many regulatory authorities issuing a warning on product information (Wang et al., 2018). This increased risk of suicidality in young people is particularly significant for paramedics when taking a history or attending a young person for a suicide attempt or other forms of self-harm, as it impacts on the risk assessment pre-hospital.

SSRIs are considered less toxic than SNRIs, and tricyclic antidepressants are the most dangerous in toxic overdose situations. While the first-line management of depression in adolescents is psychological therapies, where drugs are required, fluoxetine is recommended as it has a long half-life so it can be ceased abruptly (Anderson et al., 2017; Hopkins et al., 2015).

Serotonin toxicity

Serotonin syndrome results from increases in serotonin at the $5HT_{2A}$ receptors in the CNS, and is a potential complication associated with all drugs having a serotonergic effect. This can occur with high doses of single agents or when combinations of serotonergic agents are used or when changing from one antidepressant to another without an appropriate washout period, potential drug interactions or drug overdose. The symptoms reflect a triad of clinical features impacting the autonomic nervous system, neuromuscular activity and the central nervous system (Boyer & Shannon, 2005; Hall & Buckley, 2003), and include the following:

- neuromuscular movement disorders, such as hyperreflexia, tremors, twitching, loss of muscle coordination with hypertonia and clonus (involuntary rhythmic contractions) being symmetrical and often appearing more significant in lower limbs
- autonomic symptoms, such as hyperthermia, fever, shivering, sweating, tachycardia, hypertension, flushing, dilated pupils and diarrhoea
- cognitive effects, such as confusion, agitation, restlessness, hypomania and hyperactivity.

Severity ranges from very mild to life-threatening with a rapid onset progressing within hours. Without rapid intervention, it can cause rhabdomyolysis, renal failure and coagulopathies, all leading to fatalities. Overdoses can become life-threatening within eight hours of ingestion (Murray et al., 2015).

Management comprises supportive care with fluid replacement and correction of vital signs, along with control of autonomic instability and hyperthermia. While many cases resolve within 24 hours of instituting therapy, symptoms may persist depending on the half-life of the drug ingested or active metabolite. Moderate severity may include the following findings: tremor and hyperreflexia (greater in the lower limbs), agitation, sweating, dilated pupils, tachycardia, hypertension, diarrhoea and increased bowel sounds (Boyer & Shannon, 2005). Any patient with changes to mental status or alteration to vital signs requires hospital admission for supportive care, management with serotonin antagonist, and monitoring to prevent further deterioration.

Drug interactions with SSRIs

Administration of an SSRI with other drugs that may augment or add to the serotonin levels have the potential to increase the risk of serotonin toxicity.

Although opinions vary, this list includes the drugs implicated in moderate to severe serotonin toxicity listed in Table 18.3.

Drugs that prolong the QT interval have the potential to increase the risk of arrhythmias in combination with SSRIs, and may warrant ECG monitoring, particularly with citalopram in high doses. Citalopram and escitalopram are metabolised by CYP2C19 enzymes, and inhibitors potentially increase blood levels causing adverse effects or toxicity, whereas inducers potentially reduce efficacy (Rossi, 2019).

SEROTONIN NORADRENALINE (NOREPINEPHRINE) REUPTAKE INHIBITORS (SNRIs)

Drugs in this class include desvenlafaxine, duloxetine, reboxetine and venlafaxine, and they not only inhibit SERT like SSRIs, but also inhibit noradrenaline

Table 18.3 Common Drugs Implicated in Serotonin Toxicity

Drug Class	Drug
Antidepressant	Citalopram, clomipramine, desvenlafaxine, duloxetine, escitalopram, fluoxetine, fluvoxamine, imipramine, moclobemide, paroxetine, phenelzine, sertraline, St John's wort, tranylcypromine, venlafaxine, vortioxetine
Opioids	Dextromethorphan, fentanyl, pethidine, tramadol
Other agents	Buspirone, dapoxetine, illicit drugs (ecstasy (MDMA), hallucinogenic amphetamines, lysergic acid diethylamide (LSD), linezolid (a weak MAOI), lithium, methylene blue, methylphenidate, phentermine, tryptophan

Adapted from Buckley et al., 2014; Hall & Buckley, 2003; Rossi, 2019

(norepinephrine) transporter (NET) and can increase dopamine in the prefrontal cortex (Zastrozhin et al., 2017). This gives an additional therapeutic effect as it potentially provides another means of impacting on the neurotransmitter systems in different regions of the brain. This dual action may explain the improved efficacy of SNRIs (with the exception of reboxetine) over fluoxetine (Cipriani et al., 2009). They also appear to demonstrate a superiority in the management of pain syndromes and account for vasomotor symptoms, more so than SSRIs in perimenopause (Stahl, 2013).

Adverse effects

SNRIs can cause tachycardia, orthostatic hypotension, stress-induced cardiomyopathy and a significantly greater risk in causing hypertension, particularly venlafaxine (Wang et al., 2018). It is recommended that blood pressure be managed before commencing desvenlafaxine or venlafaxine (Rossi, 2019). As part of the paramedic assessment, close attention to blood pressure and cardiac arrhythmia monitoring is required when managing those on SNRIs.

Other adverse effects include nausea, constipation, dry mouth, weakness, impotence, loss of libido, somnolence, insomnia, headache, blurred vision, tremor, reduced appetite and hyponatraemia (SIADH) (Aronson, 2015; Rossi, 2019).

MONOAMINE OXIDASE INHIBITORS (MAOIs)

MAOIs, phenelzine and tranylcypromine have largely been superseded by newer agents with more favourable adverse-effect profiles. They irreversibly inhibit both monoamine oxidase enzymes A and B responsible for the breakdown of 5HT and noradrenaline (norepinephrine), dopamine and tyramine. This leads to higher monoamine concentrations and subsequent efficacy in depression.

Interactions: drugs and foods

A significant issue that exists with MAOIs is the effect that dietary tyramine can have on the release of noradrenaline (norepinephrine). Tyramine is produced in the fermentation process for certain foods (e.g. aged cheese, protein or yeast extracts, dried or smoked meats, red wine), and in the presence of MAOI its absorption is increased, causing sympathomimetic adverse effects, such as severe headache and acute hypertension potentially leading to hypertensive crisis. Similar interactions can occur when used in combination with many other drugs (Rossi, 2019).

Changing from one antidepressant to another

To reduce the risk of unwanted drug interactions and associated adverse effects, an adequate period between administration of the new agent and potential interacting drug is needed (Fowler, 2019).

Adverse effects of MAOIs

Common adverse effects for MAOIs include overactivity, hyper-metabolic states, hypertensive crisis, serotonin syndrome, dose-related orthostatic hypotension, sexual dysfunction, mydriasis, vasoconstriction, myoclonus, oedema of the legs, feet and hands, twitches in limbs and paraesthesias of extremities. They also cause dry mouth, constipation, weight gain, changes in libido, rashes and leucopenia.

REVERSIBLE INHIBITORS OF MONOAMINE OXIDASE A (RIMA)

Moclobamide is a reversible inhibitor of monoamine oxidase A (RIMA) and therefore selectivity has fewer potential interactions and reduces the need for dietary restrictions (Rossi, 2019). Moclobamide can be removed or displaced by the noradrenaline (norepinephrine) that has accumulated from the action of tyramine. Competition for binding MAO A re-establishes the enzyme activity, allowing the breakdown of the extra noradrenaline (norepinephrine) to proceed in the usual manner, thus decreasing the risk of the tyramine response (Stahl, 2013).

Moclobamide is indicated in major depression and social phobia, and depressed patients with comorbid phobic features and anxiety (Rossi, 2019).

Adverse effects

Moclobamide can cause nausea, dry mouth, constipation, diarrhoea, restlessness, insomnia and dizziness, but has less potential to cause sexual dysfunction than SSRIs, and is considered to have a relatively low potential for toxicity in overdose. Moclobamide can cause arrhythmias associated with QT prolongation (Murray et al., 2015; Rossi, 2019).

Interactions

Moclobamide may interact with drugs contributing to serotonin toxicity and with sympathomimetics, potentially causing hypertensive crisis.

Overdosage

Symptoms are minor and include nausea, anxiety and tachycardia. Serotonin toxicity is rarely seen with moclobemide toxicity if ingested as a sole agent, and is non-life-threatening (Murray et al., 2015).

AGOMELATINE

Agomelatine is a melatonin agonist at MT_1 and MT_2 receptors and an antagonist at $5HT_{2C}$ receptors. In depression the circadian rhythm can become desynchronised or disturbed, and agomelatine restores the circadian response by acting on the MT_1 and MT_2 receptors and blocking the $5HT_{2c}$ receptors (Stahl, 2013). This action may also set off other biological responses, such as reprogramming the sleep–wake cycle and reducing glutamate release in response to stress.

Adverse effects

Agomelatine is indicated for major depression but particularly with sleep disturbance, and has a lower risk of sexual adverse effects (Kennedy et al., 2016). It has been associated with raising aminotransferases, dizziness and abdominal pain, and although it rarely causes liver failure, monitoring is required (Rossi, 2019).

Interactions

Agomelatine is a substrate for CYP1A2 and therefore has the potential to interact with drugs that inhibit or induce this enzyme.

MIRTAZEPINE AND MIANSERIN

Both mirtazapine and mianserin are non-selective tetracyclic antidepressants inhibiting a range of monoamine receptors and are known as noradrenergic (norepinephrinergic) and specific serotonergic antidepressants (NaSSAs). They block presynaptic alpha-2 autoreceptors on the noradrenergic (norepinephrinergic) neurons, and therefore block the mechanism for noradrenaline (norepinephrine) to switch off its own release as these receptors are gatekeepers or self-regulators for noradrenaline (norepinephrine). It also halts noradrenaline (norepinephrine) from stopping serotonin release, and consequently leads to elevated levels of serotonin. This mechanism differs to that of an SNRI which blocks the monoamine transport system, and, as such, mirtazapine has been used in combination with an SNRI to enhance the response.

Mirtazepine and mianserin also act to block postsynaptic $5HT_{2A}$, $5HT_{2c}$ and $5HT_3$ receptors and histamine H_1 receptors. Mianserin, however, also has alpha-1 antagonist actions that counter its effect on enhancing serotonin neurotransmission, which may contribute to causing hypotension. The histamine H_1 receptor blockade also contributes to the relief of sleep disturbances associated with depression, and there are claims of a more rapid antidepressant effect than with some SSRIs (Aronson, 2015).

Mirtazapine is principally liver metabolised by CYP1A2, CYP2D6 and CYP3A4, and has similar tolerability to SSRIs.

Adverse effects

Adverse effects include constipation, dry mouth, drowsiness, increased appetite, weight gain and elevated liver enzymes (Aronson, 2015).

Mianserin can cause sedation and dizziness, but less dry mouth as it has fewer anticholinergic effects (Aronson, 2015). Although rare, it has been associated with causing blood dyscrasias (thrombocytopenia, agranulocytosis), hepatotoxicity and arthritis.

Both mirtazapine and mianserin are beneficial in individuals with depression who present with anxiety symptoms and sleep disturbance, and the dual action may benefit difficult-to-treat patients.

VORTIOXETINE

Vortioxetine is considered a multimodal agent with the aim to enhance efficacy for some individuals with depression by targeting several systems. This drug demonstrates activity on SERT, is an antagonist at 5HT receptor subtypes ($5HT_3$, $5HT_7$ and $5HT_{1D}$), a serotonin agonist at $5HT_{1A}$ and partial agonist at $5HT_{1B}$ increasing serotonin levels in the CNS along with increasing noradrenergic (norepinephrinergic) and dopaminergic neurotransmission (Sanchez et al., 2015). It has been shown to be beneficial in individuals with cognitive dysfunction (Sanchez et al., 2015).

Vortioxetine has demonstrated efficacy and statistically been shown to be better than agomelatine (Sanchez et al., 2015). It appears that not only the inhibitory effects on SERT are responsible for its efficacy, but also its effect on binding to $5HT_3$ receptors and their action on GABA interneurons, reinforcing the theory that tempering or moderating the neurotransmitter systems potentially impacts antidepressant efficacy (Sanchez et al., 2015).

TRICYCLIC ANTIDEPRESSANTS (TCAs)

Tricyclic antidepressants are also known as classic antidepressants, with their nomenclature based on their chemical structure having a triple carbon ring. Currently in Australia they include the following drugs: amitriptyline, clomipramine, dosulepin (dothiepin), doxepin, imipramine and nortriptyline (Rossi, 2019). They vary in their action on noradrenaline (norepinephrine) and serotonin inhibition, with most blocking NET and SERT to some extent.

In addition, most TCAs have an action on not only serotonin receptors but other receptors that include muscarinic, alpha-1 and histaminic H_1. They can affect sodium ion channels, which is particularly problematic in overdoses, leading to seizures, arrhythmias, coma and death. It is well recognised that the TCAs have the potential to cause many side effects, and it is largely these, and the potential for toxicity, that limit their use in clinical practice.

Adverse effects

Their anticholinergic effect is associated with causing dry mouth, urinary retention, blurred vision and constipation, which are typically experienced on initiation but often wane after a few weeks of therapy. The antihistaminic effect is responsible for causing sedation and potentially weight gain. By blocking alpha-1 receptors, they can cause dizziness and postural hypotension.

It is well recognised that TCAs cause many adverse effects contributing to high discontinuation rates. A meta-analysis showed fewer patients discontinued the SSRI fluoxetine due to adverse events than TCAs (Bech et al., 2000). All TCAs lower the seizure threshold, directly associated with blood levels and dosage.

About one-fifth of patients experience significant postural hypotension contributing to an increased falls risk, and tolerance to this effect doesn't develop during therapy (Aronson, 2015). However, as it is recognised to occur in individuals with raised systolic pressures demonstrating pronounced postural drops, TCAs can be avoided in those more susceptible.

Withdrawal effects with TCAs from abrupt cessation of long-term use can occur as early as the morning after a missed dose, but more frequently appear after 2 days and up to 2 weeks. These can include sweating, anxiety, restlessness, diarrhoea, hot and cold flushes, delirium or mania, and may be associated with cholinergic overactivity (Aronson, 2015).

Toxicity

TCAs have the potential to cause significant toxicity in overdose and have been associated with suicide attempts. They are some of the most frequently ingested substances in self-poisonings, which prompted the search for safer drugs for depression. In overdose their main affect is seen in the CNS and the cardiovascular system (Murray et al., 2015). TCAs, particularly dothiepin, are the most lethal antidepressants in overdose (Anderson et al., 2017).

Dothiepin has a higher incidence of convulsions and cardiac arrhythmias in overdose when compared with other TCAs (Buckley et al., 1994). The tachyarrhythmias may be associated with seizure-induced hypoxaemia possibly from increasing cardiac excitability and associated acidosis leading to increased free TCAs as pH can determine protein binding.

In the heart, they cause a widening of the QRS complex by blocking the cardiac fast sodium channels, and can cause QT prolongation blocking potassium efflux at the time of cardiac repolarisation (Murray et al., 2015). This predisposes an individual to fatal ventricular fibrillation. CNS symptoms of sedation and coma often appear before cardiovascular symptoms. Anticholinergic effects, such as agitation, restlessness, dry, warm and flushed skin, myoclonic jerks and urinary retention can occur on presentation, but may be delayed.

Self-poisoning may lead to rapid presentation of serious CNS and cardiac symptoms occurring within 1 to 2 hours following ingestion. Early response and resuscitation should continue until intubation, hyperventilation and intravenous sodium bicarbonate achieves serum pH 7.50–7.55 (Kerr et al., 2001).

Drug interactions

TCAs may interact with other drugs that have an anticholinergic action, and this additive effect may cause a central anticholinergic delirium which can be overlooked. They may also add to sympathomimetic effects of other drugs such as pseudoephedrine, phenylephrine, methylphenidate or adrenaline, and can lead to potentiation of hypertensive effects. They have also been shown to contribute to CNS depression and will potentiate CNS depression of other drugs, such as alcohol (Aronson, 2015).

Most TCAs are either metabolised by or inhibit one or more CYP450 enzymes, and therefore have the potential for many drug interactions that involve such metabolic pathways (Gillman, 2007). Overall, though, TCAs are less problematic than the SSRIs with respect to metabolic interactions, particularly in comparison to fluvoxamine and fluoxetine (Gillman, 2007).

ST JOHN'S WORT

In a systematic review, Apaydin and others found moderate evidence to support extracts of hypericum perforatum, a complementary medicine known as St John's Wort, having efficacy in mild and moderate depression with an average response of 56% compared with placebo 35% (Apaydin et al., 2016). Concern remains about the dosing, preparation variation, effect duration and potential for serious drug interactions, including serotonin toxicity (Apaydin et al., 2016).

COMPARATIVE DATA FOR EFFICACY OF ANTIDEPRESSANTS

In major depressive disorders, about 50% of patients respond to initial treatment with an antidepressant. While there is a delay in the response of 1 to 2 weeks with all antidepressants and a full response is not seen for up to 4 to 6 weeks or longer, there is a need to evaluate the response to antidepressant therapy after 2 to 4 weeks from initial treatment (Fowler, 2019). Where an adequate response is achieved, antidepressants should be continued for at least 6 months if possible, and therapy should be maintained for up to 12 months to avoid recurrence or relapse. If there is a response failure, then consideration of an alternative drug class may be appropriate.

Tolerance to antidepressants is also important to consider when treatments may appear resistant. Antidepressants may induce a relapse upon discontinuation, unfavourable long-term consequences by potentially establishing processes opposing the acute response, worsening of symptoms, withdrawal syndrome, tolerance and resistance (Fava & Offidani, 2011).

Evidence suggests that while antidepressants effectively treat an acute episode, there doesn't appear to be a protective benefit once they are ceased and are less effective at relapse prevention or treating repeated episodes (Fava & Offidani, 2011). There is also suggestion that continued drug use may establish processes that oppose their initial action or induce receptor alterations and may establish the illness to be treatment resistant.

Withdrawal syndrome

Withdrawal symptoms may appear within 3 days of antidepressant cessation and resolve within 1 or 2 weeks, and include headaches, dizziness, fatigue, reduced appetite, disturbed sleep, flu-like symptoms, and nausea or vomiting. Psychological symptoms such as agitation, anxiety, panic, confusion and worsening mood may also be seen, and occasionally more severe cognitive impairment, catatonia or psychosis (Fava & Offidani, 2011).

MOOD STABILISERS

Lithium is considered the mainstay of therapy for mania since 1949 when it was first identified by John Cade, an Australian psychiatrist, to show specific action in mania (Alda, 2015). It has a number of pharmacological effects on different signalling pathways; however, their association in therapeutic efficacy are not fully understood (Alda, 2015; Stahl, 2013).

Initial suggestions for lithium's action related to regulating cell membrane properties, cell transport, ion distribution, neurotransmitter changes and cell signalling. Early studies considered elevated sodium levels in depression and mania and normalisation seen with lithium therapy (Alda, 2015).

LITHIUM

Lithium has been shown to decrease the release of noradrenaline (norepinephrine) and dopamine from nerve terminals and possibly increase serotonin release, potentially contributing to mood-stabilising effect (Baird-Gunning et al., 2016). It may dampen excessive activity in regulatory networks to allow for stabilisation of neuronal activity (Alda, 2015). Lithium reduces the recurrence risk of manic and depressive episodes by 38% and 28% respectively, and, importantly, decreases the risk of suicide by greater than 50% (Geddes & Miklowitz, 2013).

Lithium penetrates slowly into brain tissue and the CSF, and is concentrated in the thyroid gland and bone. As lithium is eliminated by the kidneys, renal function is an important determinant with respect to monitoring plasma levels. Caution is also needed in patients with hyponatraemia as renal clearance of lithium depends on sodium ion balance and urine volume, and since almost 80% is reabsorbed in the proximal tubule of the nephron in the same manner sodium ions are reabsorbed (Rossat et al., 1999), hyponatraemia potentiates the risk of lithium toxicity. This can be an issue in elderly patients with renal impairment, particularly if they become dehydrated, significantly increasing the risk for lithium toxicity.

The therapeutic range for acute mania is 0.5 to 1.2 mmol/L, maintenance range 0.4 to 1 mmol/L (Baird-Gunning et al., 2016), and toxicity levels >1.5 mmol/L. The therapeutic concentration is close to the toxic level and, once stabilised, monitoring lithium levels is required every 3 months.

Lithium is clinically used for the management of mania and hypomania, and often in combination with an antipsychotic. It also inhibits thyroid hormone release and has been used in other conditions such as hyperthyroidism.

Toxicity

Toxicity can result either from an overdose or from chronic poisoning where lithium levels have insidiously increased from subtle changes to blood levels over time by other means. The chronic intoxication may start with unnoticed changes to kidney function along with some prodromal symptoms increasing in severity with worsening kidney function. Lithium is a metallic ion and with an acute presentation can cause irritation to the gastric mucosa. Mild to moderate toxicity presents with gastrointestinal symptoms: abdominal pain, nausea, vomiting and diarrhoea which can also lead to dehydration, potentially contributing to further lithium reabsorption. Blurred vision, muscle weakness, drowsiness and loss of muscle coordination are also mild to moderate symptoms of toxicity. With acute toxicity there is often a delay to neurological symptoms, but it can present initially as tremor. Severe toxicity symptoms include significant changes to muscle tone, leading to motor speech changes (poor articulation), hypertonia, hypotension, stupor, myoclonic jerks, seizures and coma (Murray et al., 2015).

No specific antidote exists for lithium toxicity, and management relies on resuscitation, supportive care and monitoring. Maintenance of renal perfusion with fluids is essential to ensure lithium elimination and to correct fluid and sodium levels (Baird-Gunning et al., 2016).

Drug interactions

Drug interactions that increase lithium concentration can potentiate toxicity and include angiotensin-converting enzyme (ACE) inhibitors, angiotensin receptor 2 blockers (AR2B), diuretics, NSAIDs and topirimate. As a marker for the proximal reabsorption of sodium, NSAIDs naproxen and celecoxib were shown to reduce renal clearance of lithium (Rossat et al., 1999).

Drug interactions that can decrease lithium concentration include acetazolamide, potassium citrate, sodium bicarbonate and theophylline. Lithium can also increase the risk of serotonin toxicity.

Sometimes lithium can cause neurotoxicity, which may occur in combination with other drugs such as diltiazem, carbamazepine and antipsychotics (Aronson, 2015). There is also an increased risk of extrapyramidal adverse effects when lithium is used in combination with antipsychotics (Aronson, 2015).

Adverse effects

Common adverse effects include a metallic taste, mild cognitive complaints, nausea, diarrhoea, weight gain, fatigue, headache, tremor, acne, psoriasis, leucocytosis, nephrotoxicity, hypercalcaemia and hypothyroidism (Aronson, 2015).

ANTIEPILEPTIC DRUGS (CARBAMAZEPINE, LAMOTRIGINE AND VALPROATE)

Antiepileptic drugs have fewer adverse effects and less toxicity than lithium, and have demonstrated efficacy in the management of bipolar disorder. Although not yet determined, their activity may relate to how they control seizures. They reduce electrical excitability of cell membranes by blocking voltage-dependent and use-dependent sodium channels, enhance GABA-mediated synaptic inhibition and inhibit T-type calcium channels (Rossi, 2019; Stahl, 2013).

Lithium and valproate both demonstrate neuroprotective effects against glutamate-induced excitotoxicity, and elevated levels of glutamate have been found in the frontal cortex of postmortems with major depression and bipolar disorders (Hashimoto et al., 2007).

Adverse effects

Valproate may cause hair loss, weight gain, gastrointestinal side effects, paraesthesia, drowsiness, dizziness, memory impairment, menstrual irregularities, ataxia and tremor (Aronson, 2015; Rossi, 2019). Sedation, headache, dizziness and behavioural changes appear less common than with other antiepileptic drugs (Aronson, 2015).

Carbamazepine differs as it can commonly cause dizziness, nystagmus, ataxia, fatigue and transient sedation. However, it less commonly causes nausea, vomiting, cognitive dysfunction, headache, myoclonus, worsening seizures, movement disorders, hyponatraemia and leucopenia (Aronson, 2015).

Lamotrigine can cause serious rashes including Stevens-Johnson syndrome ranging from 0.3% to 0.8% in paediatric patients and 0.08% to 0.3% in adults. It generally presents early but it can be as late as 6 months, and while the rash may present as benign, treatment should be ceased. Use of low initiating doses or slow titration reduces this risk, yet concomitant administration of valproate is a contributing risk factor (Aronson, 2015). Other adverse effects include dizziness, headache and insomnia. In overdose situations, symptoms include sedation, ataxia, visual disturbances, such as diplopia and nystagmus, nausea, vomiting, slurred speech and rarely seizures (Aronson, 2015; Murray et al., 2015).

Drug interactions

Carbamazepine is a strong inducer and a substrate for CYP3A4 enzyme and can induce its own metabolism, and its metabolic pathway can also be affected by inhibitors and other enzyme inducers. It also is an inducer of CYP2C9, CYP2C19 and CYP2B6, and so can induce the metabolism of many drugs (Rossi, 2019).

Valproate inhibits uridine diphosphate glucuronosyltransferase (UGT) enzymes, affecting glucuronidation and metabolism of lamotrigine, and is also metabolised by CYP2C9 (Rossi, 2019).

ANTIPSYCHOTICS

Psychosis is a generalised term to represent a disorder where a person affected has lost some contact with reality. They can experience delusions, disordered thoughts and disruption to thought processes. There are several different types of major psychotic disorders that include schizophrenia, schizoaffective disorders, manic episodes, bipolar affective disorder, persistent delusional disorders, and acute and transient psychotic disorders.

The clinical features for schizophrenia can be divided into two distinct categories: the positive and negative symptoms.

- **Positive symptoms** include hallucinations and delusions, and can present as disorganised communication presenting paranoid ideas. In addition to changes to thoughts and communication, abnormal motor behaviour, including disorientation, unpredictable agitation or aggression, can also occur (McGlashan & Fenton, 1992).
- **Negative symptoms**, on the other hand, relate to flattening or diminished emotional responses, poor motivation, showing little interest in social activities or pleasure, and becoming withdrawn. Diminished facial and vocal expression are also features that distinguish schizophrenia from other patient groups (Kring & Moran, 2008).

CLASSIFICATION OF ANTIPSYCHOTIC DRUGS

Antipsychotic medications, also known as neuroleptics or major tranquillisers, were first introduced in the 1950s with the advent of chlorpromazine (López-Muñoz et al., 2005). They can be divided in to two classifications: those first developed known as first-generation antipsychotics (FGAs), typical or conventional antipsychotic drugs, and those which have been developed more recently, referred to as second-generation antipsychotics (SGAs) or atypical antipsychotic drugs. To align with clinical practice guidelines, the convention used throughout this chapter will use the terms first-generation antipsychotics (FGAs) and second-generation antipsychotics (SGAs) (Fowler, 2019).

The mode of action for FGAs involves the blockade of dopamine receptors in the mesolimbic pathways (Laruelle & Abi-Dargham, 1999). This is a postsynaptic blockade of the D_2 receptors. Cortical dopamine D_2/D_3 occupancy appears to be linked with antipsychotic efficacy, and the striatal D_2/D_3 occupancy has been associated with a therapeutic role (Stone et al., 2009). Clinical potency has also been shown to have a high correlation with D_2 receptor binding (Seeman, 2002).

Pharmacological therapies remain the cornerstone in the management of schizophrenia (Miyamoto et al., 2005). Early intervention services that include both psychosocial interventions and pharmacotherapy have been shown to reduce hospital admissions, and decrease the severity of symptoms and the rates of relapse in people presenting with early psychosis (Bird et al., 2010).

NEUROCHEMICAL BASIS OF SCHIZOPHRENIA

The positive symptoms seen in schizophrenia are believed to be associated with malfunctions to the mesolimbic pathway and the negative symptoms associated with the malfunction of the mesocortical circuits, potentially involving the nucleus accumbens – part of the mesolimbic region influencing motivation and pleasure (Stahl, 2013). This region is thought to be associated with increased rates of substance use and abuse. The neural circuitry, mediating drug reward and reinforcement, is associated with abnormalities in the hippocampal formation, impacting on drug reward positive reinforcing effects and the characteristics in schizophrenia (Chambers et al., 2001).

The ventromedial prefrontal cortex is believed to be associated with affective symptoms, such as depression or anxiety, while the amygdala and orbitofrontal cortex are involved with aggressive symptoms. Cognitive symptoms involving information processing and problem solving are associated with the dorsolateral prefrontal cortex.

The main neurotransmitters, dopamine and glutamate, are thought to be involved in schizophrenia, and some of these pathways may be modulated by serotonin.

Dopamine theory

The dopamine hypothesis for schizophrenia classically suggests that the positive symptoms associated with schizophrenia are linked to hyperactivity of dopamine transmission (Carlsson & Lindqvist, 1963).

In support of this theory, psychostimulants release neuronal dopamine, producing a behavioural syndrome characteristic of schizophrenia attenuated by dopamine antagonists (Laruelle & Abi-Dargham, 1999; Lieberman et al., 1987).

Evidence suggests that the dysfunction to presynaptic dopamine, its synthesis capacity, synaptic levels and the release of dopamine, constitutes the largest dopaminergic abnormality in schizophrenia (Howes et al., 2012).

While the focus regarding dopamine theory in schizophrenia surrounds dopamine D_2 receptor activity and a correlation between clinical efficacy and dopamine receptor blockade potency, it does not explain the efficacy of the SGA clozapine, which has a poor affinity for D_2 receptors. Clozapine predominantly acts on dopamine D_4 receptors which has a high homology for human dopamine D_2 and D_3 receptor genes (Van Tol et al., 1991).

The dopamine pathways in the brain include the mesolimbic, mesocortical, tuberoinfundibular and nigrostriatal pathways, each having an impact on differing functions. Two of the dopamine pathways appear to be malfunctioning in schizophrenia:

- overactivity of the mesolimbic pathway, implicated in the development of positive symptoms of schizophrenia (Davis & Kahn, 1991)
- underactivity of the mesocortical pathway, associated with negative and some of the cognitive symptoms of schizophrenia (Davis & Kahn, 1991).

The treatment goal is to reduce the activity of hyperactive pathways mediating psychosis, and to increase the activity of the hypoactive pathways mediating negative and cognitive symptoms, while simultaneously preserving the activity of those pathways that regulate motor movement (the nigrostriatal pathway) and prolactin secretion (the tuberoinfundibular pathway).

If dopamine is blocked in the mesolimbic system, not only positive symptoms will reduce but also reward mechanisms will be blocked. Patients will appear to lack motivation and have reduced interest and less pleasure from social interactions. These are associated with the flattening or withdrawn affects linked to the negative symptoms of psychosis. With blocking D_2 receptors in the nigrostriatal pathway, movement disorders result and appear like those of Parkinson's disease. These are referred to as extrapyramidal symptoms (EPS) since the nigrostriatal pathway is part of the extrapyramidal nervous system. Over time, if these receptors are blocked continuously, they can lead to chronic complications, such as tardive dyskinesia (TD), characterised as an involuntary movement disorder involving orofacial muscles and extremity areas such as hips and trunk (Solmi et al., 2018).

Prolactin increases

The dopamine D_2 receptors in the tuberoinfundibular pathway can also be blocked by SGAs. This causes hyperprolactinaemia, an adverse effect characterised by galactorrhoea and amenorrhoea, which may impact therapy adherence and risks bone demineralisation (Montejo et al., 2017).

Cholinergic effects

An increase in acetylcholine activity is seen with dopamine antagonists. Dopamine usually suppresses acetylcholine activity, and when the D_2 receptor is blocked it can cause acetylcholine to be overly active and results in unopposed EPS (Stahl, 2013).

Glutamate theory

In addition to the dopamine theory, other receptor antagonists have been shown to produce positive, negative and cognitive deficit symptoms (Miyamoto et al., 2002). These include phencyclidine and ketamine, both non-competitive antagonists at NMDA receptors leading to psychotic symptoms such as hallucinations and disorders of thought. This has led to the hypothesis that the pathophysiology of schizophrenia may involve hypo-function of NMDA receptors supported with receptor antagonist, structural brain imaging, postmortem, genetic and therapeutic effects studies (Coyle, 2006).

Responses to glutamate at other glutamate receptors in the cortex may be excessive in schizophrenia. This may mediate glutamate excitotoxicity, oligodendrocyte cell death, loss of white matter, and decreased synaptic connections of cortical neurons attributable to schizophrenia (Davis et al., 2003).

5-HYDROXYTRYPTAMINE (5HT) RECEPTORS

Early studies noted that LSD produced schizophrenia-like symptoms and has a partial agonist action at $5HT_{2A}$ receptors (Woolley & Shaw, 1954), yet the hallucinations were considered different and therefore not directly linked to schizophrenia pathogenesis (Schmidt et al., 1995). However, newer drugs having an effect on blocking $5HT_{2A}$ receptors, such as clozapine, may in part explain reduced adverse effects, enhanced efficacy and potential use in drug-resistant schizophrenia, and have a particular benefit in managing negative symptoms due to an indirect effect on dopaminergic system (Schmidt et al., 1995). Potent SGAs, such as clozapine and risperidone, with known affinity for blocking $5HT_{2A}$ receptors, have proven to be clinically effective, particularly against negative symptoms, and importantly lack EPS (Miyamoto et al., 2005).

DRUG THERAPY

Antipsychotic drug therapy is the cornerstone for the management of schizophrenia (Fowler, 2019). Aggression or overactivity can be readily managed with antipsychotics and benzodiazepines, but prevention of relapses is essential to decrease the risk of poorer clinical outcomes and to improve prognosis.

Antipsychotics also produce a state of apathy and reduced initiative. Individuals will display minimal emotions and respond slowly to external stimuli while retaining the ability to respond to questions without the loss of intellectual functioning.

Antipsychotic therapy takes several weeks to demonstrate clinical efficacy despite immediate changes to receptor blockade. They affect neuroplasticity resulting in alterations to synaptic connections in areas of the brain that are implicated in psychotic illnesses. With continued therapy, the increase in dopaminergic activity of neurons changes to inhibition within a few weeks, and both biochemical and electrophysiological markers decrease.

Controlling positive symptoms early reduces anxiety, depression, relapse frequency and cognitive deterioration. A meta-analysis of data showed a clinical improvement in schizophrenia between the 1920s and 1970s, with a favourable outcome from 24.3% to 50.5% of cases, which has been attributed particularly to the introduction of antipsychotics from the 1950s (Hegarty et al., 1994). Prior to the availability of antipsychotics, about half of all patients had a poor long-term prognosis, and this was reduced to a quarter or a third of patients following the advent of antipsychotics (Lieberman et al., 2006). However, it is estimated that around 30% of cases are treatment resistant (failed to show adequate response to at least two different antipsychotic treatments with adequate dose and duration) and remain symptomatic with a moderate to severe impact on functioning ability (Elkis & Buckley, 2016; Howes et al., 2016). They are seen to be more severely ill and suffer more severe negative symptoms (Iasevoli et al., 2018).

FIRST-GENERATION ANTIPSYCHOTICS (TYPICAL ANTIPSYCHOTICS OR FGAs)

Included in this class are the following drugs: chlorpromazine, droperidol, flupentixol, fluphenazine, haloperidol, periciazine, trifluoperazine and zuclopenthixol.

It is estimated that between 30% and 60% of patients with acute exacerbations of symptoms fail or only partially respond to FGAs (Miyamoto et al., 2005). They are now considered second-line agents based on their potential for causing adverse effects, and are mainly used in patients unresponsive to first-line SGA therapies.

FGAs may have additional pharmacological effects – a potential action on histamine H_1 receptors, an alpha-1 adrenergic receptor blockade and muscarinic cholinergic receptors. FGAs do not differ in their therapeutic application, but have different adverse effect profiles associated with different receptor affinity (Leucht et al., 2009).

Adverse effects

The major adverse effects are the EPS and TD (Table 18.4). Haloperidol followed by chlorpromazine has the greatest potential for these effects (Leucht et al., 2013), and it is estimated that up to 70% of patients on FGAs develop acute EPS (Miyamoto et al., 2002), which can include the following:

- Acute dystonias – blocking dopaminergic nigrostriatal pathway often present rapidly and affect the face, neck and hands. Occulogyric crisis and laryngeal spasms (which can be fatal) have been reported (Dayalu & Chou, 2008; Oyewole et al., 2013). These movement disorders can be reversed with anticholinergic agents (biperidan or benztropine).
- Akathisia – agitation, restlessness and anxiety managed with benztropine and diazepam. The distinction between this adverse effect and agitation from the presentation of psychosis is important and can be readily made with an assessment of response to dose changes (Rossi, 2019).
- Tardive dyskinesia (TD) – involuntary hyperkinetic movements of mouth, lips, tongue, jaw, sucking or chewing, mouth puckering and represented as tics, but can also involve the limbs and trunk (Dayalu & Chou, 2008; Solmi et al., 2018). It is estimated that about one-third of patients will develop TD, and this should be regularly assessed. The lowest doses possible should be used to minimise TD, and consideration given to associated risk factors as these adverse effects are often irreversible (Solmi et al., 2018).

Other adverse effects of FGAs include:

- sedation
- weight gain – less than SGAs (Leucht et al., 2013)
- postural hypotension
- anticholinergic side effects
- dyslipidaemia
- hyperglycaemia
- hyperprolactinaemia
- sexual dysfunction
- neuroleptic malignant syndrome.

Chlorpromazine

Additional side effects include photosensitivity, corneal lens opacities and skin pigmentation (prolonged use) (Greiner & Berry, 1964), postural hypotension and hepatotoxicity. It also causes constipation, blurred vision, difficulty urinating and

Table 18.4 Comparative Adverse Effects of Antipsychotics

Drug	Movement (EPSE)	Sedation	Anticholinergic Effect	Orthostatic Hypotension	Weight Gain	Hyperglycaemia	Prolactin Increase	Dyslipidaemia	Other
Second-Generation Antipsychotics									
Amisulpride	+	+	-	-	++	-	+++	?	QT prolongation possible
Aripiprazole	+	+	+	+	-	-	+ (NB2)	-	
Asenapine (NB3)	+	+	+	+	+	++	+	++	QT prolongation possible
Clozapine	-	+++	+++ (NB4)	+++ (NB5)	+++	+++	+/-	+++	Blood dyscrasias, cardiotoxicity, pulmonary embolism, constipation
Lurasidone	++	+	+/-	+	+/-	+/-	+	?	Little effect on QT prolongation
Olanzepine	+/-	++	++	++ (NB5)	+++	+++	+	+++	
Paliperidone	+	+	+	++	++	+	+++	++	Sexual dysfunction
Quetiapine	+	++	+	++	++	++	+	++	
Risperidone	++	+ NB5	+	++ (NB5)	++	++	+++	++	Sexual dysfunction
Ziprasidone	+	++	+	+	+/-	+	+	-	QT prolongation possible

First-Generation Antipsychotics

								QT prolongation possible
Chlorpromazine	+++ (NB6)	++	++	++	+++ (NB6)	+++	+++	+++
Flupentixol	+	+	++	++	+	++	+++	?
Haloperidol	+ (NB6)	+	+	+	+	+	++	+
Pericyazine	+	+++	+++	+++	++	?	+++	?
Trifluoperazine	+++	+	+	+	++	+	+++	?
Zuclopenthixol	++	+++	++ (NB4)	++	+	?	+++	?

Approximate frequencies: ? = little or no information reported; - = negligible or absent; + = infrequent; ++ = moderately frequently; +++ = frequently
NB1: Information in this table is based on a combination of reported adverse effect information and expert opinion, and is only intended as a guide and interpreted in the context of individual patient circumstances and presentation (e.g. drug history, concurrent drugs, the overall health of the patient, age and individual variations to elimination half-lives) and doses of drugs
NB2: Weight loss reported and used with olanzapine to reduce weight loss
NB3: Data limited on asenapine
NB4: Hypersalivation reported
NB5: Frequency may be higher at dose initiation or with high doses
NB6: Lower incidence with depot injection
Adapted from: Fowler, 2019; Leucht et al., 2009, 2013; Rossi, 2019

dry mouth, which are attributed to its affinity for muscarinic receptors and anticholinergic action.

Chlorpromazine has an affinity for histamine H_1 receptors, and therefore is associated with causing sedation. It has a number of indications – acute and chronic psychoses, short-term management of anxiety, agitation or disturbed behaviour, intractable hiccups, and nausea and vomiting in terminal illness (Rossi, 2019).

Haloperidol

Haloperidol has indications for acute and chronic psychoses, acute mania, Tourette syndrome and hallucinations associated with alcohol withdrawal (Rossi, 2019). It can also be used in agitation, severe anxiety or non-psychiatric disturbed behaviour for short-term management.

Haloperidol is mildly sedating and can cause insomnia, headache, dry mouth and excessive sweating (Sansom, 2018). It also causes akathisia and dystonic reactions. Despite this, it is rarely associated with causing hypotension, cardiac or anticholinergic effects (Aronson, 2015). Like droperidol it also can prolong the QT interval and caution is needed if used with other drugs that can elicit this response (Aronson, 2015). Haloperidol is most noted for causing extrapyramidal effects and dystonic reactions (Sansom, 2018), which can also be associated with high-potency antipsychotics and recent amphetamine use (May et al., 2016).

Droperidol

Droperidol has similar actions to haloperidol and is used in the short-term management of acute presentations of severe anxiety, agitation or behavioural changes with psychotic episodes, mania and non-psychotic disorders (Rossi, 2019). It is sedating and typically is used in the emergency management of acutely disturbed patients. Droperidol can prolong the QT interval and has been associated with causing arrhythmias, so should be avoided in combination with other drugs prolonging QT interval (Aronson, 2015).

Zuclopenthixol

Zuclopenthixol has shown superiority to other FGAs in the acute management of altered behaviour associated with serious psychosis, yet other studies showing improvement were not seen to be statistically significant (Aronson, 2015). It is indicated for acute and chronic psychoses and acute mania (Rossi, 2019).

SECOND-GENERATION ANTIPSYCHOTICS (ATYPICAL ANTIPSYCHOTICS OR SGAs)

Included in this class are the following drugs available in Australia: amisulpride, aripiprazole, brexpiprazole, asenapine, clozapine, lurasidone, olanzapine, paliperidone, quetiapine, risperidone and ziprasidone (Rossi, 2019).

It has been shown that the SGAs have fewer adverse effects, are better tolerated and are more efficacious than FGAs (Colonna et al., 2000; Miyamoto et al., 2005).

While there are claims that SGAs are better at controlling the negative symptoms of schizophrenia in a meta-analysis study, only four SGAs – amisulpride, clozapine, olanzapine and risperidone – were more effective at treating both positive and negative symptoms of schizophrenia, whereas aripiprazole, quetiapine and ziprasidone were no more efficacious than FGAs for the negative symptoms, and olanzapine and risperidone had fewer relapses (Leucht et al., 2009). All SGAs assessed had significantly fewer extrapyramidal side effects (EPSEs) than haloperidol and clozapine, and weight gain is commonly associated with SGAs (Rossi, 2019) (Tables 18.4 and 18.5).

There is a significant increased risk for all fractures with the use of antipsychotics and, while this evidence is based on observational studies, it remains important to consider in particular patient populations with a fracture risk (Papola et al., 2018).

Amisulpride

Amisulpride binds to D_2 and D_3 dopamine receptors yet it does not block serotonin. It does, however, have greater efficacy than FGAs. In comparison with haloperidol, it is considered better for negative symptoms and appears to spare dose-related EPSE (Colonna et al., 2000). Commonly it is associated with agitation, weight gain, anxiety and insomnia, but also can release prolactin and lead to hyperprolactinaemia. In addition, it has been shown to prolong the QT interval, particularly in overdose, and can cause hypokalaemia (Isbister et al., 2010; Leucht et al., 2013).

Aripiprazole

Aripiprazole is indicated for use in schizophrenia, bipolar disorder as monotherapy, or in combination with valproate or lithium in mania. It has a favourable tolerability profile with low propensity to cause EPSEs, hyperlipidaemia, hyperprolactinaemia and sedation compared with other SGAs (Suzuki et al., 2014). Weight gain does not appear to be an issue with aripiprazole use as it has a moderate binding affinity to histamine H_1 receptors, a key correlate for weight gain (Shapiro et al., 2003), and along with quetiapine, aripiprazole has shown consistent efficacy in the management of major depression (Leucht et al., 2009).

It has partial agonist properties at dopamine D_3 and $5HT_{1A}$, $5HT_{2A}$ and $5HT_{2C}$ serotonin receptors, and has a higher affinity for dopamine D_2 receptors than other SGAs, and is similar to risperidone, which, along with $5HT_{2A}$ affinity, correlates with antipsychotic efficacy (Shapiro et al., 2003). It acts as an agonist in underactive dopaminergic pathways, and acts as an antagonist in overactive dopaminergic pathways.

Clozapine

Clozapine can significantly enhance the quality of life of individuals with treatment-resistant schizophrenia and is effective in 20% to 70% of such patients (Davydov & Botts, 2000; Miyamoto et al., 2002).

Table 18.5 Comparative Neurotransmitter Receptor Affinities for Antipsychotic Drugs at Therapeutic Doses

Receptor	Clozapine	Risperidone	Olanzapine	Quetiapine	Ziprasidone	Amisulpride	Aripiprazole	Haloperidol
D_1	+	+	++	-	+	-	-	+
D_2	+	+++	++	+	+++	+++	+++	+++
D_3	+	++	+	-	++	++	++	+++
$D4$	++	-	++	-	+	-	+	+++
$5\text{-}HT_{1A}$	-	-	-	-	+++		++	-
$5\text{-}HT_{1D}$	-	+	-	-	+++		+	-
$5\text{-}HT_{2A}$	+++	+++	+++	++	++++	-	++	+
$5\text{-}HT_{2C}$	++	++	++	-	++++		++	-
$5\text{-}HT_6$	++	-	-	-	+		+	-
$5\text{-}HT_7$	++	+++	++	++	++	-	++	++
α_1	++	+++	++	++	++	-	+	-
α_2	+	++	+	-	-		+	-
H_1	+++	-	+++	++	++	-	+	-
M_1	+++	-	+++	++	-	-	-	
DAT	++		++		-	-	-	
NAT	+		++		++		-	
SERT					++		-	

Relative affinity: Minimal to none –; low +; moderate ++; high +++; very high ++++
Adapted and modified from Miyamoto et al., 2005

As clozapine has a low dopamine D_2 receptor occupancy, it has comparatively low rates of EPSE. It also has a high affinity for binding to $5HT_{2A}$ and $5HT_5$ receptors, binds to $5HT_{2B}$, $5HT_{2C}$, and is a partial agonist at $5HT_{1A}$ receptors and binds strongly to muscarinic receptors, α_1-adrenoceptors and histamine H_1 receptors (Shivakumar et al., 2018). Clozapine's metabolite, N-desmethylclozapine is an M_1 agonist and can potentiate the NMDA receptor currents in the hippocampus, which may explain clozapine's differing therapeutic profile (Miyamoto et al., 2005).

Common adverse effects include sedation, dizziness, tachycardia, ECG changes, nausea and vomiting. It is also associated with increased weight gain, fatigue and some anticholinergic side effects such as muscular weakness, dry mouth and constipation; however, clozapine also causes hypersalivation in up to 31% of patients (Shivakumar et al., 2018) possibly associated with an opposing activation of muscarinic M_4 receptors and/or affecting the swallowing reflex through an α_2-adrenoceptor blockade (Davydov & Botts, 2000).

Clozapine can cause a range of significant adverse effects that include eosinophilia, myocarditis, cardiomyopathy and agranulocytosis. The risk for agranulocytosis of 0.8% and neutropenia 2.9% is greatest in the first 18 weeks (Latif et al., 2011), so weekly blood tests are required during this time, and monthly thereafter (Atkin et al., 1996; Latif et al., 2011).

Myocarditis, although rare, is a fatal hypersensitivity complication occurring within the first month or two of clozapine therapy (Shivakumar et al., 2018), and potentially fatal cardiomyopathy has been reported up to 3 years after initiation (Aronson, 2015).

Clozapine potentially lowers the seizure threshold, and seizures have been reported with higher doses or rapid dose escalation or concomitant epileptogenic drugs (Aronson, 2015).

Clozapine is metabolised by CYP1A2, CYP2D6 and CYP3A4 enzymes, and therefore its blood levels can be altered by drugs or substances that either inhibit or induce the activity of these enzymes (Sansom, 2018). The polycyclic aromatic hydrocarbons associated with tobacco smoking are known to induce CYP1A2 enzymes, reducing blood levels of clozapine and olanzapine. It is estimated that smoking can lower clozapine concentrations by as much as 40% than in non-smokers, and when smoking is ceased the CYP1A2 enzymes are no longer induced and levels of clozapine will rise, potentially causing toxicity (Khorassani et al., 2018). This is an important consideration in clinical practice with smoking rates as high as 60% to 90% of individuals with schizophrenia or other psychotic disorders (Crockford & Addington, 2017; Morgan et al., 2012; Tsuda et al., 2014).

Lurasidone

Lurasidone is a central dopamine D_2 and serotonin $5HT_{2A}$ receptor antagonist and partial agonist at $5HT_{1A}$ receptors with an indication for schizophrenia. It is a substrate for the CYP3A4 enzyme and potentially is subject to drug interactions with strong inducers or inhibitors of this enzyme. Lurasidone does not cause weight gain in adults compared with placebo and of all antipsychotics it has the lowest potential to prolong QTc interval (Leucht et al., 2013).

Olanzapine

Olanzapine has a wide range of receptor affinities and is relatively well tolerated, but does cause drowsiness and weight gain. It also can cause hyperglycaemia and may present complications in patients with diabetes. In rare cases it has been associated with causing neutropenia, which is reversible on cessation and can cause seizures. It is metabolised by CYP1A2, CYP2D6 and CYP3A4 enzymes, and with CYP1A2 accounting for 50% to 60% of the metabolism, it can interact with polycyclic aromatic hydrocarbons associated with tobacco smoking, and it is estimated that the daily dose should be decreased by 30% in non-smokers compared with smokers (Tsuda et al., 2014).

Quetiapine

Quetiapine has a low propensity to cause EPSE and can cause dizziness, dry mouth and hypotension. It doesn't affect prolactin levels significantly (Leucht et al., 2013), but has implications with metabolic systems and may cause increased blood glucose levels, dyslipidaemia and weight gain (Rossi, 2019). It has an indication for schizophrenia, bipolar disorder, GAD and as an adjunct in the management of treatment-resistant major depression.

Risperidone

Risperidone blocks dopamine D_2 and $5HT_{2A}$ receptors and is considered a potent serotonin antagonist. The extrapyramidal effects appear to be dose related, particularly akathisia. Moderate weight gain is seen; however, risperidone does cause significant hyperprolactinaemia and endocrine problems (Leucht et al., 2013).

Ziprasidone

Ziprasidone is indicated for schizophrenia and related psychoses and acute mania (Rossi, 2019). Intramuscularly, ziprasidone showed greater efficacy and reduced adverse events compared with haloperidol (Aronson, 2015). Ziprasidone along with lurasidone (and haloperidol) were the only antipsychotics shown to have no significant increase in weight gain compared with placebo, however ziprasidone can prolong the QTc interval (Leucht et al., 2013).

SUMMARY

While debate continues over the benefits of the different classes of antipsychotics (Hartling et al., 2012), several SGAs, including aripiprazole, quetiapine and ziprasidone, were found not to be significantly different from FGAs in their overall efficacy and symptom control, whereas four SGAs – amisulpride, clozapine, olanzapine and risperidone – were identified as having superior effectiveness, including control of positive and negative symptoms (Leucht et al., 2009). In addition, SGAs have fewer EPSEs, particularly for clozapine, risperidone and olanzapine, than FGAs, and two antipsychotics, aripiprazole and ziprasidone, have little association with weight gain and are favoured where this is an issue.

OVERDOSE

Associated toxicity is an important consideration with the use of drugs used in mental health, as they are commonly implicated in overdose presentations and deliberate self-poisonings (Australian Bureau of Statistics, 2016). It is a leading cause of death in patients under 40 years of age, and is a leading differential diagnosis in a young adult presenting with cardiac arrest (Murray et al., 2015). Unlike in the elderly, resuscitation can have good neurological outcomes in cardiac arrest associated with poisonings, even with prolonged CPR (Murray et al., 2015).

In poisonings, hypotension and altered conscious state with associated loss of protective airway reflexes are serious life-threatening consequences and require urgent initiation of basic resuscitative care measures. Morbidity of an overdose (OD) patient is understandably increased in elderly patients, likely due to other comorbid conditions (Hamad et al., 2000). It has been shown that 50% of patients over 65 years presenting with OD required intubation, compared with 19% under 65 years, and there was a five times higher mortality rate – 12.5% to the overall mortality of 2.7% (Hamad et al., 2000).

Drug overdoses with antipsychotics, antidepressants and mood-stabilising agents can cause a wide range of physiological symptoms that include seizures, delirium and agitation, anticholinergic syndrome, serotonin syndrome, neuroleptic malignant syndrome, significant cardiovascular changes, including arrhythmias, respiratory acidosis (drug-induced CNS depression), neuromuscular changes, hypothermia and specific adverse effects of individual agents (Murray et al., 2015).

Antidotes to reverse some toxic symptoms may be indicated during the resuscitative phase; however, consideration of their benefit needs to be balanced against their adverse effect profile, indication and contraindications or cautions. Intervention with sodium bicarbonate may be warranted to restore the impairment to fast sodium channel function (reverse cardiotoxicity) and change the pH to alter the drug distribution and excretion with tricyclic antidepressant poisonings (Murray et al., 2015).

While most of the symptomatology for presentations are associated with increases in the concentration of the implicated drugs, sometimes the signs and symptoms may be related to the withdrawal effects, as seen with the benzodiazepines or hypnotics.

Seizure management often is required with OD presentations (eg. antidepressants venlafaxine and bupropion), signalling severe intoxication with significant consequences. While some consider that clinical determination using the Glasgow Coma Scale (GCS) may not always correlate well in poisonings (Murray et al., 2015), Hamad and others found that the Acute Physiologic Assessment and Chronic Health Evaluation (APACHE) II scoring system and the GCS were both highly predictive within the first few hours of hospital presentation (Hamad et al., 2000). Along with mental status assessment, the GCS is considered a reliable prognostic tool for drug overdose. It is understandable that careful evaluation of cognitive features and mental alertness are important indicators, particularly as a significant number of overdoses relate to drugs used in mental health, with benzodiazepines, antidepressants and antipsychotics involved in 29.4%, 17.6% and 6.1%, respectively, of pharmaceutical overdose deaths in the United States (Jones et al., 2013).

Medications implicated in poisonings with extended-release formulations may delay the onset of seizures or other toxicity symptoms. Management of seizures may involve the use of benzodiazepines or barbiturates if refractory. However, phenytoin should be avoided in drug overdoses because it may worsen the blockade on fast sodium channels and contribute further to potential cardiotoxicity (Murray et al., 2015).

Retrieval of the poisoned patient for transfer sometimes from a rural area to a specialised or metropolitan hospital is also another complication that must be carefully managed. Poisoning transfers often occur during the most severe phase and therefore adequate preparation and planning is essential, particularly as patients can rapidly deteriorate. Patient stabilisation before retrieval is necessary, and priorities for resuscitation and supportive care need to be maintained (Murray et al., 2015).

NEUROLEPTIC MALIGNANT SYNDROME

Neuroleptic malignant syndrome (NMS) is a rare but a potentially life-threatening reaction that can be caused by dopamine antagonists and antipsychotic medications. While it is considered to be an idiosyncratic reaction, it can occur with any dopamine antagonist and can also occur from withdrawal of a dopamine agonist in a patient with Parkinson's disease (Corbett & Wilson, 2018). While it can occur with any antipsychotic, it seems to occur more often with high-potency FGAs (e.g. haloperidol) (Seitz & Gill, 2009) and with high doses or increased doses of an antipsychotic within the previous 5 days, and the use of two or more antipsychotics or depot injections of haloperidol. In addition, other risk factors include young, male, genetic predisposition, pre-existing brain disorder, dehydration and psychiatric comorbidity (Murray et al., 2015).

It is characterised as changes in altered consciousness, delirium, confusion and autonomic changes that include high fever (>38 °C), excessive sweating, muscle or lead pipe rigidity (elevated creatinine kinase [CK] levels), tremor, tachypnoea, autonomic instability (hypertension, tachycardia) and often an elevated WBC, and the condition can progress rapidly within 24 to 72 hours or it can be slower and insidious taking several days (Corbett & Wilson, 2018). Fatalities range from 5% to 20% of presentations, and severity indicators surround muscle rigidity; as muscle breaks down it releases CK, which in severe cases accumulates causing rhabdomyolysis and subsequent kidney failure (Corbett & Wilson, 2018). Severe hyperthermia can also cause multi-organ system failure (see Table 18.6).

Table 18.6 Drug-Induced Extrapyramidal Syndrome Presentations

Condition	Drugs	Onset	Neuromuscular Tone	Reflexes	Pupils	Autonomic	Skin	Mental Status
Anticholinergic syndrome	FGAs Antimuscrinics Antihistamines TCAs	Rapid <12 hours	Tremor Myoclonus	Normal	Dilated	HR↑ Flushing Dry mouth Urinary retention	Hot, red, dry	Confusion Agitation Delirium Mumbling Coma
Malignant catatonia	Antipsychotic Induced Levetiracetam, levofloxacin rimonabant	Rapid Hours to days	Rigidity Grimacing Cataplexy loss of tone Waxy flexibility	Bradyreflexia	Normal	HR↑ RR↑ Fever	Sweaty	Delirium Agitation Stupor Mutism
Dystonic	Antipsychotic Antiemetics Valproate Rivastigmine tetrabenazine	Rapid Acute: hours Subacute: days	Rigidity Abnormal posturing	Normal	Normal (exception oculogyric crisis)	Normal	Normal	Normal
Encephalitis/ Meningitis	Infection; Bacterial Viral	1–7 days	Nuchal rigidity Kernig sign Focal neurological deficits	Hyperreflexia	Photophobia	Headache Fever NV shock	Rash Mottled	Seizure Altered conscious state Behavioural changes Disorientation

Continued

Table 18.6 Drug-Induced Extrapyramidal Syndrome Presentations *Continued*

Condition	Drugs	Onset	Neuromuscular Tone	Reflexes	Pupils	Autonomic	Skin	Mental Status
Malignant hyperthermia	Halogenated anaesthetics, Depolarising neuromuscular blocking drugs	Rapid minutes to 24 hours Genetic basis	Muscle contracture	Hyporeflexia	Normal	Fever	Sweaty Mottled	Agitation
Neuromuscular malignant syndrome	Dopamine antagonist Withdrawal of Dopamine agonist	Insidious Progressive 1–3 days or longer	Lead-pipe Rigidity	Bradyreflexia	Dilated or normal	HR↑ BP↑ RR↑ Fever	Sweaty Pale	Confusion Delirium Mutism Staring Coma
Serotonin syndrome	Serotonin agonist SSRI SNRI TCA	Rapid <12 hours	Increased tone (especially in lower limbs)	Hyperreflexia and clonus	Dilated	HR↑ BP↑ Fever Diarrhoea	Sweaty	Anxiety Agitation Confusion Progress to coma
Sympathomimetic syndrome	Adrenaline dopamine Pseudoephedrine Ephedra, Ma-Huang Amphetamines Caffeine, theophylline Moclobemide SNRIs	Rapid <2 hours	Tremor	Hyperreflexia	Dilated	HR ↑ BP ↑ Fever	Sweaty Flushing Pallor	Excitation Euphoria Agitation Delirium Seizures

Adapted from: Caroff & Campbell, 2016; Fink & Taylor, 2009; Fowler, 2019; McGill et al., 2016; Murray et al., 2015

NMS diagnosis is based on good history taking, clinical assessment and differentiation from other diagnoses, such as anticholinergic syndrome, catatonia, dystonia, encephalitis, malignant hyperthermia, meningitis, serotonin syndrome, sympathomimetic syndrome and others (Corbett & Wilson, 2018; Murray et al., 2015).

NMS is managed with resuscitation, correction of abnormalities (hyperthermia, hypoglycaemia), and benzodiazepines for muscle relaxation and controlling delirium in mild to moderate presentations. In severe forms, reversal agents, such as dopamine agonists, dantrolene or electroconvulsive therapy (ECT) are used (Caroff & Campbell, 2016; Corbett & Wilson, 2018; Murray et al., 2015).

CONCLUSION: PRE-HOSPITAL CONSIDERATIONS

A comprehensive assessment of therapy and consideration to potential issues impacting patient management is needed for all patient presentations. Evaluation for potential toxicities, adverse effects, drug–drug interactions from both prescription and non-prescription medicines or other substances, including delayed responses or causal relationship, all need to be identified. In addition, patient characteristics – hydration status, medication adherence, dosage, comorbidities and age-related changes to pharmacokinetic and pharmacodynamic aspects – must also be accounted for in the management of patient presentations with mental health and associated psychopharmacological therapies.

LINKS AND RESOURCES

Australian Bureau of Statistics: http://www.abs.gov.au/ausstats/abs@.nsf/Lookup/by%20Subject/3303.0~2016~Main%20Features~Drug%20Induced%20Deaths%20in%20Australia~6

https://www.abs.gov.au/AUSSTATS/abs@.nsf/Lookup/4326.0Main+Features32007?OpenDocument

http://www.abs.gov.au/ausstats/abs@.nsf/Lookup/by%20Subject/4364.0.55.001~2014-15~Main%20Features~Mental%20and%20behavioural%20conditions~32

Australian Institute of Health and Welfare (AIHW) reports: https://www.aihw.gov.au/reports/australias-health/australias-health-2016/contents/summary

Cytochrome P450 table: https://drug-interactions.medicine.iu.edu/MainTable.aspx

REFERENCES

Airagnes, G., Pelissolo, A., Lavallée, M., et al., 2016. Benzodiazepine misuse in the elderly: risk factors, consequences, and management. Curr. Psychiatry Rep. 18 (10), 89.

Alda, M., 2015. Lithium in the treatment of bipolar disorder: pharmacology and pharmacogenetics. Mol. Psychiatry 20 (6), 661–670.

Anderson, J., Mitchell, P.B., Brodaty, H., 2017. Suicidality: prevention, detection and intervention. Aust. Prescr. 40 (5), 162–166.

Apaydin, E.A., Maher, A.R., Shanman, R., et al., 2016. A systematic review of St. John's wort for major depressive disorder. Syst. Rev. 5 (1), 148.

Aronson, J.K., 2015. Meyler's Side Effects of Drugs: The International Encyclopedia of Adverse Drug Reactions and Interactions, sixteenth ed. Elsevier, Oxford.

Atkin, K., Kendall, F., Gould, D., et al., 1996. Neutropenia and agranulocytosis in patients receiving clozapine in the UK and Ireland. Br. J. Psychiatry 169 (4), 483–488.

Australian Bureau of Statistics (ABS), 2016. Causes of Death, Australia, 2015. Australian Bureau of Statistics, Canberra. Online. Available: https://www.abs.gov.au/ausstats/abs@.nsf/Lookup/by%20Subject/3303.0~2016~Main%20Features~Drug%20Induced%20Deaths%20in%20Australia~6.

Baird-Gunning, J., Lea-Henry, T., Hoegberg, L.C.G., et al., 2016. Lithium poisoning. J. Intensive Care Med. 32 (4), 249–263.

Bech, P., Cialdella, P., Haugh, M., et al., 2000. Meta-analysis of randomised controlled trials of fluoxetine v. placebo and tricyclic antidepressants in the short-term treatment of major depression. Br. J. Psychiatry 176 (5), 421–428.

Bighelli, I., 2018. Antidepressants versus placebo for panic disorder in adults. Cochrane Database Syst. Rev. (4), CD010676.

Bird, V., Premkumar, P., Kendall, T., et al., 2010. Early intervention services, cognitive–behavioural therapy and family intervention in early psychosis: systematic review. Br. J. Psychiatry 197 (5), 350–356.

Boyer, E.W., Shannon, M., 2005. The serotonin syndrome. N. Engl. J. Med. 352 (11), 1112–1120.

Brett, J., Murnion, B., 2015. Management of benzodiazepine misuse and dependence. Aust. Prescr. 38 (5), 152–155.

Buckley, N., Dawson, A., Whyte, I., et al., 1995. Relative toxicity of benzodiazepines in overdose. BJM 310 (6974), 219–221.

Buckley, N.A., Dawson, A., White, I., et al., 1994. Greater toxicity in overdose of dothiepin than of other tricyclic antidepressants. Lancet 343 (8890), 159–162.

Buckley, N.A., Dawson, A.H., Isbister, G.K., 2014. Serotonin syndrome. BMJ 348 (1626), 10–1136.

Carlsson, A., Lindqvist, M., 1963. Effect of chlorpromazine or haloperidol on formation of 3-methoxytyramine and normetanephrine in mouse brain. Acta Pharmacol. Toxicol. (Copenh.) 20 (2), 140–144.

Caroff, S.N., Campbell, E.C., 2016. Drug-induced extrapyramidal syndromes: implications for contemporary practice. Psychiatr. Clin. North Am. 39 (3), 391–411.

Chambers, R.A., Krystal, J.H., Self, D.W., 2001. A neurobiological basis for substance abuse comorbidity in schizophrenia. Biol. Psychiatry 50 (2), 71–83.

Cipriani, A., Furukawa, T.A., Salanti, G., et al., 2009. Comparative efficacy and acceptability of 12 new-generation antidepressants: a multiple-treatments meta-analysis. Lancet 373 (9665), 746–758.

Colonna, L., Saleem, P., Dondey-Nouvel, L., et al., 2000. Long-term safety and efficacy of amisulpride in subchronic or chronic schizophrenia. Amisulpride Study Group. Int. Clin. Psychopharmacol. 15 (1), 13–22.

Corbett, B., Wilson, M.P., 2018. Neuroleptic malignant syndrome. In: Nordstrom, K.D., Wilson, M.P. (Eds.), Quick Guide to Psychiatric Emergencies: Tools for Behavioral and Toxicological Situations. Springer, Cham, pp. 259–264.

Coyle, J.T., 2006. Glutamate and schizophrenia: beyond the dopamine hypothesis. Cell. Mol. Neurobiol. 26 (4–6), 363–382.

Crockford, D., Addington, D., 2017. Canadian schizophrenia guidelines: schizophrenia and other psychotic disorders with coexisting substance use disorders. Can. J. Psychiatry 62 (9), 624–634.

Davis, K.L., Kahn, R.S., 1991. Dopamine in schizophrenia: a review and reconceptualization. Am. J. Psychiatry 148 (11), 1474–1486.

Davis, K.L., Stewart, D.G., Friedman, J.I., et al., 2003. White matter changes in schizophrenia: evidence for myelin-related dysfunction. Arch. Gen. Psychiatry 60 (5), 443–456.

Davydov, L., Botts, S.R., 2000. Clozapine-induced hypersalivation. Ann. Pharmacother. 34 (5), 662–665.

Dayalu, P., Chou, K.L., 2008. Antipsychotic-induced extrapyramidal symptoms and their management. Expert Opin. Pharmacother. 9 (9), 1451–1462.

De Kloet, E.R., Joëls, M., Holsboer, F., 2005. Stress and the brain: from adaptation to disease. Nat. Rev. Neurosci. 6 (6), 463–475.

Elkis, H., Buckley, P.F., 2016. Treatment-resistant schizophrenia. Psychiatr. Clin. North Am. 39 (2), 239–265.

Fava, G.A., Offidani, E., 2011. The mechanisms of tolerance in antidepressant action. Prog. Neuro-Psychopharmacol. Biol. Psychiatry 35 (7), 1593–1602.

Fink, M., Taylor, M.A., 2009. The catatonia syndrome: forgotten but not gone. Arch. Gen. Psychiatry 66 (11), 1173–1177.

Fowler, P.R., 2019. eTG complete, the complete Therapeutic Guidelines in electronic format. Online. Available: https://tgldcdp.tg.org.au/topicTeaser?guidelinePage=Psychotropic&etgAccess=true. 2 February 2020.

Geddes, J.R., Miklowitz, D.J., 2013. Treatment of bipolar disorder. Lancet 381 (9878), 1672–1682.

Geulayov, G., Ferrey, A., Casey, D., et al., 2018. Relative toxicity of benzodiazepines and hypnotics commonly used for self-poisoning: an epidemiological study of fatal toxicity and case fatality. J. Psychopharmacol. 32 (6), 654–662.

Gillman, P., 2007. Tricyclic antidepressant pharmacology and therapeutic drug interactions updated. Br. J. Pharmacol. 151 (6), 737–748.

Gravielle, M.C., 2016. Activation-induced regulation of GABAA receptors: is there a link with the molecular basis of benzodiazepine tolerance? Pharmacol. Res. 109, 92–100.

Greiner, A.C., Berry, K., 1964. Skin pigmentation and corneal and lens opacities with prolonged chlorpromazine therapy. Can. Med. Assoc. J. 90 (11), 663–665.

Hall, M., Buckley, N., 2003. Serotonin syndrome. Aust. Prescr. 26 (3).

Hamad, A.E., Al-Ghadban, A., Carvounis, C.P., et al., 2000. Predicting the need for medical intensive care monitoring in drug-overdosed patients. J. Intensive Care Med. 15 (6), 321–328.

Hartling, L., Abou-Setta, A.M., Dursun, S., et al., 2012. Antipsychotics in adults with schizophrenia: comparative effectiveness of first-generation versus second-generation medications: a systematic review and meta-analysis. Ann. Intern. Med. 157 (7), 498–511.

Hashimoto, K., Sawa, A., Iyo, M., 2007. Increased levels of glutamate in brains from patients with mood disorders. Biol. Psychiatry 62 (11), 1310–1316.

Hegarty, J.D., Baldessarini, R.J., Tohen, M., et al., 1994. One hundred years of schizophrenia: a meta-analysis of the outcome literature. Am. J. Psychiatry 151 (10), 1409–1416.

Hopkins, K., Crosland, P., Elliott, N., et al., 2015. Diagnosis and Management of Depression in Children and Young People: Summary of Updated NICE Guidance, vol. 350. p. h824.

Howes, O.D., Kambeitz, J., Kim, E., et al., 2012. The nature of dopamine dysfunction in schizophrenia and what this means for treatment: meta-analysis of imaging studies. Arch. Gen. Psychiatry 69 (8), 776–786.

Howes, O.D., McCutcheon, R., Agid, O., et al., 2016. Treatment-resistant schizophrenia: Treatment Response and Resistance in Psychosis (TRRIP) working group consensus guidelines on diagnosis and terminology. Am. J. Psychiatry 174 (3), 216–229.

Huynh, A., Cairns, R., Brown, J.A., et al., 2018. Patterns of poisoning exposure at different ages: the 2015 annual report of the Australian Poison Information Centres. Med. J. Aust. 209 (2), 74–79.

Iasevoli, F., D'Ambrosio, L., Francesco, D.N., et al., 2018. Clinical evaluation of functional capacity in treatment resistant schizophrenia patients: comparison and differences with non-resistant schizophrenia patients. Schizophr. Res. 202, 217–225.

Isbister, G.K., Balit, C.R., Macleod, D., et al., 2010. Amisulpride overdose is frequently associated with QT prolongation and torsades de pointes. J. Clin. Psychopharmacol. 30 (4), 391–395.

Jones, C.M., Mack, K.A., Paulozzi, L.J., 2013. Pharmaceutical overdose deaths, United States, 2010. JAMA 309 (7), 657–659.

Jones, C.M., Paulozzi, L.J., Mack, K.A., 2014. Alcohol involvement in opioid pain reliever and benzodiazepine drug abuse-related emergency department visits and drug-related deaths – United States, 2010. MMWR Morb. Mortal. Wkly. Rep. 63 (40), 881–885.

Kennedy, S.H., Lam, R.W., McIntyre, R.S., et al., 2016. Canadian Network for Mood and Anxiety Treatments (CANMAT) 2016 clinical guidelines for the management of adults with major depressive disorder: section 3, pharmacological treatments. Can. J. Psychiatry 61 (9), 540–560.

Kerr, G., McGuffie, A., Wilkie, S., 2001. Tricyclic antidepressant overdose: a review. Emerg. Med. J. 18 (4), 236–241.

Khorassani, F., Kaufman, M., Lopez, L.V., 2018. Supatherapeutic serum clozapine concentration after transition from traditional to electronic cigarettes. J. Clin. Psychopharmacol. 38 (4), 391–392.

Kring, A.M., Moran, E.K., 2008. Emotional response deficits in schizophrenia: insights from affective science. Schizophr. Bull. 34 (5), 819–834.

Küçükibrahimoğlu, E., Saygın, M.Z., Çalışkan, M., et al., 2009. The change in plasma GABA, glutamine and glutamate levels in fluoxetine-or S-citalopram-treated female patients with major depression. Eur. J. Clin. Pharmacol. 65 (6), 571–577.

Laruelle, M., Abi-Dargham, A., 1999. Dopamine as the wind of the psychotic fire: new evidence from brain imaging studies. J. Psychopharmacol. 13 (4), 358–371.

Latif, Z., Jabbar, F., Kelly, B.D., 2011. Clozapine and blood dyscrasia. Psychiatrist 35 (1), 27–29.

Leucht, S., Cipriani, A., Spineli, L., et al., 2013. Comparative efficacy and tolerability of 15 antipsychotic drugs in schizophrenia: a multiple-treatments meta-analysis. Lancet 382 (9896), 951–962.

Leucht, S., Corves, C., Arbter, D., et al., 2009. Second-generation versus first-generation antipsychotic drugs for schizophrenia: a meta-analysis. Lancet 373 (9657), 31–41.

Lieberman, J., Kane, J., Alvir, J., 1987. Provocative tests with psychostimulant drugs in schizophrenia. Psychopharmacology (Berl) 91 (4), 415–433.

Lieberman, J.A., Stroup, T.S., Perkins, D.O., 2006. Textbook of Schizophrenia. American Psychiatric Publishing, London.

Liu, B., Liu, J., Wang, M., et al., 2017. From serotonin to neuroplasticity: evolvement of theories for major depressive disorder, Review. Front. Cell. Neurosci. 11, 305.

López-Muñoz, F., Alamo, C., Cuenca, E., et al., 2005. History of the discovery and clinical introduction of chlorpromazine. Ann. Clin. Psychiatry 17 (3), 113–135.

May, R., Al-Taie, A., Garg, V., 2016. Acute laryngeal dystonia: a persisting psychiatric emergency. Australas. Psychiatry 24 (5), 497–498.

McGill, F., Heyderman, R., Michael, B., et al., 2016. The UK joint specialist societies guideline on the diagnosis and management of acute meningitis and meningococcal sepsis in immunocompetent adults. J. Infect. 72 (4), 405–438.

McGlashan, T.H., Fenton, W.S., 1992. The positive-negative distinction in schizophrenia: review of natural history validators. Arch. Gen. Psychiatry 49 (1), 63–72.

Milhorn, H.T., 2018. Sedative-hypnotic dependence. In: Milhorn, H.T. (Ed.), Substance Use Disorders. Springer, Cham, Switzerland, pp. 59–76.

Miyamoto, S., Duncan, G.E., Goff, D.C., et al., 2002. Therapeutics of schizophrenia. In: Davis, K.L., Charney, D., Coyle, J.T., et al. (Eds.), Neuropsychopharmacology: The Fifth Generation of Progress. Lippincott Williams & Wilkins, Philadelphia, pp. 775–807.

Miyamoto, S., Duncan, G.E., Marx, C., et al., 2005. Treatments for schizophrenia: a critical review of pharmacology and mechanisms of action of antipsychotic drugs. Mol. Psychiatry 10 (1), 79–104.

Montejo, Á.L., Arango, C., Bernardo, M., et al., 2017. Multidisciplinary consensus on the therapeutic recommendations for iatrogenic hyperprolactinemia secondary to antipsychotics. Front. Neuroendocrinol. 45, 25–34.

Morgan, V.A., Waterreus, A., Jablensky, A., et al., 2012. People living with psychotic illness in 2010: the second Australian national survey of psychosis. Aust. N. Z. J. Psychiatry 46 (8), 735–752.

Murray, L., Little, M., Pascu, O., et al., 2015. Toxicology Handbook, third ed. Elsevier Australia, Chatswood.

Olfson, M., Mojtabai, R., Merikangas, K., et al., 2017. Reexamining associations between mania, depression, anxiety and substance use disorders: results from a prospective national cohort. Mol. Psychiatry 22 (2), 235–241.

Oyewole, A., Adelufosi, A., Abayomi, O., 2013. Acute dystonic reaction as medical emergency: a report of two cases. Ann. Med. Health Sci. Res. 3 (3), 453–455.

Pagliaccio, D., Luby, J.L., Bogdan, R., et al., 2015. Amygdala functional connectivity, HPA axis genetic variation, and life stress in children and relations to anxiety and emotion regulation. J. Abnorm. Psychol. 124 (4), 817–833.

Papola, D., Ostuzzi, G., Thabane, L., et al., 2018. Antipsychotic drug exposure and risk of fracture: a systematic review and meta-analysis of observational studies. Int. Clin. Psychopharmacol. 33 (4), 181–196.

Park, T.W., Saitz, R., Ganoczy, D., et al., 2015. Benzodiazepine prescribing patterns and deaths from drug overdose among US veterans receiving opioid analgesics: case-cohort study. BMJ 350, h2698.

Penninga, E.I., Graudal, N., Ladekarl, M.B., et al., 2016. Adverse events associated with flumazenil treatment for the management of suspected benzodiazepine intoxication – a systematic review with meta-analyses of randomised trials. Basic Clin. Pharmacol. Toxicol. 118 (1), 37–44.

Reinhold, J.A., Rickels, K., 2015. Pharmacological treatment for generalized anxiety disorder in adults: an update. Expert Opin. Pharmacother. 16 (11), 1669–1681.

Risch, N., Herrell, R., Lehner, T., et al., 2009. Interaction between the serotonin transporter gene (5-HTTLPR), stressful life events, and risk of depression: a meta-analysis. JAMA 301 (23), 2462–2471.

Riss, J., Cloyd, J., Gates, J., et al., 2008. Benzodiazepines in epilepsy: pharmacology and pharmacokinetics. Acta Neurol. Scand. 118 (2), 69–86.

Rosmond, R., Björntorp, P., 2000. The hypothalamic–pituitary–adrenal axis activity as a predictor of cardiovascular disease, type 2 diabetes and stroke. J. Intern. Med. 247 (2), 188–197.

Rossat, J., Maillard, M., Nussberger, J., et al., 1999. Renal effects of selective cyclooxygenase-2 inhibition in normotensive salt-depleted subjects. Clin. Pharmacol. Ther. 66 (1), 76–84.

Rossi, S. (Ed.), 2019. Australian Medicines Handbook 2019, twentieth ed. Australian Medicines Handbook, Adelaide.

Sanacora, G., Treccani, G., Popoli, M., 2012. Towards a glutamate hypothesis of depression: an emerging frontier of neuropsychopharmacology for mood disorders. Neuropharmacology 62 (1), 63–77.

Sanchez, C., Asin, K.E., Artigas, F., 2015. Vortioxetine, a novel antidepressant with multimodal activity: review of preclinical and clinical data. Pharmacol. Ther. 145, 43–57.

Sansom, L. (Ed.), 2018. Australian Pharmaceutical Formulary and Handbook, twenty-fourth ed. Pharmaceutical Society of Australia, Canberra.

Schildkraut, J.J., 1965. The catecholamine hypothesis of affective disorders: a review of supporting evidence. Am. J. Psychiatry 122 (5), 509–522.

Schmidt, C.J., Sorensen, S.M., Kenne, J.H., et al., 1995. The role of 5-HT2A receptors in antipsychotic activity. Life Sci. 56 (25), 2209–2222.

Seeman, P., 2002. Atypical antipsychotics: mechanism of action. Can. J. Psychiatry 47 (1), 29–40.

Seitz, D.P., Gill, S.S., 2009. Neuroleptic malignant syndrome complicating antipsychotic treatment of delirium or agitation in medical and surgical patients: case reports and a review of the literature. Psychosomatics 50 (1), 8–15.

Shapiro, D.A., Renock, S., Arrington, E., et al., 2003. Aripiprazole, a novel atypical antipsychotic drug with a unique and robust pharmacology. Neuropsychopharmacology 28 (8), 1400–1411.

Shivakumar, K., Amanullah, S., Shivakumar, R., et al., 2018. The role of clozapine in treatment-resistant schizophrenia. In: Shivakumar, K., Amanullah, S. (Eds.), Complex Clinical Conundrums in Psychiatry. Springer, Cham, pp. 115–122.

Sigel, E., Ernst, M., 2018. The benzodiazepine binding sites of GABAA receptors. Trends Pharmacol. Sci. 37 (7), 659–671.

Solmi, M., Pigato, G., Kane, J.M., et al., 2018. Clinical risk factors for the development of tardive dyskinesia. J. Neurol. Sci. 389, 21–27.

Stahl, S.M., 2013. Stahl's Essential Psychopharmacology: Neuroscientific Basis and Practical Applications, fourth ed. Cambridge University Press, Cambridge.

Stone, J.M., Davis, J.M., Leucht, S., et al., 2009. Cortical dopamine D2/D3 receptors are a common site of action for antipsychotic drugs – an original patient data meta-analysis of the SPECT and PET in vivo receptor imaging literature. Schizophr. Bull. 35 (4), 789–797.

Suzuki, T., Mihara, K., Nakamura, A., et al., 2014. Effects of genetic polymorphisms of CYP2D6, CYP3A5, and ABCB1 on the steady-state plasma concentrations of aripiprazole and its active metabolite, dehydroaripiprazole, in Japanese patients with schizophrenia. Ther. Drug Monit. 36 (5), 651–655.

Tsuda, Y., Saruwatari, J., Yasui-Furukori, N., 2014. Meta-analysis: the effects of smoking on the disposition of two commonly used antipsychotic agents, olanzapine and clozapine. BMJ Open 4 (3), e004216.

Van Tol, H.H., Bunzow, J.R., Guan, H.C., et al., 1991. Cloning of the gene for a human dopamine D4 receptor with high affinity for the antipsychotic clozapine. Nature 350 (6319), 610–614.

Wang, S.M., Han, C., Bahk, W.M., et al., 2018. Addressing the side effects of contemporary antidepressant drugs: a comprehensive review. Chonnam Med. J. 54 (2), 101–112.

Woolley, D.W., Shaw, E., 1954. A biochemical and pharmacological suggestion about certain mental disorders. Proc. Natl. Acad. Sci. USA 40 (4), 228–231.

Zastrozhin, M.S., Brodyansky, V.M., Skryabin, V.Y., et al., 2017. Pharmacodynamic genetic polymorphisms affect adverse drug reactions of haloperidol in patients with alcohol-use disorder. Pharmgenomics Pers. Med. 10, 209–215.

Zhang, H., Li, L., Wu, M., et al., 2016. Brain gray matter alterations in first episodes of depression: a meta-analysis of whole-brain studies. Neurosci. Biobehav. Rev. 60, 43–50.

Glossary

Acceptance and commitment therapy (ACT) Focuses on helping individuals to behave more consistently with their own values, and to be able to apply mindfulness and acceptance skills to responses to uncontrollable experiences.

Active and reflective listening A way of engaging with another person's verbal and non-verbal communication and cues. Involves listening with full concentration, and includes micro skills such as paraphrasing, summarising and clarifying.

Addiction No longer considered a medical term because of critical or judgmental connotations, it has been replaced by 'substance dependence' or 'substance use disorder' (severe).

Affect The outward or observable expression of feeling or emotion.

Affect regulation The ability of an individual to modulate their emotional or feeling state in order to adaptively meet the demands of their environment.

Ageism Prejudicial attitudes towards a group of people in a certain age group.

Aggression An act or a threat to commit an act that is intended to cause harm to another person.

Alcoholism Not a medical term, it is used by the public to describe the state of alcohol dependence.

Anhedonia An inability to feel pleasure in normally pleasurable activities.

Antipsychotics A group of medications shown to be effective in managing psychotic symptoms and acute agitation. Can be used both short and long term, depending on the presentation of symptoms and underlying psychotic disorder.

Anxiety disorders Conditions in which intense feelings of apprehension are long-standing and disruptive. For example, generalised anxiety disorder and panic disorder.

Arousal The physiological and psychological state of being awoken or reactive to stimuli.

Assertiveness In a paramedic context, this entails displaying high levels of empathy while setting limits on the behaviour presented to you.

Attachment theory The idea that children form a close bond and attachment to their earliest caregivers, and that this attachment pattern may influence aspects of the child's later life.

Automatic negative thoughts (ANTs) Exaggerated or unhelpful thoughts individuals have about themselves, others, their future or the world around them that can predispose them to interpret situations in a way that fits their perspective, as opposed to changing their perspective to fit the situation.

Avoidance The act of staying away from stressors rather than dealing with them.

Biopsychosocial An interdisciplinary approach that considers the interconnection between biological, psychological and socio-environmental factors.

Bipolar disorders Affective disorders in which a person alternates between the emotional extremes of mania and depression.

Burnout A state of emotional, physical, psychological and behavioural exhaustion in response to exposure to prolonged stress.

Capacity The ability of a person to understand the nature, purpose and consequences of a decision. See also: competence.

Categorical model of personality Aims to define 'types' of personalities by clusters of characteristics that often occur together, rather than the expression of specific traits.

Challenging behaviour An umbrella term which encompasses a range of behaviours which may include violence, sexual disinhibition, self-harm and manipulative, high-need or demanding behaviour (Brunero & Lamont, 2016).

Chronic conditions Long-lasting conditions with persistent effects; for example, cancer, diabetes and heart disease.

Classical conditioning A procedure in which a neutral stimulus is repeatedly paired with a stimulus that elicits a reflex or other response until the neutral stimulus alone comes to elicit a similar response.

Clinical recovery Synonymous with cure, it refers to the resolution of mental health problems and experiences regarded diagnostically as symptoms (for example, auditory hallucinations), and a resumption of the life led prior.

Closed-ended questions Questions that elicit very short or single-word responses. Useful for clarifying specific points. For example, 'It sounds like you are feeling horrible at the moment, are you thinking about harming or killing yourself?'

Cognitive The mental process of comprehension, judgment, memory and reason; in contrast to emotional and behavioural processes.

Cognitive behavioural therapy (CBT) Looks at problem solving the present reality rather than the past, with an emphasis on personal responsibility and unhelpful thoughts and behaviours. Involves the identification and challenging of negative thoughts to modify behaviour.

Cognitive impairment Loss of memory or attentiveness, and confusion or difficulty with comprehension and recall. The individual may have difficulty with learning new things, concentrating or making decisions that affect their daily life.

Collateral history Gathering information about an individual from other sources; for example, friends and family, old reports from school or the general practitioner.

Community mental healthcare Mental healthcare provided by both government and non-government organisations in various community- and hospital-based ambulatory services; for example, outpatient and day clinics.

Comorbidities The coexistence of two or more illnesses in the same individual.

Competence Building on 'capacity', it is the ability to form action and translate understanding into practice.

Complex developmental trauma Exposure to multiple traumatic events – often of an invasive, interpersonal nature – and the wide-ranging, long-term effects of this across key components of young people's development.

Compulsions Repetitive behaviours that interfere with an individual's daily functioning, but are repeated in an attempt to prevent dangers, risks or events associated with an obsession.

Consumer Used to refer to those receiving mental health services. The term was adopted to empower people experiencing mental health problems and support their agency in terms of their treatment by mental health services. Adopted widely in government policy, the term is rejected by many with a lived experience as misrepresenting their lived experience of disempowerment.

Controlled breathing An umbrella term that includes a number of systematic breathing techniques that can be used to focus attention on drawing air into and expelling air out of the body to reduce anxiety or panic. For example, counting breaths, inhaling and exhaling for a certain amount of time, or deep abdominal breathing.

Coping mechanisms An individual's usual means of dealing with stress or trauma.

Crisis When a stressor overwhelms a person's capacity to cope.

Cultural safety A place or environment where a person's cultural needs are respected and acknowledged.

Culture Shared social norms, values, everyday practices and beliefs.

De-escalation The active adoption of a range of psychosocial techniques, with an aim to reduce disruptive or aggressive behaviour (NICE, 2005). Aligns with the philosophy of person-centred care using the least restrictive means available. Also referred to as 'talking down', defusion or diffusion.

Defensive behaviour An instinctive and protective trait that is activated when an individual perceives a threat.

Delirium A transient organic psychiatric syndrome characterised by acute onset, fluctuating course, altered level of consciousness, global impairment in cognition, perception and memory, and widespread derangement of cerebral metabolism and behaviour. Also referred to as metabolic encephalopathy, acute confusional state and toxic psychosis.

Delusions False beliefs, based on incorrect inference about external reality. Firmly held despite contradictory evidence or proof (Sadock et al., 2015).

Dementia Covers a variety of disorders that lead to deterioration in brain function. For example, Alzheimer's disease, vascular dementia and dementia with Lewy bodies.

Diagnostic and Statistical Manual of Mental Disorders, **Fifth Edition (*DSM-V*)** A reference work published by the American Psychiatric Association that provides guidelines and criteria for diagnosing and classifying mental disorders. Currently on the fifth edition.

Dialectical behaviour therapy (DBT) Built on the principles of CBT, dialectical philosophy and mindfulness. Focuses on helping individuals find a balance between acceptance and change, and finding a life worth living.

Discrimination Behaviours or actions that are unfavourable towards and actively exclude a targeted individual or group.

Dysthymia Chronic depressed mood, with persistent mild symptoms of depression.

Early remission When an individual has stopped or reduced their substance use intake, and the criteria for 'abuse' would no longer be met, for a period of between 3 and 12 months.

Eating disorders Severe and persistent disturbance in eating, and associated distressing thoughts and behaviours in relation to food and body image; for example, anorexia nervosa, binge eating disorder and bulimia nervosa.

Electroconvulsive therapy (ECT) The induction of a seizure under controlled conditions and under anaesthesia. Done via the application of a gentle electrical current to the cranium.

Emergency A life-threatening or imminently harmful situation requiring an immediate response to protect the health of a patient or others.

Emotional lability Instability of emotional experiences and mood.

Empathy The ability to tune into a patient's inner experience and emotions, and attempt to create connection by demonstrating curiosity about them and their subjective experience.

Family and systemic therapy (FT) Aims to explore and resolve conflict within the family unit. The emphasis of the therapy is not on any particular individual within the family, but rather on the family structure as a whole by examining the interacting dynamics of family members and situations.

Grounding A technique to de-escalate individuals who are overwhelmed by what may be happening to them, by encouraging them to 'slow down', ground themselves and reorientate their focus back to the present moment.

Hallucinations False sensory perception, whereby individuals perceive voices or other stimuli when no stimuli are present.

Holistic healthcare Support that looks at the whole person – including their physical, emotional, social and spiritual wellbeing – not just their mental health needs.

Impairment Any loss or abnormality of psychological, physiological or anatomical structure of function.

Intentional and suicidal self-harm (ISSH) Deliberate physical harm to oneself, but not necessarily with the intention of dying.

Interpersonal therapy (IPT) Time-limited therapy that aims to relieve symptoms of distress and improve interpersonal functioning in individuals who are depressed and/or suffering problems with relationships or significant life changes.

Lived experience In the field of mental health, it refers to people's accounts of their own mental health problems and knowledge of treatments, interventions and the consequences of this. Increasingly, the experience of living with mental health problems is regarded as a source of particular expertise.

Mandatory notification Alerting a governing body about concerns that a health practitioner may be putting public safety at risk.

Means restriction Minimising a suicidal person's access to lethal means of suicide.

Melancholic depression Characterised by the presence of multiple neurovegetative features and psychological symptoms of depression. Also referred to as 'biological' or 'endogenous' depression.

Mental disorder Significant impairment of an individual's cognitive, affective and/or relational abilities that may require intervention and may be a recognised, medically diagnosed illness or disorder.

Mental health An integrated state of physical, emotional, psychological and social well-being. Individuals are able to realise their own abilities, cope with the normal stresses of life, work productively and are able to make a contribution to their community.

Mental health assessment Focuses on an individual's emotional and cognitive state, how they are interacting and behaving within their environment and with others, how they view their circumstances, their thought patterns, flow and content at that time, how they view their mental state, and their ability to make decisions regarding their actions and care needs.

Mental health carers People who voluntarily provide support and assistance to those with mental ill-health.

Mental illness A condition or medical condition that severely affects, impairs or disturbs a person's thoughts, mood, perception, behaviour, cognition, memory and ability to function.

Mentalisation-based treatment (MBT) Therapeutic approach designed to treat people with borderline personality disorder (BPD) by helping people to separate their own thoughts and feelings from those around them. Focuses on creating a well-managed attachment relationship between an individual and a therapist to stabilise their emotional expression, allow them to consider internal representations and reinstate lost mentalisation.

Microaggression Everyday slights, indignities, put-downs and insults that members of marginalised groups experience in day-to-day interactions with individuals who are often unaware that they have engaged in an offensive or demeaning way.

Micro-skills Subtle verbal and non-verbal action used to help develop rapport and elicit information. For example, phrases to show active listening (e.g. 'mmm', 'okay', 'aha' or 'yes').

Mindfulness-based cognitive therapy (MBCT) Theory-driven therapeutic approach developed to prevent the relapse and recurrence of major depression. MBCT emphasises mindfulness meditation as the primary therapeutic approach (APS, 2018), and in doing so encourages individuals to see emotions and cognitions as merely 'mental events' – as opposed to aspects of the self or accurate reflections of reality.

Mobility The ability to move or be moved.

Modifiable risks Risk factors that influence health, and that individuals can take measures to change; for example, high alcohol use.

Mood Subjective experience of emotion as reported by an individual.

Mood disorders Conditions that disturb an individual's mood to the point that it interferes with their ability to function; for example, depression and bipolar disorder. Also referred to as affective disorders.

Motivational interviewing (MI) A directive, client-centred communication approach that enhances an individual's reasons to change by exploring and helping them to resolve ambivalence.

Neurocognitive disorders Reduced mental function due to a medical disease other than a psychiatric illness. Involves impairments in cognitive abilities such as memory, problem-solving and perception.

Neurodevelopmental disorders Characterised by developmental deficits that produce impairments in personal, social, academic or occupational functioning. For example, intellectual disability, communication disorders and autism spectrum disorders (ASD).

Non-suicidal self-injury (NSSI) Deliberate, self-inflicted injuries without suicidal intent; for example, cutting and scratching.

Non-verbal cues The transmission of messages or signals through non-verbal platforms; for example, gestures, posture, facial expression and spatial distance.

Normalising Assists individuals to realise that their distressing thoughts and erratic behaviours may just be the body's normal response to stressors; for example, the 'fight, flight or freeze' response.

Open-ended questions Questions that invite expanded expression. Useful when commencing assessment and for building rapport. For example, 'I see that what you're going through is very distressing … Can you tell me more about what has been happening for you?'

Paraverbal cues The messages that individuals transmit through the tone, pitch, volume and pacing of their voice.

Person-centred care Care that is centred on the needs, preferences, values and circumstances of the recipients. It ensures that those receiving healthcare are treated with dignity and respect.

Personal recovery An individual's journey to a self-reconciliation with the challenges and features of mental health problems and incorporation into that individual's new self-image. It does not require the resolution of the mental health problems, but rather reaching an accommodation with these problems such that the person's life is not defined by these problems alone.

Personality The pattern of psychological and behavioural qualities that form an individual's unique character.

Personality disorders Long-term and inflexible patterns of behaviour, thinking and emotion that lie outside the norm and cause significant distress and dysfunction; for example, borderline personality disorder, antisocial personality disorder and narcissistic personality disorder.

Positive reinforcement A therapy method that uses rewards to strengthen desirable behaviours and outcomes.

Protective factors Characteristics, attributes or conditions that occur at an individual, family, community or society level that buffer against risk in otherwise adverse circumstances; for example, engagement at school, supportive peers, self-understanding, positive peer connections.

Psychoanalytic therapy (PT) Positions psychological problems as stemming from the unconscious mind, and aims to help people understand how these are related. The focus in PT is on past experiences and emotions, with the assumption that people hold painful and distressing feelings, memories and experiences in their unconscious mind by using defensive mechanisms such as denial, repression and rationalisation.

Psychosis An altered mental state, with gross impairment in reality testing. Symptoms may include delusions, hallucinations, thought disorder or incoherent speech.

Psychotic depression Considered to be a particularly severe form of melancholic depression, or a similar depressive subtype. Frequently characterised by the same psychic and neurovegetative symptoms of depression, together in the presence of mood-congruent psychotic symptoms: delusions of guilt, poverty, persecution, worthlessness, punishment, inadequacy and nihilism.

Psychotropic A type of medication that affects mental functioning. These medications fall into four different categories: antipsychotics (also called major tranquillisers), antidepressants, mood stabilisers and minor tranquillisers.

Reasonable force Force that is proportionate to the exercise of the function.

Recovery A reworking of one's self-understanding to live a meaningful life with or without continuing mental health problems.

Recovery-orientated care Person-centred care that involves sensitivity to individuals' particular needs, preferences, safety, vulnerabilities and wellbeing. It recognises lived experience and empowers people to genuinely participate in decision making.

Reflective practice Commonly viewed as the process of learning through and from experience, of gaining new insights into yourself and your practice (Boud et al., 1985; Finlay, 2008). It often involves examining our assumptions of everyday practice, being self-aware and critically evaluating our own responses to practice situations (Finlay, 2008).

Resilience The ability to adjust to changes and secure positive outcomes.

Restrictive practice Limiting an individual's movement. In the paramedic context it can refer to physical, mechanical and/or chemical restraint. Restrictive practices should be used only as a last resort to prevent harm to self or others.

Reward circuit Areas of the brain involved with addictive drug effects. It is activated during intoxication and rewards the user with pleasant feelings.

Risk-taking Engagement in dangerous or potentially self-damaging activities, with limited or no regard to risk or consequences.

Safety planning A prioritised list of strategies and sources of support that people can use to alleviate a suicidal crisis. The fundamental aim is to help an individual in suicidal crisis live with being suicidal rather than die from being suicidal.

Self-care The practice of consciously undertaking acts to improve one's own physical, mental and emotional health; for example, exercise and mindfulness.

Self-determination An individual's ability to make decisions about themselves, for themselves.

Self-harm Refers to a range of behaviours an individual does to themselves to cause harm, regardless of motive or if there was suicidal intent.

Socratic questioning A questioning technique to guide individuals' thoughts from the 'concrete' (or what they perceive as absolute) to the 'possible', in order for them to generate a stronger problem-solving ability. For example, 'What do you mean by …?', and 'What would happen if …?'

Solution-focused brief therapy (SFBT) Seeks to explore an individual's own solutions to their problems, rather than focusing on the problems themselves. Achieves this by looking to the future and asking the individual what would be different in their life if a 'miracle' had occurred and steps had been taken to move towards their preferred future.

Somatisation The conversion of mental states or experiences into bodily symptoms, presenting as multiple physical complaints with no objective evidence of organic impairment.

Stereotypes A false assumption that all members of a group share the same characteristics or traits.

Stigma A discrediting attribute that reduces an individual or a group to undesirable characteristics.

Stress An essential and characteristic response to challenging or threatening situations that can affect the body's physical, mental or emotional wellbeing and homeostasis. Stress can be external (environmental, psychological, social) or internal (illness, medical situation). It can trigger the sympathetic arm of the autonomic nervous system, preparing the body for a fight, flight or freeze response. Chronic stress can lead to a range of medical issues, including mental ill-health.

Structural model of personality Relies on a theoretical basis of human development, and subsequent structure of personality and behaviour. Both psychoanalytic and cognitive behavioural theories approach personality in this way.

Substance abuse Not a diagnostic term, but is used as a description that applies to taking an illicit substance that has the potential to cause harm to the individual. Historically (*DSM-IV*) it was used to describe 12 months of harmful substance use that did not meet the criteria for substance dependence.

Substance dependence An ICD-11 diagnosis – characteristics include a strong drive to use the substance and impaired ability to control use, as well as increased priority given to the substance over other activities. There are often features of physiological dependence such as tolerance and withdrawals. Use continues despite harms, and the pattern has been present for at least 12 months, although in some situations it can arise in a shorter period of time. The *DSM-V* equivalent is substance use disorder, severe. This replaces use of the term 'addiction'.

Suicidal ideation Thinking about, considering or planning suicide. Also referred to as suicidal thoughts.

Suicide The act of intentionally causing one's own death.

Suicide attempt An attempt to end one's own life, which may lead to one's death.

Sustained remission When an individual has stopped or reduced their substance abuse intake, and the criteria for abuse or dependence would no longer be met for periods of greater than 12 months.

Therapeutic relationship The relationship between a healthcare professional and a patient. Established to meet the needs and health outcomes of the patient.

Thought disorder An impaired capacity to sustain coherent discourse, usually apparent in an individual's communication, most often in their speech.

Trait model of personality Attempts to identify certain characteristics or behaviours that are present in individuals to different extents. Each trait is expressed on a spectrum, with some people possessing it strongly, and others more weakly.

Transcranial magnetic stimulation (TMS) The application of magnetic stimuli to the cranium, done without anaesthesia.

Trauma- and stressor-related disorders A group of psychiatric disorders that arise following a stressful or traumatic event; for example, post-traumatic stress disorder (PTSD), acute stress disorder and adjustment disorders.

Trauma-informed care Trauma-informed services are aware of and sensitive to the dynamics of trauma that are prevalent throughout society. It seeks to promote healthcare environments that are healing and recovery-focused, rather than provide services that may risk inadvertently re-traumatising individuals. It acknowledges that all individuals have a past history and current circumstances that have led to their current behaviour and physiological response.

Traumatic event(s) Experiencing, witnessing or being confronted by an event(s) that involved actual or threatened death or serious injury, or threat to the physical integrity of self or others. It differs from regular life stressors because it causes a sense of intense fear, terror and helplessness that is beyond the normal range of typical experiences (Perry, 2002).

Verbal cues A spoken prompt that stimulates a response.

Workplace violence (WPV) The experience of violence towards, and the witnessing of violence in, paramedic practice encompasses verbal assault, intimidation, physical assault, sexual harassment and sexual assault – the perpetrators of violence are predominantly patients, family members of patients and bystanders (Bigham et al., 2014; Boyle & McKenna, 2017; Maguire, 2018; Palmer, 2017; Ross et al., 2017).

REFERENCES

Australian Psychological Society (APS). 2018. Evidence-based psychological interventions in the treatment of mental disorders: a review of the literature, fourth ed. Online. Available: https://www.psychology.org.au/getmedia/23c6a11b-2600-4e19-9a1d-6ff9c2f26fae/Evidence-based-psych-interventions.pdf. 12 October 2018.

Bigham, B., Jensen, J., Tavares, W., et al., 2014. Paramedic self-reported exposure to violence in the Emergency Medical Services (EMS) workplace: a mixed-methods cross-sectional survey. Prehosp. Emerg. Care 18 (4), 489–494.

Boud, D., Keogh, R., Walker, D., 1985. Promoting reflection in learning: a model. In: Boud, D., Keogh, R., Walker, D. (Eds.), Reflection: Turning Experience Into Learning. Kogan Page, London.

Boyle, M., McKenna, L., 2017. Paramedic student exposure to workplace violence during clinical placements – a cross-sectional study. Nurse Educ. Pract. 22, 93–97.

Brunero, S., Lamont, S., 2016. Challenges, risks and responses. In: Evans, K., Nizette, D., O'Brien, A. (Eds.), Psychiatric and Mental Health Nursing, fourth ed. Elsevier, Sydney.

Finlay, L., 2008. Reflecting on 'reflective practice'. The Open University (January), 1–27.

Maguire, B., 2018. Violence against ambulance personnel: a retrospective cohort study of national data from Safe Work Australia. Public Health Res. Pract. 28 (1), e28011805–e28011805.

National Institute for Health and Clinical Excellence (NICE). 2005. Violence: the short-term management of disturbed/violent behaviour in in-patient psychiatric and emergency departments. National Collaborating Centre for Nursing and Supportive Care, London.

Palmer, S., 2017. Intoxication and violence during ambulance call-outs. J. Paramed. Pract. 9, 483–485.

Perry, B., 2002. Stress, Trauma and Posttraumatic Stress Disorders in Children: Caregiver Education Series. ChildTrauma Academy, Houston, TX, p. 9.

Ross, L., Adams, T., Beovich, B., 2017. Methamphetamine use and emergency services in Australia: a scoping review. J. Paramed. Pract. 9 (6), 244–257.

Sadock, B., Sadock, V., Ruiz, P., 2015. Kaplan & Sadock's Synopsis of Psychiatry, eleventh ed. Wolters Kluwer, Philadelphia. electronic book.

Index

Page numbers followed by "*f*" indicate figures, "*t*" indicate tables, and "*b*" indicate boxes.